Inhomogeneous Superconductors-1979
(Berkeley Springs, W.V.)

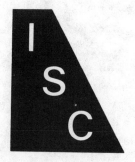

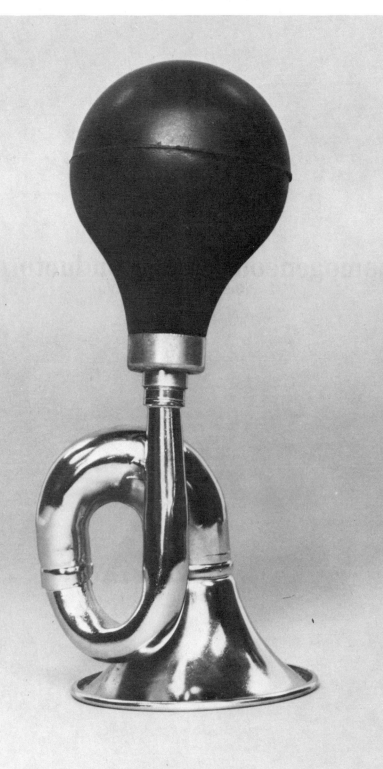

AIP Conference Proceedings
Series Editor: Hugh C. Wolfe
Number 58

Inhomogeneous Superconductors-1979

(Berkeley Springs, W.V.)

Editors

D.U. Gubser, T.L. Francavilla, S.A. Wolf
Naval Research Laboratory
and
J.R. Leibowitz
Catholic University of America

American Institute of Physics
New York   1980

L.C. Catalog Card No. 79-57620
ISBN 0–88318–157–6
DOE CONF- 791151

PREFACE

The editors in conceiving the idea for the Inhomogeneous Superconductors Conference (ISC) in early 1979, were struck by the timeliness and exciting ferment of a field which was, at the same time, not yet well represented in the published literature. It was eminently evident that the subject was now in such a state that its development would be necessarily aided by an intimate conference which promoted informal, direct interaction among those researchers actively engaged in the diverse aspects of inhomogeneous superconductivity. It is hoped the reader will agree that the papers which appear in these Proceedings serve at once to identify significant areas of current interest in inhomogeneous superconductivity, solidify basic areas of understanding, indicate some of the fundamental problems which remain, and point up some directions which hold promise for further progress.

This Conference benefitted from the help of many organizations and individuals. We sincerely appreciate the support provided by the Naval Research Laboratory, the Office of Naval Research, and the National Science Foundation, and are grateful for the good offices of the Catholic University of America. The project has profited from the many suggestions of the Organizing Committee: M. Beasley (Stanford University), J. Clem (Iowa State University), G. Deutscher (Tel Aviv University), C. Falco (Argonne National Laboratory), T.L. Francavilla, D.U. Gubser, and S.A. Wolf, (Naval Research Laboratory), A. Goldman (University of Minnesota), A. Hebard (Bell Laboratories), J.R. Leibowitz (Catholic University of America) and P. Lindenfeld (Rutgers University).

We want to thank Edgar Edelsack of ONR and Dr. Robert Hein of NSF for their interest, suggestions, and help prior to, during, and after the Conference. These Proceedings could not have been published so rapidly without the prompt and competent job done by the referees: J.H. Claassen, E.J. Cukauskas, J.L. Feldman, A.K. Ganguly, R.E. Glover, III, B.M. Klein, J.R. Leibowitz, M. Nisenoff, D.A. Papaconstantopoulos, W.E. Pickett, F.J. Rachford, and M.R. Skokan.

We also acknowledge with pleasure the congenial and efficient performance of the Coolfont Conference Center and its representative, Mr. Andrew Michael, in serving the physical needs of the conferees during the Conference. Finally, we are most indebted to our staff, headed by Lahni Blohm: Gay Priode, Melanie McDonald, Teresa Hileman, Frances Hambleton, Reyna Tosta, and L. David Jones.

D.U. Gubser
T.L. Francavilla
J.R. Leibowitz
S.A. Wolf

Washington, DC, December 1979

TABLE OF CONTENTS

INTRODUCTION TO INHOMOGENEOUS SUPERCONDUCTORS

M. Tinkham

Harvard University, Cambridge, Mass. 02138

ABSTRACT

After a brief historical perspective on the motivation for study of inhomogeneous superconductors, the formulation of Ginzburg-Landau equations suitable for such systems is reviewed. Attention is given to the important role of boundary conditions on ψ and $\nabla\psi$ at interfaces and to the connection with Josephson effect coupling between discrete elements, as in layered compounds and granular superconductors. Finally, the resistive properties of composite wire containing finite length superconducting filaments in a normal metal matrix are discussed in more detail, with emphasis on proximity effect coupling and on the critical behavior of resistance and maximum supercurrent near the percolation threshold.

INTRODUCTION

When I agreed to present this opening paper, I did so with considerable trepidation, basically because the field of inhomogeneous superconductivity is, itself, so inhomogeneous! This concern was reinforced when I saw the diversity of topics to be covered in the papers to be presented here. There seemed to be no way for me to "introduce" all of this material in a single talk, even if I were uniformly knowledgeable about it all, which I am not. Given this situation, I have decided to emphasize historical perspective in addressing the set of questions: Inhomogeneous superconductors: why, what, and whither? Perhaps this will be helpful in orienting participants who have come to this Conference from diverse backgrounds.

EARLY HISTORY

Previous to 1957 we had neither the BCS theory nor the Abrikosov theory of type II superconductors, just the London theory of superconducting electrodynamics, as generalized by Pippard. Then bulk 3-D superconductors were characterized by $T_c \lesssim 10K$, $H_{cb} \lesssim 10^3$ oe, and $J_c \sim H_c/\lambda \lesssim 10^7 A/cm^2$. Already in 1913 Kamerlingh Onnes had recognized that the existence of such a low critical field precluded the magnet applications he had anticipated; one also had to recognize that J_c could flow only in a surface skin layer of thickness $\lambda \sim 500 \overset{\circ}{A}$, so that the current carrying capacity of a macroscopic wire increased only with its perimeter, not its cross-sectional area.

These restrictions could apparently be eased if one considered a thin film with thickness d less than the penetration depth λ, thus entering the realm of 2-D systems. Because the magnetic field penetrates such a film (since $d < \lambda$), the diamagnetic energy which makes superconductivity energetically unfavorable in strong fields is reduced. As a result, one has an enhanced critical field $H_{c||} \sim H_{cb} \lambda/d$, which can be many times the bulk critical field H_{cb} if the film is thin enough. However, although the entire thickness of such a thin film can carry J_c, the total critical current $\sim J_c d$ decreases as (d/λ) is reduced. These facts made it appear attractive to consider a synthetic 3-D material made of a stack of thin 2-D films isolated from each other to let the magnetic field in, to retain the high $H_{c||}$, but capable of carrying a large total critical current. Instead of 2-D films, one could also consider a bundle of 1-D filaments, with $d \ll \lambda$, to achieve the same goal. Some laboratory efforts along these lines were made, including some interesting work[1] on porous glass impregnated by superconducting metal. Still, it seemed clear that this was not a very promising approach to practical materials, in part because of the difficulty of working with metallic and insulating layers or filaments on a thickness scale $\lesssim 100$ Å. These difficulties could be reduced by going to an entirely metallic composite, using normal metal layers (rather than insulators) between the superconducting layers to allow the field to penetrate. But thin layers of superconductor in electronic contact with normal metal have their superconductivity weakened or destroyed by the proximity effect, so this approach also had problems.

Rather than consider such synthetic composite materials, an alternate approach was to work with so-called "hard superconductors". These were metallurgically hard materials, in which internal structural defects did not readily anneal out, so that they were microscopically inhomogeneous. Such materials were found to remain partially superconducting and carry significant supercurrents in relatively high fields, exceeding the thermodynamic critical field of the bulk material. This behavior suggested that there was an internal sponge-like network of fine filamentary connections along grain boundaries, etc., which remained superconducting even after the bulk of the material had gone normal. This "Mendelssohn sponge" model of high-field superconductors was, of course, later superseded by our more modern understanding in terms of type II superconductors in which the role of structural inhomogeneity was only to introduce flux pinning.

GINZBURG-LANDAU THEORY FOR INHOMOGENEOUS SUPERCONDUCTORS

To go beyond this qualitative level of discussion, one needed a theory of superconductivity general enough to handle spatial inhomogeneity. This was offered in 1950 by the Ginzburg-Landau (GL) theory.[2] Originally introduced phenomenologically, the GL theory was shown by Gor'kov[3] in 1959 to be a rigorous consequence of the microscopic BCS theory in the limit near T_c, and it has proved qualitatively useful over a considerably wider range of temperatures. This theory is based on an expansion of the free energy density in powers of $|\psi|^2$ and $|\nabla\psi|^2$, where ψ is a macroscopic wavefunction describing the superconducting electrons, whose density $n_s \propto |\psi|^2$. The condition for minimization of this free energy reduces to two equations, which can be written

$$\alpha \psi + \beta |\psi|^2 \psi + \frac{1}{2m^*} \left(\frac{\hbar}{i} \nabla - \frac{2e\vec{A}}{c}\right)^2 \psi = 0 \qquad (1)$$

and

$$\vec{J}_s = 2e |\psi|^2 \vec{v}_s \qquad (2)$$

where

$$\vec{v}_s = (\hbar \nabla \phi - 2e\vec{A}/c)/m^* \qquad (3)$$

is the superfluid velocity, m^* is the mass of a pair, and $\psi = |\psi|e^{i\phi}$ is the macroscopic wavefunction. The parameter β is a positive constant, while $\alpha = -\hbar^2/2m^*\xi^2(T) = -\hbar^2(1 - T/T_c)/2m^*\xi^2(0)$ is negative below T_c. The operational significance of $|\psi|^2$ is that it determines the strength of the superfluid response, the penetration depth being given by

$$\lambda = \left(\frac{m^* c^2}{16\pi e^2 |\psi|^2}\right)^{\frac{1}{2}} \qquad (4)$$

From the microscopic theory we know that $|\psi|$ also has the significance of being proportional to the energy gap Δ. Within a homogeneous material the relation is simply

$$\psi = \frac{\xi(0)}{\hbar} \left[m^*N(0)\right]^{\frac{1}{2}} \Delta \qquad (5)$$

where $N(0)$ is the single-spin density of states at the Fermi energy. Hence Δ obeys an equation of the same form as ψ, namely,

$$\frac{T-T_c}{T_c} \Delta + \frac{7\zeta(3)|\Delta|^2}{8\pi^2 \left(k_B T_c\right)^2} \Delta + \xi^2(0) \left(\frac{\nabla}{i} - \frac{2\pi\vec{A}}{\phi_0}\right)^2 \Delta = 0 \qquad (6)$$

$$\vec{J}_s = \left[m^* \xi^2(0) N(0)/\hbar^2\right] 2e |\Delta|^2 \vec{v}_s \qquad (7)$$

where $7\zeta(3)/8\pi^2 = 0.107$, $\phi_0 = hc/2e$ is the flux quantum, and $\xi^2(0) \approx 0.55 \xi_0^2$ for pure materials and $0.73 \xi_0 \ell$ in the dirty limit.

Here $\xi_o = \hbar v_F/\pi\Delta(0)$, where v_F is the Fermi velocity, $\Delta(0)$ is the energy gap at $T = 0$, and ℓ is the electronic mean free path.

In either form these equations provide a powerful method for treating <u>inhomogeneous states</u> of superconductivity within <u>homogeneous materials</u>. For example, in the initial GL paper the interface energy between normal and superconducting laminas in the intermediate state of type I superconductors was calculated. Subsequently, in 1957, Abrikosov[4] discovered the mixed state solution for type II superconductors (i.e., those for which $\kappa \equiv \lambda/\xi > 1/\sqrt{2}$), in which a regular vortex array exists, each containing a single quantum of flux. This state is only weakly diamagnetic because of the penetrating flux tubes, and hence it can remain superconducting to high magnetic fields. In this way, the high critical fields of "hard superconductors" were explained without needing the thin filamentary structure of the Mendelssohn sponge. Still, structural inhomogeneity is required to "pin" the vortex lattice against the Lorentz force $\vec{J} \times \vec{B}$ in order that a resistanceless supercurrent can be carried in the presence of penetrating flux. This inhomogeneity can be due to dislocations, grain boundaries, voids, second phases, etc., and the metallurgical optimization of this sort of inhomogeneity is a subject of great technical importance.

If one wishes to extend the application of GL theory to grossly inhomogeneous systems, complications arise. Two limiting cases are reasonably tractable. If the parameters $N(0)$, $\xi(0)$, and T_c change slowly enough on the scale of $\xi(T)$, presumably one can take the usual GL equations as being locally valid, with slowly varying coefficients. Even here there are problems, however, since the equations are only strictly valid near T_c where Δ is small; if the local T_c varies considerably, even if slowly, this requirement cannot be met simultaneously over the whole sample. In the other simple limit, there is a sharp interface between each material and the next, so that one can piece together solutions of the equations for homogeneous materials by use of suitable boundary conditions on the macroscopic wave function ψ derived[5] from the underlying microscopic theory. Mooij and Dekker[6] have proposed a scheme for dealing with variation of parameters on an intermediate length scale, by breaking the variation into a sequence of small discrete steps and applying the boundary conditions at each step to arrive at a limiting form for continuous variation. In this way, they found it necessary to include an explicit term proportional to $\nabla\psi \cdot \nabla\ell$ in the GL equation with position-dependent mean free path. This procedure seems to be a reasonable way to improve on the approximation of simply using (1) with position-dependent coefficients, but no GL type of approximation can be reliable for treating variation on a length scale of $\xi(0)$ or smaller.

These macroscopic boundary conditions can be derived only by use of microscopic theory, but one can get some understanding of them in a more elementary way. The argument seems more transparent if couched in the language of Δ rather than ψ. We know from the Anderson theory of dirty superconductors[7] that Δ is essentially independent of ℓ; hence we expect Δ to be continuous at an interface where only ℓ changes. Given the relation (5) this implies that $\psi/\xi(0)$ is continuous, so ψ changes in proportion to $\xi(0)$, or $\ell^{\frac{1}{2}}$ in the dirty limit. Applying also the condition of continuity of supercurrent, we find that $\xi^2(0)v_s$ is continuous; hence v_s or grad Δ must change as $1/\xi^2(0)$, or $1/\ell$ in the dirty limit; correspondingly, $\nabla\psi$ changes as $1/\xi(0) \sim 1/\ell^{\frac{1}{2}}$. These simple considerations show why boundary conditions of the sort introduced by Zaitsev[5] are required to supplement the differential equations (1) and (6) in dealing with inhomogeneous superconductors.

The argument is less simple when the adjoining materials have different T_c values and other material parameters. However, if we take the interface to be completely transparent to electrons, the electronic state occupancies specified by the BCS coherence factors u and v for a given energy must be continuous across the interface, since any discontinuity would raise the energy unduly. If that is the case, the condensed electron density per state, namely,

$$\frac{F}{N(0)} = \int u(E)v(E)\left[1-2f(E)\right] dE = \frac{\Delta}{N(0)V} \tag{8}$$

will be continuous. Here V is the BCS average electron-phonon matrix element. This equation is essentially the one defining Δ in the BCS theory in terms of the u's and v's, but here the u's and v's are not required to have the value appropriate to the local gap. Although this argument is only heuristic, the conclusion that $F/N(0) = \Delta/N(0)V$ is continuous across a boundary with intimate electronic contact is in agreement with that given by the microscopic theory.[8]

If one of the metals is normal, and has V = 0, to take an extreme case, this condition implies that in the normal metal Δ will also be zero, but F will not be, and F determines the effective superconducting electron density. The boundary condition on derivatives is that (in dirty materials) D dF/dx is continuous, where $D = 1/3 \ v_F\ell$ is the diffusion constant. This relation is necessary for conservation of current at the interface, as follows by generalization of the result in the preceding paragraph. Away from the boundary F is expected to fall off in the normal metal with a characteristic length scale given by $\hbar v_F/2\pi k_B T$ if it is clean and by

$$\xi_N = \left(\frac{\hbar v_{FN}\ell_N}{6\pi k_B T}\right)^{\frac{1}{2}} \tag{9}$$

if it is dirty. If the "normal" metal is really a superconductor above its T_{cN}, ξ_N will diverge at T_{cN}. These remarks summarize the most elementary results concerning the "proximity effect". These simple considerations describe only the linearized response, and hence are most reliable near a second-order transition of the composite to the normal state. Nonetheless, we have the result that the superconducting electron density $|\psi|^2 \sim 1/\lambda^2 \sim \xi^2(0)F^2$ will in general suffer a discontinuity in slope and value at an interface between different materials, and then vary over a length scale characterized by a suitably generalized coherence length $\xi(T)$. Computer calculations are required to treat all but simple special cases.

If the elements in the inhomogeneous system are small in dimension, $d \ll \xi(T)$, then the variation of $\psi(r)$ within each element is small, and ψ is specified by a single value of $|\psi|e^{i\phi}$ for each element, apart from the internal phase gradients needed to drive any supercurrent. In that case, the problem can be reduced to a discrete set of interelement boundary conditions. If the coupling between elements is not too strong, it is often helpful to view this as a type of Josephson effect coupling. For example, this provides a way of modeling the properties of granular superconductors, a topic to be covered in detail in the next paper.

The superconducting layered compounds comprise another class of systems in which this type of modelling is useful. An example is TaS$_2$ with pyridine intercalated between the atomic layers of metallic material. The properties of these materials were analyzed in detail by Beasley and co-workers[9], treating the layers as 2-D superconductors with a Josephson coupling through the interleaved layers of intercalate. In elementary terms, these systems can be viewed as a realization of the idealized 3-D material made of a stack of very thin 2-D films, which was alluded to in an earlier section of this paper. As might be expected from this picture, these materials have very high parallel critical fields but more modest perpendicular critical fields; none the less, they show 3-D superconducting coherence, at least in weak fields and not too far from T_c. Since Beasley will be discussing these materials later in the Conference, I shall not go into more detail here. Rather, I shall now turn to another class of inhomogeneous superconductors which my group has studied in recent years.

TSUEI WIRE AND PERCOLATIVE SUPERCONDUCTIVITY

An important practical example of inhomogeneous superconductivity is the multifilamentary composite wire developed for making stable superconducting magnets. This is inhomogeneous on two characteristic length scales: First, it must have metallurgical inhomogeneity on the scale of ξ or the intervortex spacing (typically ~ 200 Å) to provide strong pinning of the vortex lattice against the $\vec{J} \times \vec{B}$ Lorentz force, and hence a high critical current density. Secondly, the superconductor must be finely divided into filaments of diameter d $\lesssim$ 50 µm embedded in a highly conductive normal metal matrix (usually Cu) to provide stability[10] against thermal fluctuation. Since the filament diameters are much larger than ξ, their properties are essentially the same as bulk material, and they present no interesting problems appropriate to this Conference.

For our purposes here, it is more interesting to move on to a discussion of "Tsuei wire"--a composite material[11] which resembles a commercial multifilamentary conductor except that the filaments are produced metallurgically, and hence can be made much finer, but they are not continuous. This raises non-trivial questions about conduction in a heterogeneous medium in which the scale of subdivision is not much greater than the superconducting coherence length or the range of proximity effect coupling, so that there is no longer a clearcut distinction between superconducting and normal regions. Moreover, the spread of long-range coherent superconductivity over macroscopic regions of the sample appears to be governed by percolation over the random array of filamentary segments.

Let me first briefly describe the process which produces the wire. If one wants Nb_3Sn filaments in Cu, one melts Nb, Sn, and Cu together and quenches the melt into an ingot. The Nb precipitates out in dendritic particles on a scale depending on the cooling rate. This material is then drawn into wire, which deforms the original Nb particles into long filaments. Finally, a heat treatment reacts the Sn out of the Cu matrix to form Nb_3Sn. To a first approximation, the deformation of the Nb particle follows that of the macroscopic ingot. If the cross-sectional area is reduced by a reduction factor Re, the length also increases by Re to conserve volume, so that the length to diameter ratio scales up as $Re^{3/2}$. For the representative value Re = 600, $Re^{3/2} \sim 10^4$, so the originally isotropic inclusions become very long and thin. Typical lengths are up to 1 cm, while diameters are typically only 1 µm. Thus, there will typically be 10^5 filaments passing through any cross section of a sample wire, while the current need make only a few jumps from filament to filament to get from one end of the sample segment to the other.

In assessing the potential usefulness of such materials, one is particularly interested in whether the resistance will be zero or at least close enough so that it could be used to make cheap magnet wire. Given the notion of a percolation threshold[12] at some volume fraction (~15% in 3-dimensions, ~50% in 2-dimensions) one might expect strictly zero resistance above that fraction, and finite (but small) resistance at smaller volume fractions. But the effective superconducting volume fraction will depend on temperature, current density, and magnetic field because of the "proximity effect", which allows superconducting electrons to diffuse a normal metal coherence length ξ_N [See (9)] out from the superconducting filaments themselves. This length will be of the order of a fraction of a micron under typical conditions. But because the coherence energy of the wavefunction only falls exponentially, as e^{-x/ξ_N}, <u>some</u> superconductive coupling will continue until this energy falls below the thermal noise level. Thus, at low temperatures and with small measuring currents, one expects to find true perfect conductivity, as in a bulk superconductor, and one does.

But the technically interesting case is one of <u>high</u> current densities, $T \gtrsim 4^\circ K$, and in the presence of strong magnetic fields. All these influences reduce the proximity effect coupling, effectively shrinking the superconducting volume fraction. In fact, if the superconducting filament diameter is comparable to ξ, the superconducting volume fraction may be even less than the nominal one, since the finest filaments will be normal. Although the detailed variation of T_c depends on the geometry and the interface conditions, roughly one has

$$\frac{T_c}{T_{cb}} = 1 - \left(\frac{\pi\xi(0)}{d}\right)^2 \tag{10}$$

so that if $\xi(0) \sim 1000$ Å and $d \sim 1$ μm, a 10% reduction of T_c might be expected. This effect will be important for pure Nb in Cu, but in Nb_3Sn, $\xi(0)$ is so small that the effect should be negligible.

It is useful to consider first a simple limit, in which one assumes that the proximity effect is completely suppressed (by current or field), and that the superconductive volume fraction f_s consists of a collection of long thin cylinders of length L and diameter d formed by the drawing process, and hence aligned along the wire. The rest of the volume is assumed filled with a completely normal Cu matrix.

It is intuitively clear that these long aligned filamentary fragments will be much more effective in reducing the resistance of the wire than would an equal volume fraction in the form of isotropic inclusions, or of randomly oriented filamentary fragments. I gave an elementary treatment[13] of this problem several years ago, the result being that the remnant resistivity should be reduced below that of the matrix by the factor

$$\frac{\rho_{rem}}{\rho_0} \approx \frac{1}{1 + f_s L^2/d^2} \approx \frac{1}{f_s}\frac{d^2}{L^2} \approx \frac{1}{f_s}\frac{1}{R_e^3} \tag{11}$$

which can readily reach 10^{-7}. Since the matrix itself is Cu at low temperatures, the reduced resistance could be so small as to be detectable only with superconducting instrumentation. The physical reason for this result is that the resistance stems from the spreading resistance around the superconductive filaments as the current fans out to pass from one to an adjacent one. The spreading resistance per cell decreases as $1/L$, while the effective

"Maxwell-Garnett cell" is deforming to a length L and diameter $\sim d/f_s^{\frac{1}{2}}$. A conclusion similar to (11) for extremely elongated filaments was reached by Callaghan and Toth,[14] apart from numerical factors. By contrast with this physically reasonable result, conventional effective medium theory applied to this case leads to a prediction of zero resistance for all f_s exceeding the depolarization factor of the inclusions. For the usual isotropic case this would be the reasonable magnitude of 1/3, but for these filaments it would be an unreasonable value of order $d^2/L^2 \approx 10^{-8}$!

Proceeding phenomenologically, it seems reasonable to build the critical behavior near the percolation threshold concentration f_c for perfect conductivity into (11) by an additional factor $(1-f_s/f_c)^s$. As noted above, one expects $f_c \sim 0.15$ in 3-dimensions and $f_c \sim 0.5$ in 2-dimensions, while theoretical estimates[15] of the critical exponent s yield ~ 0.7 in 3-dimensions and range from 1 to 1.4 in 2-dimensions. Taking the long-filament limit of (11), we expect then that

$$\frac{\rho_{rem}}{\rho_o} \approx \frac{1}{f_s} \frac{d^2}{L^2} \left(1 - \frac{f_s}{f_c}\right)^s \qquad f_s < f_c \qquad (12)$$

$$= 0 \qquad\qquad\qquad f_s > f_c$$

where f_s will depend smoothly on current, temperature, and magnitude field.

What is the experimental situation? Davidson's early experiments on samples containing Nb_3Sn in a Cu matrix appeared to confirm the existence of a percolation threshold near 15% by volume: a 7 1/2% sample showed the predicted plateau of resistance reduced by a factor of $\sim 10^5$ from the normal state, whereas the 15% sample resistance dropped directly to zero when the Nb_3Sn became super-conducting. Further experiments by Lobb et al[17] on Nb filaments in a matrix of Cu or of a Cu-rich alloy revealed a more complex picture. His samples with pure Cu matrix showed no plateau of reduced resistance, instead losing all resistance at the Nb transition, even with a Nb concentration of only 10%. This result indicated the presence of a far-reaching proximity effect coupling giving an enhanced f_s. To test this interpretation, Lobb diffused Zn into the very same sample, to shorten the mean free path and weaken the proximity coupling. The result was a small plateau at the expected resistance level of $\sim 10^{-5}$ that of the normal state, before the final plunge to zero resistance at a lower temperature. To further reduce proximity coupling, Lobb made a series of samples with various concentrations of Nb in a Cu matrix containing 3% Ni. (Magnetic impurities are particularly effective in weakening the superconductive pairing in the normal metal.) In all cases, there was a drop in resistance of several orders of magnitude just below the T_c of Nb, as expected from (11), followed by a drop to zero resistance at a lower (current-dependent) temperature T_{c1} as implied by (12). This drop was interpreted in terms of an approach to the percolation threshold as the proximity effect increased the effective superconducting volume fraction with decreasing temperature. With this interpretation, the resistance was fitted to the expected critical behavior, namely

$$R = R_o \left(\frac{T}{T_{c1}} - 1\right)^s \qquad (13)$$

Fitted values of s were in the range 1-1.15, which are reasonably consistant with estimates for 2-D percolation, but contrast with the estimated 3-D values. This seemed not unreasonable, since the aligned superconducting filaments make the medium highly anisotropic, the resistance of the wires below T_c arising primarily from current flow in the transverse plane between filaments.

It can be shown[18], however, that as f_s approaches arbitrarily close to f_c (or T to T_{c1}), the measured value of s should approach the isotropic value for the appropriate physical dimension, regardless of any finite anisotropy. This raises interesting questions of what to expect for effective measured exponents, and how close to T_{c1} one must be in order to measure the true limiting value. We have approached this problem in several different ways.

The most obvious approach is to make measurements on undrawn (isotropic) Cu-Nb alloy samples. When this was done, we found a much smaller drop in resistance when the Nb became superconducting than in the drawn samples, as expected from (12). Unfortunately, these particular samples had sufficient compositional inhomogeneity that reliable estimates of s could not be made. Further work along this direction is planned.

A second approach has been study[18] of a 2-D physical model system consisting of photolithographically produced metallic images of laser speckle patterns. This system allows us to systematically vary the aspect ratio of metal islands on an insulating substrate. The measured results, plus numerical simulations and renormalization group calculations on anisotropic random resistor lattices confirm the notion that highly anisotropic systems have very narrow critical regions, i.e., regions in which the isotropic value for s is measured.

Another physical quantity which should exhibit percolative critical behavior is the maximum supercurrent density, J_c. By analogy with (12), one expects that

$$J_c \propto (f_s - f_c)^v \qquad (14)$$

where v is another critical exponent. Large cell renormalization group calculations by Lobb and Frank,[19] reported elsewhere at this

Conference, suggest that $v = 1.343 \pm 0.016$ in two dimensions, a value in good agreement with the experimental value of $v = 1.3 \pm 0.1$ reported by Deutscher and Rappaport.[20] Lobb and Frank[21] used a similar method to calculate s in two dimensions, with the result $s = 1.35 \pm 0.02$. Different experiments and theories still give a wide range of estimates for s. With improved experimental techniques and increased attention to finite size effects, it should be possible to gain a better understanding of the extent of the critical region in anisotropic systems, and of the values of the transport critical exponents that hold therein.

ACKNOWLEDGEMENTS

This research was supported in part by the NSF, both directly and through the Harvard MRL. It is a pleasure to acknowledge the assistance of C.J. Lobb, T.M. Klapwijk, and W.J. Skocpol in the preparation of this manuscript.

REFERENCES

1. C.P. Bean, M.V. Doyle, and A.G. Pincus, Phys. Rev. Lett. 9, 93 (1962); J.H.P. Watson, Phys. Rev. 148, 223 (1966).
2. V.L. Ginzburg and L.D. Landau, Zh. Eksperim. i Teor. Fiz. 20, 1064 (1950).
3. L.P. Gor'kov, Zh. Eksperim. i Teor. Fiz. 36, 1918 (1959). [Sov. Phys.-JETP 9, 1364 (1959)]
4. A.A. Abrikosov, Zh. Eksperim. i Teor. Fiz. 32, 1442 (1957); [Sov. Phys.-JETP 5, 1174 (1957)]
5. R.O. Zaitsev, Zh. Eksperim. i Teor. Fiz. 48, 1759 (1965); 50, 1055 (1966). [Sov. Phys.-JETP 21, 1178 (1965); 23, 702 (1966)]. Also, P.G. deGennes, Superconductivity in Metal and Alloys, W.A. Benjamin, New York, 1966, Chapter 7.
6. J.E. Mooij and P. Dekker, J. Low Temp. Phys. 33, 551 (1978).
7. P.W. Anderson, J. Phys. Chem. Sol. 11, 26 (1959).
8. See, for example, G. Deutscher and P.G. de Gennes, Chapter on "Proximity Effects" in Superconductivity, ed. by R.D. Parks, M. Dekker, New York, 1969.
9. D.E. Prober, M.R. Beasley, and R.E. Schwall, Phys. Rev. B 15, 5245 (1977).
10. See, for example, M. Tinkham, Introduction to Superconductivity, McGraw-Hill, New York, 1975, p. 184.
11. C.C. Tsuei, Science 180, 57 (1973); J. Appl. Phys. 45, 1385 (1974).
12. See, for example, V.K.S. Shante and S. Kirkpatrick, Adv. Phys. 20, 325 (1971); H. Scher and R. Zallen, J. Chem. Phys. 53, 3759 (1970); R. Zallen and H. Scher, Phys. Rev. B4, 4471 (1971).
13. A. Davidson, M.R. Beasley, and M. Tinkham, IEEE Trans. Magnetics, Vol. MAG-11, p. 276, 1975.
14. T.J. Callaghan and L.E. Toth, J. Appl. Phys. 46, 4013 (1975).

15. J. Bernasconi, Phys. Rev. B18, 2185 (1978), and references cited therein.
16. A. Davidson and M. Tinkham, Phys. Rev. B 13, 3261 (1976).
17. C.J. Lobb, M. Tinkham, and W.J. Skocpol, Sol. State Comm. 27, 1273 (1978).
18. L.N. Smith and C.J. Lobb, Phys. Rev. B, to be published Nov. 1, 1979.
19. C.J. Lobb and D.J. Frank, to be published in these Proceedings.
20. G. Deutscher and M.L. Rappaport, J. Physique Lett. 40, L-219 (1979).
21. C.J. Lobb and D.J. Frank, J. Phys. C., to appear.

THEORY OF SUPERCONDUCTIVITY IN
GRANULAR COMPOSITES

Bruce R. Patton, W. Lamb, and D. Stroud
The Ohio State University, Columbus, Ohio 43210

ABSTRACT

The nature of superconductivity in granular composite materials is discussed, starting from a microscopic Hamiltonian. The Ginzburg-Landau free energy arising from the Hamiltonian is presented. For weak enough intergranular coupling, the superconducting transition splits into two parts, a single grain ordering temperature T_{co}, and a long-range phase ordering temperature T_c. Numerical results are presented for the order parameter and specific heat in three dimensions. Calculations of the conductivity and susceptibility are also presented.

INTRODUCTION

Much interest has been focused recently on the general class of inhomogeneous materials with superconducting properties.[1-5] In addition to being of technological importance because of their high critical fields, the nature of the superconducting state in such systems is a fundamental theoretical question. Among the basic issues that arise are the relation of the superconducting transition to percolation in an ordinary random system, the behavior of the superconducting transition as the minimum metallic conductivity[6] is approached, and to what extent superconductivity can exist in a system in which the states are localized at $T = 0$. Previous work has emphasized the importance of fluctuations in granular systems, and the role of Josephson coupling in producing superconductivity.[5]

In this report we describe our calculations which start from a microscopic Hamiltonian for an inhomogeneous superconducting system, derive the form of the Ginzburg-Landau free-energy functional, separate the solution into a single grain part and a phase-ordering part for weak enough coupling, and derive a new Ginzburg-Landau free-energy functional appropriate to the phase-ordering transition. We have made comparative numerical calculations for periodic and aperiodic systems for the (phase) order parameter and the specific heat. From the time dependent Ginzburg-Landau equation and the simplest effective medium description of the normal conduction, we find it is possible to describe a wide variety of typical experimental data. We find a cross over from a concave downward resistive transition (foot structure) to concave upward transition (tail structure) as the fraction of superconducting component is increased through the percolation fraction ($f = f_c$). In the case of the foot, the conductivity diverges with an exponent which, in the mean field limit, is $\mu = 2 - d/2$ while in the more relevant case of critical fluctuations is $\mu = \nu(4 - d)$, to a good approximation. Finally, the susceptibility is derived from the solution of the phase-order

Ginzburg-Landau free-energy plus an argument relating the permeability to the percolation of flux through the insulating component.

MICROSCOPIC THEORY

The essential feature of granular superconductivity is the existence of superconducting regions separated by non-superconducting or even insulating regions. Experiments have been done on a wide variety of materials, but the basic features seem to be contained in a microscopic Hamiltonian of the following form

$$H = \sum_i H_i + \sum_{i,j} (M_{ij} + U_{ij}) \tag{1}$$

where the indices i and j run over the grains. The single grain Hamiltonian H_i includes a one body part plus the intra-grain Coulomb and electron-phonon interactions. The finite size of the grain introduces a discreteness into the single body energy level spacing $\Delta E = 1/N(0)\Omega$, where $N(0)$ is the density of states at the Fermi surface of the granular material and Ω is the volume of the grain. As long as the level spacing is much smaller than the temperature, the discreteness has little effect; however when $\Delta E \sim k_B T$ the superconducting transition becomes greatly smeared.[10] The finite size of the grain may also change the relative magnitudes of the phonon-induced attraction and the Coulomb repulsion between electrons within a grain, thus causing the single grain transition temperature to vary. However, there appear to be a number of superconductors whose properties are stable enough that small grains have essentially the same transition as the bulk, and thus we specialize to that case for simplicity in the following.

The second term in Eq.(1) involves the mixing of electron states on different grains and is proportional to the overlap of wave functions from adjoining grains. In the tunneling limit M_{ij} is given by

$$M_{ij} = \sum_{pp'} (V\, a_{ip}^+ a_{jp'} + h.c.). \tag{2}$$

For large values of V the electron states become delocalized and the effects of the discrete intra-grain energy level spacing are reduced.

The last term in Eq.(1) involves the inter-grain Coulomb interaction and the phonon-mediated interaction of electrons on different grains. Although these terms may in principle give rise to interesting effects, they are not pursued in the following. Thus we will drop these terms for present. We do note however, that although it was originally pointed out that the inter-grain Coulomb interaction could lead to a strong suppression of superconductivity,[7] recently, it has been argued that the criterion for suppression is actually much weaker.[8] In addition, on physical grounds one expects the phonon exchange between grains to tend to cancel the Coulomb interaction as the coupling M_{ij} becomes large.

Even without the last term, the microscopic Hamiltonian (1) (and its generalization to finite electromagnetic fields) is sufficiently rich to lead to a variety of interesting effects dependent on the phase coherence properties of the system. As one example of this computable from (1) we mention the optical absorption of a superconducting composite. In addition, numerous other effects are most easily obtained by deriving from the Hamiltonian (1) the appropriate form of the Ginzburg-Landau free energy functional for the superconducting transition.

GINZBURG-LANDAU THEORY

The Ginzburg-Landau (G-L) free-energy is obtained from Eq.(1) via the standard procedure.[9] Basically, the total degrees of freedom in (1) are reduced to a position dependent pair wave function by integrating out over the electronic degrees of freedom. The two particle term gives rise to the quadratic and gradient pieces, while the four particle term gives the quartic interaction of the G-L expression. If the grains in one spatial direction are small compared to the coherence length, then the M_{ij} in that direction play the role of the (discrete) gradient terms. Although we could just as easily consider one or two dimensional "grains," we will examine here the zero-dimensional grain case, meaning the size of the grain in all three directions is smaller than the bulk coherence length. In this case the pair wave function on a grain is a spatially constant complex number ψ_i and the G-L free energy functional is

$$\mathfrak{F} = \sum_i \left(a|\psi_i|^2 + b|\psi_i|^4/2 \right) + \sum_{i,j} c_{ij}|\psi_i - \psi_j|^2 \tag{3}$$

where[1] the free energy $F = -T \int_i \Pi \, d^2\psi_i \exp(-\mathfrak{F}/T)$ and $(k_B = 1)$

$$a = N(0)\left(\frac{T - T_{co}}{T_{co}}\right)$$

$$b = N(0)\,\frac{7\zeta(3)}{8\pi^2 T_{co}^2}$$

$$c_{ij} = \frac{(\pi N(0)V)^2}{4T_{co}} = \frac{\pi}{8T_{co}}\,\frac{\hbar}{e^2 R_{ij}} \; . \tag{4}$$

In Eq.(3) the order parameter is measured in units of energy, while in (4), R_{ij} is the normal state resistance between grains. As discussed before, the a's and b's could be random in addition to the c_{ij}'s, however for simplicity we take them constant. To generalize

Eq.(3) to finite magnetic fields one must add a quadratic shift of T_{co} to the a term, while the c_{ij} terms between grains are multiplied by the phase factor associated with the line integral of the vector potential between grains i and j.

For relatively weak coupling, the free-energy (3) leads to a phase transition to a zero-resistance state at a temperature T_c considerably below the single-particle transition T_{co}. This result is understood qualitatively as follows. If we ignore the coupling term in (3), the phases of the wave functions vary randomly from site to site. Even including the Josephson coupling term, one expects the phases to remain random since the _effective_ coupling is of the order of $\langle |\psi_i|^2 \rangle c_{ij}$, which is small near T_{co}. As T drops, the tendency to phase order increases as $\langle |\psi_i|^2 \rangle$ grows until a phase transition characterized by long-range phase coherence sets in at a temperature $T_c \approx Z \langle |\psi_i|^2 \rangle c$, where Z is an effective number of nearest neighbors and c a typical nearest-neighbor Josephson coupling.

For T well below T_{co}, amplitude fluctuations are expected to be small and $|\psi_i|^2$ can be well approximated by its most probable value, $|\psi_i|^2 = |a|/b$. In such a case the free-energy involves an integral over phases. Writing $\psi_i = |\psi_i| e^{i\phi_i}$, we can express the partition function in this phase-only limit as

$$Z = \int (\prod_i d\phi_i) \exp \left\{ +\beta \sum_{i>j} J_{ij} \cos(\phi_i - \phi_j) \right\}, \tag{5}$$

with $J_{ij} = |\psi_i|^2 c_{ij}$. Eq. (5) is recognized as formally identical to a ferromagnetic x-y model with random coupling strengths, and we shall refer to the corresponding reduced free-energy functional as the "x-y limit."

To illustrate some of the behavior to be expected of the model (3), we have solved for the partition function within a random mean-field approximation. We have modelled the granular system by 125 identical spherical grains, arranged quasi-amorphously in a cubic unit cell in such a fashion that the volume fraction f occupied by the spheres equaled 0.45. The configuration was generated by a Monte-Carlo program in which the particles were assumed to interact like hard spheres of the appropriate diameter and which allowed periodic repetition of the unit cell. The constants c_{ij} were taken to depend exponentially on particle separation.

The relevant mean-field equations are:

$$F = -k_B T \ln \prod_{i=1}^{N} \int_0^\infty \int_0^\pi |\psi_i| d|\psi_i| d\phi_i \exp \left\{ -\beta \left[\mathcal{F}_{sp}(|\psi_i|) - H_i^{eff} \cos\phi_i \right] \right\}$$

$$H_i^{eff} = \sum_j \langle |\psi_j|^2 \rangle_{sp} c_{ij} \langle \cos\phi_j \rangle \tag{6}$$

with $\langle \cos\phi_j \rangle = -(\partial F/\partial H_j^{eff})_{\beta, H_i^{eff}}$. Here $\langle |\psi_i^2| \rangle_{sp}$ is the mean-square single-particle density of Cooper pairs, as obtained from the single-particle partition function.[10] Results for the phase order parameter $\eta = \langle \cos\phi \rangle_{av}$ are shown in Fig. 1, for c_{ij}'s of various ranges.

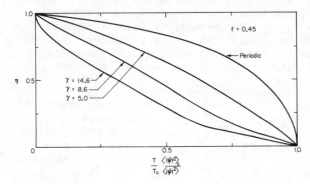

Fig. 1 The phase order parameter versus a temperature scale normalized by the single particle order parameter for various values of the inverse fall off length γ of the c_{ij} ($\gamma \to 0$ reproduces the periodic case).

Next, we note a relationship between the two transition temperatures and the inter-grain resistance, for the model of Eq. (3). For a lattice, the mean field expression for T_c is $k_B T_c = Z\, c_{ij} |\psi_i|^2$. Using Eq. (4) plus the standard microscopic expression for the order parameter in which $|\psi_i|^2 \propto (T_{co} - T)$, we obtain

$$T_{co}/T_c = 1 + R_{ij}/R_o \qquad (7)$$

where $R_o = 1.17 Z \hbar/e^2 \cong 4500 Z\Omega$. (In two dimensions $R_{ij} = R_\square$, the resistance of a square sample.) We have checked this relationship within the numerical calculations described above, for different size grains, measured in units of the dimensionless energy level spacing $\delta = \Delta E/k_B T_{co}$. Figure 2 shows the results for various values of δ; note that $\delta = 0$ is the case for Eq. (7).

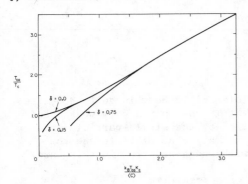

Fig. 2 The ratio of the single grain transition temperature to the phase-ordering transition temperature plotted versus a measure of the effective resistance, $k_B T_{co} K_c/\langle c \rangle$, where K_c is a dimensionless coupling constant of order unity, and $\langle c \rangle$ is the average of the distribution of Josephson couplings c_{ij}.

The mean-field model, Eq. (6), will give a jump in the specific heat at $T = T_c$ whereas a weak divergence is expected in reality. Nevertheless, the approximation should give a qualitatively reasonable

18

idea of the relative sizes of the specific heat anomalies at T_{co} and T_c. Some of our model specific heat calculations are shown in Fig. 3 for both periodic and aperiodic systems made up of particles of several different sizes, as well as for bulk systems. In all the figures shown, two peaks can be distinguished in the specific heat, one corresponding to the single-particle transition near T_{co}, which is rounded due to the finite size of the particles, the other (a discontinuity in this approximation) arising from the onset of long-range superconductivity at T_c. In the case of relatively

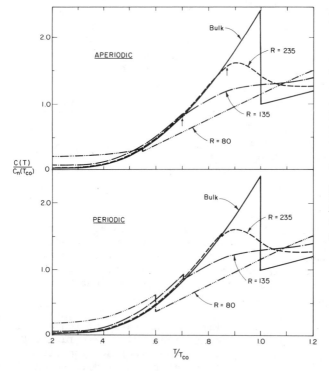

Fig. 3 The specific heats for periodic and aperiodic configurations in units of the normal specific heat per grain at T_{co} are plotted versus temperature in units of the single grain transition T_{co} for various values of grain radius R in Å. The periodic configuration corresponded to a simple cubic array.

large particles the single-particle specific heat is quite BCS-like and the phase-ordering transition at T_c has only a very weak specific heat signature. For small particles, the single-particle transition is very much broadened and it may be possible to see the specific heat anomaly associated with phase-ordering in this case.

CONDUCTIVITY AND SUSCEPTIBILITY

The behavior of the conductivity is one of the extremely interesting properties of a superconducting composite, since it is in general sensitive to the transition of the individual grains at T_{co}, their relative fraction, and the phase-ordering transition at T_c.

If the two temperatures T_c and T_{co} are reasonably well separated, then it is possible to develop a straightforward quantitative expression for the conductivity. In general we may distinguish four types of behavior, depending on a) whether $T_c \sim T_{co}$ or $T_c \ll T_{co}$; and on b) whether the component that goes superconducting is above or below its critical threshold f_c for ordinary percolation in the composite.

Case I. If $f > f_c$ and $T_c \sim T_{co}$ as with strongly coupled grains, then the resistive transition occurs essentially at T_{co}, with a small exponential tail down to T_c.

Case II. If $f > f_c$, but $T_c \lesssim 0.7\ T_{co}$, as in a normal metal composite, then the resistance drops mainly at T_{co}, but with a longer tail down to T_c. Except near T_c, the shape of the tail is determined by fluctuations into the normal state on each grain plus the nature of the percolative behavior of the medium as discussed below.

Case III. If $f < f_c$ with $T_c \gtrsim 0.5\ T_{co}$, as in a high resistance composite, then the resistance drops to a clearly defined plateau value between T_c and T_{co}, which is the classical effective resistance of the material when one component has zero resistance. The transition to zero total resistance then occurs at T_c with concave <u>downward</u> slope in three dimensions.

Case IV. As the normal resistance is increased, we eventually obtain the case $f < f_c$ with $T_c \ll T_{co}$. In this situation only a small change in the resistance occurs at T_{co}, the details of which depend on the conduction mechanism. If the Josephson coupling is weak enough, other effects may predominate, leading to $T_c \rightarrow 0$, in which case the resistance may continue to increase as T decreases.

We construct a theory of the resistive transition in two stages. Since long-range phase correlations are unimportant near T_{co}, the resistance close to T_{co} is controlled by the classical percolation of a two component medium. This is described by $\sigma_{eff}(f, \sigma_a, \sigma_b)$, which denotes the exact classical conductivity of a medium consisting of a fraction f of a superconducting metal with conductivity σ_a, and a fraction $1 - f$ of non-superconducting component with conductivity σ_b. We strongly emphasize that percolation ideas are not adequate or appropriate for the transition near T_c, which is a true thermodynamic transition with broken phase symmetry and not a geometric transition.

As $T \rightarrow T_c$, long-range Josephson phase correlations develop, which give an increase in conductivity σ_J analogous to the fluctuation conductivity of a homogeneous superconductor. The total conductivity may therefore be written

$$\sigma = \sigma_J(T) + \sigma_{eff}(f, \sigma_a(T), \sigma_b) \qquad (8)$$

where the effective conductivity σ_{eff} depends on the temperature through $\sigma_a(T)$, which increases strongly at T_{co}.

In the model calculations of the conductivity presented in Fig. 4, σ_{eff} was calculated from the effective medium approximation (EMA) for $d = 3$, the simplest approximation which preserves the percolation transition from a state of finite resistance to one of

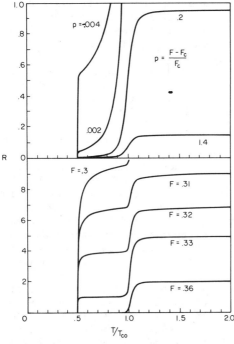

Fig. 4 Resistivity R versus temperature T for a model granular composite containing a volume fraction F of superconducting grains, where the critical percolation fraction F_c =1/3 in the EMA and T_c = 0.5 T_{co}.

zero resistance.

The Josephson fluctuation conductivity was calculated using the time-dependent Ginzburg-Landau equation and expanding Eq.(3) in terms of fluctuations about T_c. The details will be presented elsewhere. Near T_c the conductivity is found to vary with temperature as $\sigma_J \sim (T - T_c)^{-\mu}$, where, as in the case of a homogeneous d-dimensional superconductor, the exponent $\mu = (4 - d)/2$ in the mean field limit of weakly interacting fluctuations. In the more applicable case of critical fluctuations, a dynamic scaling argument[1] for this type of theory leads to the more general behavior $\mu = \nu(4 - d)$, where ν is the critical exponent for the coherence length (the small critical exponent η has been set equal to zero). As seen from Fig. 4, for $f < f_c$, a clear foot structure is discernable and in this case critical fluctuations would give an exponent in d = 3 of $\mu \cong \frac{2}{3}$, in agreement with the experiments on thick films.[3] As d → 2, the exponent ν is expected to diverge. Thus the resistance should go to zero near T_c with zero slope, in sharp contrast to the case in three dimensions. Again, this general behavior is in good agreement with experiment.[2]

The zero-field magnetic susceptibility of a composite superconductor can be described in a manner closely paralleling the conductivity. For a superconductor exhibiting a double transition, one expects three regimes of behavior: (i) for $T > T_{co}$, a normal paramagnetic state, with increasing single-grain diamagnetic fluctuations as T approaches T_{co} from above, followed by a drop in the effective permeability at T_{co}; (ii) for $T_c < T < T_{co}$, a plateau in the effective permeability μ_{eff}, followed by a further drop near T_c associated with diamagnetic fluctuations arising from transient loops of super-current; (iii) for $T < T_c$, perfect diamagnetism ($\mu = 0$). The regime of perfect diamagnetism is expected to exist at $H = 0$ only if $f > f_c'$, where f_c' is the concentration at which the <u>non-superconducting</u> fraction of the composite forms a connected path throughout the sample. In $d = 3$, one expects, in general, that $f_c' > f_c$, and therefore that there may exist a regime of concentration and temperature in which the sample will have zero resistance but will not be perfectly diamagnetic even in zero applied field. The physical reason for this possible effect may be that the non-superconductor acts as a conductor of magnetic <u>flux</u>, and as long as this component forms an infinite connected cluster the sample could be penetrated by flux even if it had zero resistance.

We have computed the permeability of a model granular super-conductor including both the single-grain and the current-loop susceptibility and taking care to treat local field effects correctly within the EMA. Details of the method will be presented elsewhere. Some of our results are shown in Fig. 5. For large particles (radius R much larger than the zero-temperature penetration depth λ_0), μ drops sharply at T_{co}, (then to zero at $T = T_c$) for $f > f_c'$ but not for $f < f_c'$ ($f_c' = \frac{2}{3}$ in the EMA, which was used in these calculations). For smaller particles, this effect is considerably blurred. It would be most interesting to see if the zero-field mixed state behavior exists in a real composite as is predicted here. Indications of diamagnetic fluctuations above T_c have been seen in several experiments.

In conclusion, we have developed a simple and relatively unified picture of superconductivity in granular composites. The picture involves a single-particle transition at T_{co} followed by a collective phase-ordering transition at a lower temperature T_c at which a zero-resistance state sets in. We have carried out approximate model calculations of a variety of properties, including the specific heat, ratio of transition temperatures T_c/T_{co}, conductivity, and zero-field magnetic susceptibility, and predict a variety of novel behavior, some of which have been experimentally observed.

The authors gratefully acknowledge numerous discussions with Joseph Straley and Michael Lee, and support from NSF (DMR 78-11770 and DMR 77-22929).

22

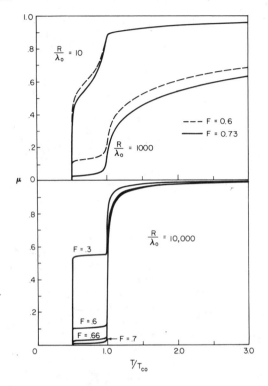

Fig. 5 Effective permeability μ versus temperature T for a model granular composite containing volume fraction F of superconductor. The curves correspond to superconducting particles of three different ratios R/λ_0, where R is the particle radius and λ_0 its zero-temperature penetration depth.

REFERENCES

1. B. R. Patton, W. Lamb, and D. Stroud, Bull. Am. Phys. Soc. 24, 356 (1979), and to be published.
2. D. U. Gubser and S. A. Wolf, J. Phys. (Paris), Colloq. 39, C6-579 (1979), and these proceedings.
3. A. M. Goldman, K. Epstein, B. D. Dahlberg, and R. Mikkelson, these proceedings and to be published.
4. G. Deutscher and M. L. Rappaport, J. Phys. (Paris), Colloq. 39, C6-581 (1978).
5. G. Deutscher, Y. Imry, and L. Gunther, Phys. Rev. B 10, 4598 (1974).
6. D. J. Thouless, Phys. Rev. Lett. 39, 1167 (1977).
7. B. Abeles, Phys. Rev. B 15, 2828 (1977).
8. W. L. McLean and M. J. Stephen, Phys. Rev. B 19, 5925 (1979).
9. N. R. Werthamer in Superconductivity, Ed. R. D. Parks (Marcel Dekker, N.Y., 1969), p.321.
10. B. Mühlschlegel, D. J. Scalapino, and R. Denton, Phys. Rev. B. 6, 1767 (1972).
11. To compute C_V, we use the G-L coefficients suggested by M. Tinkham, Introduction to Superconductivity, (McGraw-Hill, N.Y., 1975), p.110.

CRITICAL BEHAVIOR OF PERCOLATING SUPERCONDUCTORS

G. Deutscher, O. Entin-Wohlman, M. Rappaport and Y. Shapira
Tel Aviv University, Ramat Aviv, Tel Aviv, Israel

ABSTRACT

The properties of granular superconductors are reviewed, with emphasis on the specific properties that result from their inhomogeneous structure at the grain-size scale. Percolation theories are shown to provide a useful basis for the understanding of critical current and heat capacity data.

INTRODUCTION

Granular superconductors have been known since 1966, when Abeles et al.[1] discovered that aluminum thin films evaporated in a poor vacuum had unusual superconducting properties. Most noticeable among them was the fact that their critical temperature was significantly larger than that of bulk aluminum (typically a factor of two higher). Unfortunately up to this day no satisfactory explanation has been found to this interesting effect, although this enhancement was shown to be correlated with the small grain size observed in these films[1,2] - an observation which was at the origin of the interest in "granular superconductivity".

Another unusual property of these films was their very high upper critical field[3], which was interpreted in terms of an extreme type II behavior. The very small normal state conductivity observed in these films would indeed correspond to high κ values - of the order of 100 in the most dirty films - according to the Gorkov-Goodman formula. The origin of the unusually low conductivity was again to be found in the granular structure of the film, which electron micrographs show as consisting of small aluminum grains, of the order of one hundred $\mathring{A}$ in diameter or less, and amorphous aluminum oxide. The low conductivity was interpreted as being due to the presence of oxide barriers between the grains, resulting in a low tunneling probability, an electron being scattered back and forth several times in a grain before it could jump over to the nearest neighbor. This low tunneling probability can result in an effective mean free path much shorter than the grain size, and even shorter than the interatomic distance in the metal. It was shown by Parmenter that this effective mean free path is indeed the one that determines the κ value of the material. The high critical field is therefore a consequence of the granularity of the system.

Similar observations - granular structure, low conductivity, increased critical temperature and critical field - were later observed in many different superconductor-insulator (or semiconductor) eutectic systems[4]. It could be argued however that the discrete character of the structure of these films, as opposed to the homogeneous structure of truly amorphous materials, is not really that important. Indeed, amorphous superconductors also have high critical fields and often enhanced critical temperatures[5]. The purpose of this paper is precisely to review more recent experiments, in which the discrete character of the structure of the composite results in novel and sometimes striking properties. We first discuss in Section I recent critical field and critical temperature measurements which illustrate the role played by the granularity of the structure (as opposed to amorphicity). We then turn in Section II to the behavior of the critical current and of the specific heat, for which disorder in the structure plays an essential role: recent measurements can indeed be interpreted quantitatively within the framework of percolation theories, and even shed some light on the details of the percolation process. In Section III we discuss briefly the question of localization near the superconductor - insulator transition, and in Section IV some possible device applications of granular superconductors.

SECTION I - GRANULARITY EFFECTS

The effects of the weak intergrain Josephson coupling are best revealed by experiments in which this coupling can be varied without changing the chemical composition and/or the structure of the sample. For instance, this coupling can be varied by changing the temperature or by applying a magnetic field of appropriate strength. If the intergrain coupling is achieved through a photo-conductor, it can also be varied by shining light onto the sample[6]. The superconducting transition of discontinuous In films deposited on a CdS[7] layer is shown in Fig. 1. Here the large size of the In grains, about 2000 Å (Fig. 2), guarantees that they behave like bulk In. The transition is seen to occur in two steps. A first drop in resistance occurs at the critical temperature of bulk In ($T_c = 3.4K$), where the In grains or clusters of grains become superconducting. This drop is followed by a plateau until the resistance finally drops gradually to zero at a temperature which is significantly smaller than that of pure In. Similar double transitions have been reported for other granular superconductors with fairly large grains[8] and inter-preted as resulting from increased intergrain Josephson coupling as the temperature is reduced. The coupling energy becomes then larger than kT for a sufficiently large number of intergrain junctions to ensure the existence of a continuous superconducting path. What is particularly nice, however, in the In/CdS experiment is that i) the initial drop in resistance occurs at the critical temperature of bulk In and ii) the lower end of the transition can be changed by shining light onto the sample. This results in increased Josephson coupling and, as expected, in a higher transition temperature. Although the lower end of the transition is quite broad, due presumably to a broad range of

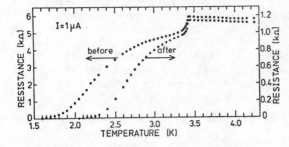

Fig. 1

Resistive transition of an In/CdS sample before and after illumination.

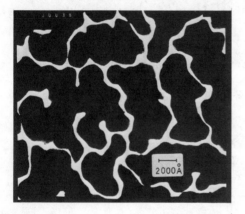

Fig. 2

Electron micrograph of In/CdS sample (dark areas are In islands).

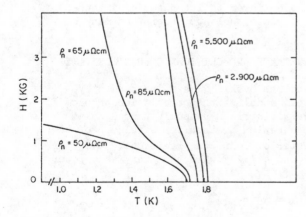

Fig. 3

Critical fields of Al-Ge coevaporated films - note the upturn in the critical field below the decoupling temperature.

junction resistances, there is, in fact, a temperature range where the sample can be turned from a finite resistance state to zero resistance state by shining light onto it.

Another way to modify the intergrain Josephson coupling is to apply a magnetic field of appropriate strength. The idea here is that by forcing vortex lines between grains, one can in effect "disconnect" them. This will be achieved when the average vortex spacing will be of the order of the grain size, i.e. when

$$H = \frac{\phi_0}{2\pi\xi^2(T)} \gtrsim \frac{\phi_0}{2\pi d^2}$$ where $\xi(T)$ is the coherence length that

describes the intergrain order parameter correlation and d is the grain size. Since $\xi(T)$ decreases as the temperature is lowered if $\xi(T=0) \lesssim d$ there will be a temperature below which the critical field of the sample will in fact be that of the isolated grains, resulting in an upturn of the critical field[9]. For very weak intergrain coupling (small $\xi(T=0)$ this temperature will be very close to T_c, so that the critical field of the sample will be that of the isolated grains in most of the temperature range. This is precisely the behavior observed in granular Al-Ge films (Fig. 3), as a direct result of the granularity of the film: the critical field in the weak coupling limit becomes exactly that of the isolated grains, as can be calculated from the measured value of the grain size without any adjustable parameter.

These experiments are clear indications that the granular structure can give rise to special properties that are not observed in bulk or amorphous structures.

SECTION II - DISORDER EFFECTS

Some of the properties of granular superconductors cannot be understood without introducing theoretical models that take explicity disorder effects into account. Fortunately, since we are dealing here with disorder at a macroscopic scale (at least for large enough grains, and compared to interatomic distances), percolation models are appropriate tools to understand many of these properties.

IIa) NORMAL STATE CONDUCTANCE AND CRITICAL CURRENT DENSITY

DeGennes[10] and Skal and Shklovskii[11] have independently proposed a simple geometrical model of the percolation problem[12]. If we consider for instance resistors R randomly placed on a lattice with probability occupation p, then for a value $p>p_c$ there will exist an infinite cluster of connected resistors. Computer experiments show that the conductivity will then vary as a power law

$$\sigma = \sigma_0 (p-p_c)^t \tag{1}$$

where the exponent t $\simeq$ 1.7 in 3D systems and t $\simeq$ 1.0 in 2D. The de Gennes model is a geometrical description of the infinite cluster as consisting of macrobonds of physical length $\mathcal{L}$ interconnecting at nodes, the distance between nearest nodes being the coherence length ξ for the percolation problem. Both lengths diverge at $p = p_c$

$$\xi = \xi_o (p-p_c)^{-\nu}$$
$$\mathcal{L} = \mathcal{L}_o (p-p_c)^{-(\nu+\delta)} \qquad (2)$$

where $\delta \gtrsim 0$ is the exponent that describes the twistedness of the macrobonds. In this model the lengths ξ and $\mathcal{L}$ control, respectively, the number of macrobonds per unit cross-section of the sample and the length of the macrobonds per unit length of the sample. The conductivity is then given by

$$\sigma = \sigma_o (p-p_c)^{(d-1)\nu+\delta} \qquad (3)$$

In the superconducting state, however, the critical current density is controlled only by the number of macrobonds per unit cross section of the sample, i.e. by ξ[13]. Since

$$j_c = j_{co} (p-p_c)^{(d-1)\nu} \qquad (4)$$

a measurement of j_c as a fimctopm pf $(p-p_c)$ provides a direct determination of the critical exponent of the coherence length. In addition, by comparing the behavior of σ and j_c one can obtain a determination of the twistedness exponent δ.

By performing this simple analysis on experimental data for Al-Ge and Pb-Ge films[13] values for the critical exponent ν and δ were obtained: $\nu = 0.87$; $\delta_{3D} = 0$; $\nu_{2D} = 1.35$; $\delta_{2D} < 0$. Similar values were obtained by S. Kirkpatrick from computer experiments[14]. The result $\delta_{2D} < 0$ indicates that deGennes' model is not applicable to the 2D case. The reason for that seems to be that this model neglects the fact that a fairly large number of macrobonds are interconnected around the nodes of the infinite cluster, thus significantly increasing the conductivity of the infinite cluster and compensating (3D) or even overcompensating for the twistedness effect. The computer experiments of Kirkpatrick[14] do indicate that this effect exists with $\delta_{2D} \simeq .03$.

Since the deGennes model does not give such a good description of the percolating cluster after all, one may question whether it is legitimate to use it to extract values for ν from experimental data. We think that this is, in fact, appropriate for the following reasons: i) critical current measurements are sensitive not to the more multiply connected regions around the nodes, but only to the weaker parts of the percolating network; and ii) these weaker parts seem to consist on the average

of approximately only one macrobond thread running between nodes,
for all values of the coherence length (concentration). So the
deGennes model seems in fact to be more valid for the description
of the critical current behavior than for that of the normal state
conductance. As a consequence, the values for ν_{3D} and ν_{2D} obtained
from the analysis of experimental data[13] should be fairly reliable.

IIB) HEAT CAPACITY TRANSITION

Measurements of the heat capacity transition in granular
films are of particular interest in view of the prediction[15] that
very different behavior should be observed, depending on the
grain size and the intergrain coupling. If the intergrain
resistance is R (in the normal state) then i) for $R << \hbar/e^2$ (i.e.
for a normal resistivity $\rho << \hbar d/e^2$ where d is the grain size)
the granular material should exhibit the regular BCS jump for
any grain size, while ii) for $R >> \hbar/e^2$, no resistive and no heat
capacity transitions should be observed at small grain sizes
$d << d_c$, and a BCS jump in the heat capacity (but no resistive
transition) for $d >> d_c$. For $R >> \hbar/e^2$ and intermediate grain
sizes $d \gtrsim d_c$, the BCS jump should be smeared by OD fluctuation
effects[16]. The value of the characteristic size d_c corresponds
to a volume V such that the superconducting condensation energy
at T = 0 is of the order of $k_B T_c$. It is of the order of 50Å.

Results on small grains $(d\sim30Å)$[17] agree fairly well with
these predictions. For values of the resistivity $\rho \gtrsim 10^{-2}\Omega cm$,
no heat capacity transition is observed. However, up to
$\rho \sim 3\times10^{-2}\Omega cm$ a resistive transition is still observed at a
temperature not much lower than the mean field critical temperature
of granular aluminum $(T_c\sim2.3K)$. This does not quite correspond
to the predictions of ref. 15. For intermediate grain sizes,
$d \gtrsim d_c$ and $\rho >> \hbar d/e^2$, exactly the opposite behavior has been
observed[18]. As shown in fig. 4, the heat capacity transition
is quite visible while there is no sign of a resistive transition:
the resistivity of the sample increases by several decades as
the temperature is reduced from 7K down to 1K. This result is
in agreement with theoretical expectations. It proves that the
disappearance of the resistive transition at high resistivities
is not due to the total disappearance of superconductivity, but
rather to the quenching of the Josephson intergrain coupling,
which gives confidence in the granular description of the
material. Moreover, the smearing of the BCS jump as shown in
Fig. 4 does fit with the grain size of these samples $(d \simeq 150Å)$
and the calculations of Mühlschlegel et al.[16]

What remains to be understood is the detailed behavior of
the heat capacity measured in the small grain limit[17], and,
in particular, the fact that these samples can have a resistive
transition without a heat capacity transition. Clearly, what is
missing in the model of ref. 15 are the effects of the disorder
certainly present in the samples. In other terms, there is not

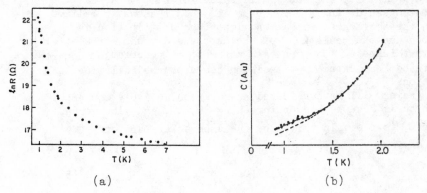

Fig. 4   Insulating behavior (a) and heat capacity transition (b)
of a large grain (d ∿ 150 Å) Al-Ge sample.

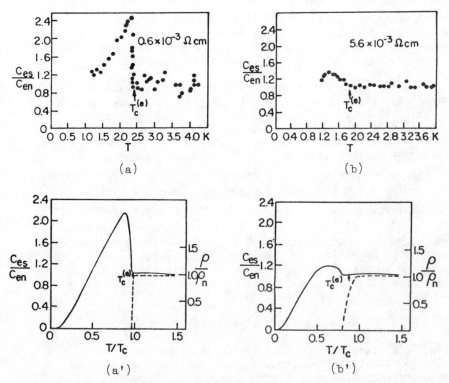

Fig. 5   Experimental (a and b) and theoretical (a' and b') heat
capacity transitions of Al-Al$_2$O$_3$ films.   The
theoretical curves have been calculated using the
experimental values of the resistivity.

just one grain size and one single value for R, but rather distributions $n(d)$ and $n(R)$. There are good reasons to believe that in the small grain limit the important distribution is $n(R)$, because the resistance of the barriers depends exponentially on their thickness. One can then attempt[19] a percolation description of the heat capacity transition based on the following two assumptions:

i) Two grains will be considered as superconductively connected when their Josephson coupling energy $E_j > kT$, and vice versa. Here E_j is the value given by the Ambegaokar-Baratoff expression,

$$E_j \propto [\Delta(T)/R]\tanh[\Delta(T)/kT] \qquad (5)$$

where $\Delta(T)$ is the BCS value for the energy gap.

ii) When a grain is connected to the infinite superconducting cluster, it contributes the BCS heat capacity $C_{es}(T)$. When it is not connected to the infinite cluster, it contributes the value of the 0-D behavior[16] according to its size. In the small grain case, this contribution is completely smeared and has no anomaly around the BCS critical temperature.

This model assumes that the thermodynamic fluctuations are completely quenched as soon as the grains are connected to the infinite cluster. This is the only way in which superconducting coherence is taken into account. Contrary to what is expected for a system with uniform E_j, there will not be a sharp transition at a temperature $T < T_{BCS}$ but rather a smeared transition as the temperature is reduced below T_{cBCS}. The number of grains with $E_j > kT$ increases progressively because of the temperature dependence of the energy gap. The resistive transition occurs at the temperature $T_c^{(e)}$ at which the infinite cluster is formed; below $T_c^{(e)}$ it "fattens up" and a (smeared) BCS like jump appears. This model fits very well the experiment, including the existence of samples with a resistive transition and no heat capacity transition for small grain sizes and high resistivity (see fig. 5).

III - THE SUPERCONDUCTOR-INSULATOR TRANSITION

The model described in the previous section takes into account the effect of thermodynamic fluctuations and disorder on the superconducting transition. It does not, however, take into account the effect of localization on superconductivity. Experimentally, it is observed that the superconducting transition goes down rapidly when the insulator volume fraction is increased to the point where the samples become strongly semiconducting in the normal state, suggesting that localization effects may play an important role in the destruction of superconducting coherence, in addition to thermodynamic fluctuations (which would in principle always allow a low but finite critical temperature, contrary to what seems to be observed experimentally).

In granular materials the localization transition takes place because of the electrostatic energy E_c necessary to add an electron to a grain surrounded by an insulating barrier[4]. A spin 1 model suggested by deGennes[20] predicts that in an ordered array of grains the superconducting coherence is quenched when $E_c > z E_j$ where z is the number of nearest neighbors. A similar result has been obtained by McLean and Stephen[21] and Simanek[22]. A value for E_c can, in principle, be obtained by analyzing the temperature dependence of the normal state conductivity using the expression derived by Sheng and Abeles[4]

$$\sigma = \sigma_0 \exp[-(T_0/T)^{\frac{1}{2}}] \qquad (6)$$

where T_0 is proportional to E_c. The problem, however, is that the conductivity of weakly semiconducting samples (with a depressed but finite T_c) does not fit this expression[23,24], which unfortunately makes a quantitative check of the $\delta = 1$ model impossible. The exact nature of the localization in these samples is for the moment unclear. Slightly dirtier samples (not superconducting) have a conductivity that follows eq. (6), and the value of E_c that is obtained through the conductivity analysis is indeed larger than zE_j.

IV - DEVICE APPLICATIONS

It has been observed that the small initial current densities attainable near the superconductor-to-insulator transition are very favorable for SQUID application because the condition $LI_c = \phi_0$ is then easily achieved in a granular weak-link SQUID[25], and good RF SQUID behavior has indeed been observed in granular aluminum SQUIDS[25] and later in granular Nb and NbN SQUIDS[26]. They also appear to be promising as radiation detectors[27].

It should however be noticed that the excellent properties observed in the granular weak links (sinusoidal current-phase relationship; Shapiro steps observed up to high voltages) run contrary to the generally accepted view that coherent behavior in a weak link can only be achieved if its length is of the order of the superconducting coherence length. The device applications of granular weak links look very promising, but more work will have to be done to understand exactly how they work.

ACKNOWLEDGEMENT

This research was supported by the Israel Council for Research and Development and by the Karlsruhe Nuclear Research Center.

REFERENCES

1. B. Abeles, R. W. Cohen and G. W. Cullen, Phys. Rev. Lett. 17, 632 (1966).

2. G. Deutscher, M. Gershenson, E. Grünbaum and Y. Imry, J. Vac. Sci. Technol. 10, 697 (1973).

3. R. W. Cohen and B. Abeles, Phys. Rev. 168, 444 (1968); R. H. Parmenter, Phys. Rev. 154, 353 (1967).

4. B. Abeles, Applied Solid State Science, Vol. 6, 1976.

5. W. Buckel and R. Hilsch, Z. Phys. 131, 420 (1952).

6. I. Giaever, Phys. Rev. Lett. 20, 1286 (1968).

7. G. Deutscher and M. Rappaport, Phys. Lett. 71A, 471 (1979).

8. G. Deutscher and M. Rappaport, J. de Phys. C6, Vol. 39, 581 (1978)

9. G. Deutscher and S. Dodds, Phys. Rev. B16, 3936 (1977) and Y. Shapira, to be published.

10. P. G. de Gennes, J. Physique Lett. 37, L-1 (1976).

11. A. S. Skal and B. I. Shklovskii, Sov. Phys. Semicond. 8, 1029 (1975).

12. S. Kirkpatrick, AIP Conf. Proc. 40, 99 (1978) and J. P. Straley ibid p. 118.

13. G. Deutscher and M. Rappaport, J. Physique Lett. 40, L219 (1979).

14. S. Kirkpatrick this volume.

15. G. Deutscher, Y. Imry and L. Gunther, Phys. Rev. B10, 4598 (1974).

16. B. Mühlschlegel, D. J. Scalapino and R. Denton, Phys. Rev. B6, 1767 (1972).

17. T. Worthington, P. Lindenfeld and G. Deutscher, Phys. Rev. Lett. 41, 316 (1978).

18. Y. Shapira, Ph.D. Thesis Tel Aviv 1979 and to be published.

19. G. Deutscher, O. Entin-Wohlman, S. Fishman and Y. Shapira, to be published.

20. P. G. de Gennes, private communication as referred to in ref. 17.

21. W. L. McLean and M. J. Stephen, Phys. Rev. B19, 5925 (1979).

22. E. Simánek, Solid State Comm. 31, 419 (1979).

23. W. L. McLean, T. Chui, B. Bandyopadhyay, and P. Lindenfeld, this volume.

24. G. Deutscher, B. Bandyopadhyay, T. Chui, P. Lindenfeld, W. L. McLean, and T. Worthington, submitted for publication.

25. G. Deutscher and R. Rosenbaum, Appl. Phys. Letters 27, 366 (1975).

26. S. A. Wolf, E. J. Cukauskas, F. J. Rachford and M. Nisenoff, IEEE Trans. on Magnetics MAG-15, 595 (1978).

27. R. B. Laibowitz, A. N. Broers, J.T.C. Yeh, and J. M. Viggiano, to be published; J. H. Claassen, E. J. Cukauskas, and M. Nisenoff, this volume.

PHASE ORDERING AND STRUCTURAL DISORDER
IN BULK GRANULAR SUPERCONDUCTORS

J. Rosenblatt, P. Peyral and A. Raboutou
Institut National des Sciences Appliquées
B.P.14A., 35043 Rennes Cedex France

ABSTRACT

A bulk granular superconductor, obtained by compacting a metallic powder in epoxy resin, displays coherence properties only below
a certain temperature, lower than the superconducting transition
temperature of individual grains. We discuss the effects of disorder
on the coherence transition and more particularly those due to
random orientation of individual contacts in the sample. A non-
linear differential equation is obtained for the analog of
Josephson's phase difference in a single junction. It shows the
existence of a coherent penetration depth of the whole sample, due
to Josephson coupling between grains and allows a calculation of
the field dependence of critical currents. These effects are well
confirmed by experiments. Percolation contributions to the current
are also discussed.

INTRODUCTION

We refer to bulk granular superconductors (BGS)[1] as three-
dimensional assemblies of bulk (i.e. of dimensions $a \gg \lambda(T)$, $\xi(T)$)
superconducting grains coupled to each other through Josephson
contacts. In granular films, where grains are usually much smaller,
charging energy effects [2,3] tend to destroy Josephson coupling
and complicate the overall picture. On the other hand our samples
do not admit a continuum description [4] where the superconducting
phase is assumed to vary slowly from one grain to the next.
In fact, if the Josephson interaction were switched off, superconducting phases in different grains could be perfectly random
(it takes no energy, but a gauge transformation to assign them
arbitrarily) and the corresponding order parameters or condensation amplitudes would form a set of vectors randomly oriented
in the complex plane. Assume now that a coupling energy

$E_J = \Phi_o I_J / 2\pi$ (I_J being the critical current of a junction)

exists between nearest neighbors. If the temperature is such
that $k_B T \gg E_J$ the vectors will still be oriented at random. But

when $k_B T \ll E_J$, one would expect that all vectors will tend to

align themselves about a particular orientation, resulting in
overall phase coherence in the sample. On this basis we have
assumed[4] that a transition from a paracoherent to a coherent
state would take place at a certain temperature $T_o < T_c$, $k_B T_o \simeq E_J$.

Actually, we have found quite good agreement between a calculation combining Bethe's version of the mean field theory of phase transitions[5] and Ambegaokar and Halperin's[6] expression for the noise-induced voltage in a single junction, and our data on the temperature dependence of the resistance in BGS in the paracoherent region[4] Our experimental research was initially prompted out by Tilley's[7] prediction of superradiance, that is emission of electromagnetic radiation of power proportional to n^2 by an assembly of n junctions. However phase coherence as described above is a static phenomenon and in this sense opposed to superradiance which requires synchronisation of phase motion in individual junctions. The extent to which the two effects are interdependent is still an open question. Turning back to static behavior, a description[8], based on Wallace and Stavn's treatment of the tunneling hamiltonian in terms of pseudo spin operators[9] shows that a translationally invariant system whould indeed display a phase transition to coherence. In fact, the interaction can be seen to be formally the same as that of the X-Y model[10] of anisotropic ferromagnets. The appropriate order parameter for this transition is $\psi = \langle e^{i\phi} \rangle$ where the brackets denote a thermal average and ϕ is the (fluctuating) superconducting phase in a grain. But the problem here is that granular superconductors are far from being translationally invariant. The coupling strength may vary from one junction to the next, grains are not all of the same size and shape, etc. One particular feature of structural disorder has been suggested to us by the experimental observation[11] that the modulation of critical current by an external field was essentially the same irrespective of whether the field was perpendicular or parallel to the impressed current. We concluded that this simply expressed the fact that individual junctions were oriented at random in the sample and therefore made no distinction between various directions of the field. In what follows we shall develop an idealised model of this effect. It will allow us to define a "pseudophase" playing a role similar to Josephson's phase difference and satisfying a non linear differential equation. This equation provides an expression for the coherent penetration depth of the sample and gives a description of the effects of a field on the critical current. At high fields, the latter can be understood in terms of a percolation problem, also due to randomness in contact orientation.

A MODEL OF ORIENTATIONAL DISORDER

Of the many sources of disorder in our systems, we shall focus our attention here on random junction orientation. That is, we shall assume that I_J is the same for all junctions. If $\vec{a}$ is the vector joining the centers of two neighboring grains, we consider it constant in modulus but ascribe to it a probability $P(\theta)\, d\theta = \sin\theta\, d\theta$ of forming an angle between θ and $\theta + d\theta$ with a given direction. When an external field $\vec{H}$ is applied, a "microscopic" field $\vec{h}(\vec{r})$, meandering around and into the grains down to a superconducting penetration depth, develops in the sample. We consider instead $\vec{B}(\vec{r}) = \overline{\vec{h}} = \nabla \wedge \vec{A}$, where the bar indicates an average over a volume small compared with the sample, but large enough to countain many grains. In the absence of Josephson coupling, $\vec{B} = \mu \vec{H} \simeq (1 - f) \vec{H}$, where f is the filling factor of grains in the sample[12]. Fig.1 depicts these approximations. To them we add the

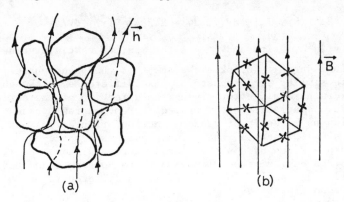

Fig. 1 (a) "Realistic" granular system. (b) Simplified model.

following physical assumption :
     In the presence of fields and currents, the free energy per unit volume may be written :

$$F = \overline{F}_0 + \overline{F}_1 + B^2/(8\pi\mu) \qquad (1)$$

where F_0 is the free energy in the absence of fields and currents. Consider now the form of F_1. If the order parameter $\psi = <e^{i\phi}> = |\psi|e^{i\phi}$ has $|\psi| \to 1$ each junction should contribute to it with Josephson's free energy $E_J \left(1 - \cos(\vec{a} . \nabla\tilde{\phi})\right)$. On the other hand, when $|\psi| \to 0$, a Ginsburg-Landau form, $F_1 \propto |\nabla\psi|^2$, is plausible. We therefore write, in gauge invariant form,

$$\overline{F}_1 = n_J E_J \int_0^{\pi/2} \left(1 - \cos|\vec{a}.(i\nabla - 2\pi\vec{A}/\Phi_0)\psi|\right) \sin\theta d\theta, \qquad (2)$$

where $n_J = z/2a^3$ is the number of junctions per unit volume with z the number of first neighbors of a grain. This choice is admittedly far from being unique. But it may at least show how collective effects should modify individual junction behavior. Furthermore, away from possible vortices, we expect $|\psi|$ to change slowly compared with $\overset{\sim}{\phi}$. If such is the case, the argument of the cosine in Eq. (2) becomes $|\psi|\ \vec{a}.\vec{k}$, where $\vec{k} = \nabla\overset{\sim}{\phi} - 2\pi\vec{A}/\Phi_o$ is a gauge invariant phase gradient. Defining now the vector quantity $\vec{\gamma} = |\psi|a\vec{k}$, minimisation of Eqs.(1) and (2) with respect to $\vec{A}$ gives for the average current density

$$\vec{j} = (z/2a^2)(\vec{\gamma}/\gamma)I_J|\psi|dV(\gamma)/d\gamma = 2.294j_{co}(\vec{\gamma}/\gamma)dV/d\gamma \qquad (3)$$

where $V(\gamma) = 1 - \gamma^{-1}\sin\gamma$ and j_{co} is the maximum absolute value of $\vec{j}$, attained when $\gamma = 0.6626\pi$. We see that the pseudophase $\vec{\gamma}$ plays a role similar to Josephson's phase difference, although it is a tridimensional vector giving the direction of the current and its modulus satisfies a somewhat different current-phase relationship as a result of random junction orientations. As phase in a single junction, the pseudophase has a space- and time-dependence given by a non linear differential equation. This can be obtained easily if one invokes phase coherence and therefore fluxoid quantisation in the system. In differential form the latter condition reads :

$$\nabla \wedge \vec{k} = 2\pi \left[\Sigma\ \delta(\vec{r} - \vec{r_i})\ \vec{B}/B - \vec{B}/\Phi_o \right] \qquad (4)$$

where the δ-functions are two-dimensional and indicate vortices located at $\vec{r_i}$. Away from vortices, i.e. for $\vec{r} \neq \vec{r_i}$, we apply the curl operator, take into account Maxwell's equations, Josephson's phase-voltage relation $\vec{E} = (\Phi_o/2\pi c)\ \partial\vec{k}/\partial t$ and Eq.(3) to obtain :

$$\nabla^2\vec{\gamma} - (\mu\epsilon/c^2)\ \partial^2\vec{\gamma}/\partial t^2 = (3/\lambda_c^2)\ V'(\gamma)\vec{\gamma}/\gamma \qquad (5)$$

where $V'(\gamma) = dV(\gamma)/d\gamma$, and

$$\lambda_c^2 = 3c\Phi_o a/(4\pi^2\mu z I_J|\psi|^2) \qquad (6)$$

is the coherent penetration depth squared for $\gamma \to o$, that is for very weak fields. We may point out here that Eq.(5) is of the type admitting soliton solutions[13] propagating with constant velocity. Their proper treatment requires the addition of dissipative terms not included in Eq.(5).

MAGNETIC FIELD EFFECTS

We shall be concerned here with static problems where $\vec{\gamma}$ depends on a single variable, x, say. Then Eq.(5) admits a first integral for the absolute value of $\vec{\gamma}$:

$$\gamma'^2 = (d\gamma/dx)^2 = (6/\lambda_c^2) V(\gamma) + \gamma_o'^2, \tag{7}$$

with γ_o' an integration constant. Consider a semiinfinite sample occupying the half space $x > 0$, with an applied field H along the z-axis. Then $\vec{\gamma}$ has the single component $\gamma_y = \gamma$. If there are no fields or currents far inside the sample $\gamma'(\infty) = \gamma(\infty) = \gamma_o' = 0$ according to Eq.(7), which gives, on the surface,

$$\gamma_s' = 2\pi a|\psi|\mu H/\Phi_o = \sqrt{6}(1 - \gamma_s^{-1} \sin\gamma_s)^{1/2} /\lambda_c \tag{8}$$

This has a maximum value when γ_s is the smallest non-zero root of the trascendental equation $\gamma_s = \tan\gamma_s$, i.e. $\gamma_s = 1.43\pi$. We conclude that the Meissner effect exists in the sample up to a maximum field

$$H_1 = 1.103\sqrt{6} \Phi_o/(2\pi\mu\lambda_c a|\psi|) = 1.103\left[2zI_J\Phi_o/(\mu ca^3)\right]^{1/2} \tag{9}$$

It may be verified that, apart from a numerical factor close to unity, $\mu H_1^2/8\pi$ is just the coupling energy density of the z/2 junctions per grain. For a typical coupling energy of the order of liquid He temperature (which implies that the paracoherence-to-coherence transition can be observed)$I_J \simeq 2 \times 10^{-7}$A, giving $H_1 \simeq 1$mG from Eq.(9) and $\lambda_c \simeq 0.4$ mm from Eq.(6) with z = 6 and a = 50μm. We describe a measurement of λ_c confirming this estimate in another communication to this conference[14]. Let us point out here that such measurements are delicate particularly because of the high sensitivity of the effective penetration depth

$$\lambda = B_s^{-1} \int_0^\infty B dx = \gamma_s/\gamma_s' = \gamma_s\lambda_c \left(6(1 - \gamma_s^{-1} \sin \gamma_s)\right)^{-1/2} \tag{10}$$

to external fields. For example, when H = H_1, $\lambda = 1.66 \lambda_c$.

Similar sensitivity to magnetic fields can be found in critical currents. Let us first calculate the maximum supercurrent in the absence of field. Assume that the current is parallel to the z-axis. Again $\vec{\gamma}$ has a single component, $\gamma_z = \gamma$. We remark from the right-hand side of Eq.(5) that γ'' is proportional to the current density and therefore $\gamma_s' - \gamma_o' \propto \int \vec{j}\, dx = J(0)$, the current per unit length along the y-axis. From (7) it is found that $\gamma_s' - \gamma_o'$ has a maximum value when $\gamma_o' = 0$, which gives for the maximum supercurrent once the constants have been worked out :

$$J_c(0) = 2.066 j_{co}\lambda_c \tag{11}$$

We remark that $H_1 = 8.26\pi \, j_{co}\lambda_c/c = 4\pi J_c(0)/c$, which is just Silsbee's rule.

When both a current and a field are applied, the situation is more complicated because we are led to consider two components of $\vec{\gamma}$. Furthermore, the possibility of quantum interference when the field is parallel to the current appears. Consider for example a slab occupying the region $-d \leq x \leq d$ ($d \gg \lambda_c$) with current and field both applied along the z-axis. Taking $\vec{A} = (0, A_y, 0)$ gives a y-component for γ, while the current provides the z-component. The situation is somewhat simplified if $H \gg H_1$. Then screening currents can be neglected and $B \simeq \mu H$, $A_y = \mu Hx$ and $\gamma_y = \gamma'_{yo} x$ with

$$\gamma'_{yo} = - a|\psi| 2\pi B/\Phi_o = -2.7 \, \lambda_c^{-1} \, H/H_1 \quad \text{from Eq.(9). Furthermore}$$

$$\gamma = (\gamma_y^2 + \gamma_z^2)^{1/2} \gg 1 \text{ over most of the sample, except for a small}$$

region where $x < \lambda_c$, contributing negligibly to the total current. We solve the equation for γ_z

$$\frac{d^2\gamma_z}{dx^2} = \frac{1}{2} \frac{d\gamma'^2_z}{d\gamma_z} = \frac{3}{\lambda_c^2} \frac{\gamma_z}{\gamma} \frac{dV}{d\gamma} \tag{12}$$

by taking into account that, for $\gamma \gg 1$

$$x = \int_0^\gamma \left(6V/\lambda_c^2 + \gamma'^2_o\right)^{-1/2} d\gamma \simeq \gamma \, (1 - 3/\gamma'^2_o \lambda_c^2) \, /\gamma'_o \tag{13}$$

$$\gamma' \simeq \gamma'_o \, (1 + 3/\gamma'^2_o \lambda_c^2), \tag{14}$$

to lowest order, and that

$$\frac{d\gamma_z}{d\gamma} = \frac{(\gamma - \gamma'^2_o x \,/\gamma')}{\gamma_z} \simeq \frac{\gamma}{\gamma_z} \frac{6}{\gamma'^2_o \lambda_c^2}, \tag{15}$$

where $\gamma'(0) = \gamma'_o = \gamma'_{yo}$ results from the condition of maximum supercurrent $\gamma'_z(0) = 0$. Finally $\gamma'_z\lambda_c = 6 \sqrt{V(\gamma)} /\gamma'_o\lambda_c$, which, by steps similar to those leading to Eq.(11) gives us

$$J_c(H)/J_c(0) = 0.822(1 - \gamma_s^{-1}\sin\gamma_s)^{1/2} \, H_1/H \tag{16}$$

where γ_s is found from Eq.(13) with $x = d$. Eq.(16) predicts a rather sharp peak centered at $H = 0$ with superimposed oscillations. Our measurements do show a central peak but, contrary to Eq.(16), they suggest a non-zero value for $J_c(H)$ when $H \to \infty$. This led us to study another mechanism, i.e., percolation[15], to explain the persistence of supercurrents up to high fields.

SUPERCURRENT PERCOLATION

In the framework of our model, the current effectively going through a junction is

$$I = I_J \sin(\gamma \cos\theta), \tag{17}$$

that is, for a given γ, I depends on orientation. Actually $|I| = I_J$ for orientations θ_ℓ such that $\cos\theta_\ell = \pm (\ell + 1/2)\pi/\gamma$ with $\ell = 0,1,\ldots,N-1$ and N = Int. Part $(\gamma/\pi + 1/2)$. This is just the well-known fact that maximum supercurrent is attained when the junction contains a half integral number of flux quanta. Consider now the sets $\{I_o\}$ of all junctions with orientations such that $I_J \geqslant I \geqslant I_o$ and probability of occurence $P(I_o)$ high enough so that they form a cluster spanning the whole system. If I_o is chosen such as to make total current carried by the set a maximum (say $I_o = I_1$), other sets will be "saturated" as the critical current is approached. We expect then critical current to be determined by this particular set. Of course, $I_1 < I_m = \max(I_o)$ and $P(I_1) > P_c = P(I_m)$ where P_c is the percolation threshold. Let δ be defined by $|I| \geqslant I_o$ for $\cos\theta_\ell + \delta \geqslant \cos\theta \geqslant \cos\theta_\ell - \delta$, so that :

$$I_o = I_J |\sin(\gamma(\cos\theta_\ell \pm \delta))| = I_J |\cos(\gamma\delta)| \tag{18}$$

The conditional probability that a contact at point $\vec{r}$ with a pseudophase $\gamma(\vec{r})$ will carry a current $I \geqslant I_o$ will then be :

$$p(\gamma/2N ; I_o) = \sum_{\ell=0}^{N-1} \int_{\cos\theta_\ell - \delta}^{\cos\theta_\ell + \delta} d(\cos\theta) = 2N\delta = 2N\gamma^{-1} \cos^{-1}(I_o/I_J) \tag{19}$$

Now $\gamma/2N$ is a piecewise continuous variable in intervals $(1 - 1/2N)\pi/2 \leqslant \gamma/2N < (1 + 1/2N)\pi/2$. Then the probability of finding junctions carrying current $I > I_o$ is :

$$P(I_o) = 2 \int_{\pi/2}^{\gamma_s} p(\gamma/2N ; I_o) g(\gamma) \, d\gamma$$

$$= \gamma_s^{-1} \cos^{-1}(I_o/I_J) \left\{ \sum_{N=1}^{N_s-1} 2N \int_{2N-1}^{2N+1} du/u + 2N_s \int_{2N_s-1}^{2\gamma_s/\pi} du/u \right\} \tag{20}$$

where $g(\gamma) \simeq (2\gamma_s)^{-1}$ is the probability density for a junction to have a pseudophase γ and $N_s = N(\gamma_s)$. Finally, by approximating $\ln(2N+1)/(2N-1) \simeq 1/N$:

$$I_o = I_J \cos(\alpha P\pi/2) \qquad (21)$$

where $\alpha^{-1} = 2N_s/(2N_s-1) - \pi\gamma_s$. We now argue that near the percolation threshold current is carried by a rather low density of chains of favorably oriented contacts. The maximum current per chain is that of the weakest link, given by Eq.(21). Total current will then be proportional to I_o and to the density of percolation paths, itself approximately proportional to the conductivity of the equivalent bond percolation problem, i.e. to $(P-P_c)^\xi$, with $\xi \simeq 1.5 - 1.6$[15]. It should be also proportional to the average number of percolation bonds per site, zP, since this measures the number of parallel-connected junctions arriving to a site[16]. The percolation current thus obtained is :

$$I_p = I_{po} P(P-P_c)^\xi \cos(\alpha P\pi/2) \qquad (22)$$

where I_{po} is a proportionality constant. The critical percolation current will be given by that value of P which makes I_p a maximum, that is by the roots of the trascendental equation :

$$\xi = (u - u_c)(\tan u - 1/u) \quad ; \quad u = \alpha P\pi/2 \qquad (23)$$

The results of such a calculation are shown in Fig.2, together with the predictions of Eq.(16) for the coherent contribution. We have taken $\gamma_s \simeq 2.7 dH/\lambda_c H_1$ with $\lambda_c \simeq 0.4mm$ and $H_1 \simeq 10^{-3} Oe$, $\xi = 1.5$ and $P_c = 0.25$. The percolation current is quite insensitive to the precise values of the last two parameters, but displays rather pronounced oscillations for small values of γ_s.

A detailed comparison with experiment is given in ref.14. We just point out that, as $H \to \infty$, $\gamma_s \to \infty$ and $\alpha \to 1$, giving a finite value of I_p from Eqs.(22) and (23).

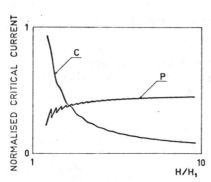

Fig.2 Coherent (C) and percolation (P)
       contributions to the current.

DISCUSSION

The model described here seeks to explain a few features of our experimental work on BGS[14] : (1) independence of quantum interference effects upon the relative orientations of current and field, (2) the existence of a central peak followed by (3) a rather long tail in the critical current, with a finite limit at high fields and (4) the appearence of many small oscillations in the $J_c(H)$ curves. All these features are qualitatively, but not quantitatively, reproduced by the model. Feature (1) is a consequence of the random orientation of junctions in the sample ; (2) is due to the establishment of phase coherence while (3) results from percolation effects. Finally (4) is explained by the intrinsic non-linearity of the Josephson effect which is preserved, albeit modified by the different types of disorder present in the sample. The model is admittedly oversimplified, in the sense that types of disorder like spread in the coupling energies, for example, are neglected. This makes the qualitative agreement obtained with the data of Ref.14 ever more encouraging.

REFERENCES

1 - J. Rosenblatt, H.Cortès, P. Pellan Phys. Lett. A33, 143 (1970).
2 - B. Abelès, Phys. Rev. B15, 2828 (1977).
3 - E. Simanek, preprint
4 - P. Pellan, G. Dousselin, H. Cortès and J. Rosenblatt, Sol. State Comm. 11, 427 (1972).
5 - H.A. Bethe, Proc. Roy. Soc. A216,45 (1935) ; C. Domb, Advan. Phys. 9, 149 (1960).
6.- V. Ambegaokar and B.I. Halperin Phys. Rev. Lett. 22, 1364 (1969)
7 - D.R. Tilley, Phys. Lett. 33A, 205 (1970).
8 - J. Rosenblatt, A. Raboutou, P. Pellan, Proc. 14th Int. Conf. Low Temp. Phys. 2, 361 (1975).
9 - P.R. Wallace and M.J. Stavn, Can. J. Phys. 43, 411 (1965).
10- See, for example D.D. Betts in Phase Transitions and Critical Phenomena, C. Domb and M.S. Green, Academic Press London 1974.
11- P. Peyral and J. Rosenblatt Proceedings of LT15 J. Phys. C6-583 (1978)
12- J. Rosenblatt, Rev. Phys. Appl. 9, 217 (1974).
13- A.C. Scott, F.Y.F. Chu and D.W. McLaughlin, Proc. I.E.E. 61, 1443 (1973).
14- A. Raboutou, P. Peyral and J. Rosenblatt, Communication to this Conference
15- S. Kirkpatrick, Rev. Mod. Phys. 45, 574 (1973).
16- V.K. Shante, Phys. Rev. B16, 2597 (1977).

THE NORMAL-STATE CONDUCTION PROCESSES OF GRANULAR SUPERCONDUCTORS

W. L. McLean, T. Chui, B. Bandyopadhyay, and P. Lindenfeld
Serin Physics Laboratory, Rutgers University
New Brunswick, N. J. 08903

ABSTRACT

We discuss the dependence of the normal-state electrical resistivity on temperature and magnetic field for granular aluminum near the metal-insulator transition. For specimens with sufficiently high room-temperature resistivities the temperature dependence is similar to that of hopping conduction, suggesting that at absolute zero they may be insulators in the normal state. In specimens with a negative temperature coefficient of resistance there is an unexpectedly large negative magnetoresistance. We consider the evidence which the results provide for the possibility that superconductivity can exist in a system of localized electron states.

INTRODUCTION

In our recent work on granular superconductors we have concentrated on the region near the percolation threshold. A variety of interesting effects occur there, related to the fact that the grains are almost independent of each other.

The superconducting properties can be described by a model in which adjacent grains are considered to be weakly coupled by Josephson tunneling.[1] Percolation through the junctions and their superconducting electrodes, the grains, allows long-range phase coherence to be established throughout the system.[2] However, as the average grain separation is made larger, phase coherence is eventually lost,[3,4] even at absolute zero, as a result of zero-point oscillations.[5]

Since the overlap of electron wave functions on adjacent grains falls off exponentially with the separation of the grains, the electrical resistivity changes rapidly in a narrow range of metal-fraction concentrations in the vicinity of the percolation threshold. According to this model, just before the demise of superconductivity, conduction in the normal state is possible only by thermal activation,[6] so that the resistivity becomes infinite at absolute zero. The model suggests that the system can then be described as being a superconducting insulator, since normal-state conduction disappears at absolute zero.

In addition, recent theoretical work[7] on the Hubbard model, with attractive U-centers and finite coupling between neighbors, leads to the conclusion that a long-range pair-correlated phase can exist even when the conductivity at higher temperatures is dominated by thermally activated hopping of single electrons.

The theoretical situation is far from decisive and we turn to the experiments for further guidance. We first review some relevant theoretical results, and then consider those aspects of our work which are related to the existence of superconductivity in a system of states which, apart from phonon coupling, are truly localized.

THEORETICAL REVIEW

Experimental studies of the temperature dependence of the normal state conductivity of granular metals have not all shown agreement with any single universal law - perhaps because of macroscopic inhomogeneities. There is a large amount of evidence[6] in support of the form $\sigma = \sigma_o \exp[-(T_0/T)^{\frac{1}{2}}]$ for which an explanation has been given by Sheng and Abeles.[8] Cases have also been found[9] where the conductivity follows Mott's formula for variable range hopping,[10] $\sigma = \sigma_o \exp[-(T_0/T)^{\frac{1}{4}}]$. In earlier measurements on granular aluminum[11] we found that neither of these forms fitted the data, but that the conductivity between 1.2 and 4.2K could be fitted by either $\sigma = \sigma_m + \sigma_o \exp[-(T_0/T)^{\frac{1}{2}}]$ or $\sigma = \sigma_m + \sigma_o \exp[-(T_0/T)^{\frac{1}{4}}]$, where σ_m is independent of T.

It may be worth recalling the origin of the fractional powers of the inverse temperature in the exponents. Conduction by hopping from one potential well to another as in Mott's theory, or from grain to grain as in Sheng and Abeles' theory, is possible because of overlap of the electron wavefunctions centered on adjacent sites. If the amplitude of the wavefunction falls off as $\exp(-\alpha r)$, this leads to a factor $\exp(-2\alpha R)$ in the transition rate between the sites; here R is the separation of the well or grain edges. In Mott's theory, disorder causes a mismatch ΔE between the energy eigenvalues on the two sites and so phonon absorption or emission is needed to assist the transition. This introduces an additional factor $e^{-\Delta E/kT}$. For hopping of range R, Mott assumes that ΔE is given by the smallest spacing between levels in a spherical volume of radius R and is approximately $3/4\pi R^3 N(0)$, where $N(0)$ is the density of states. In Sheng and Abeles' theory a similar activation factor arises in the following way. Suppose that two adjacent grains are initially uncharged. After an electron has been transferred from one to the other the system has gained an electrostatic energy ("charging energy") $E_c = e^2/2C$, where C is the intergrain capacitance. This leads to the activation factor $\exp(-E_c/2kT)$, analogous to the factor $\exp(-E_g/2kT)$ in a semiconductor with a gap E_g.

Two further assumptions are made in this theory. The first is that hopping occurs preferentially along paths in the system for which the charging energy is constant. The second is that in a given sample with a uniform volume fraction of metal but with a variety of grain diameters, the ratio R/d is a constant, where R is the shortest distance between two neighboring grains of the same diameter d. The result is then that $E_c = K/R$, where K is a constant.

In both the Mott and the Sheng-Abeles theories it is assumed that the bulk conductivity is dominated by the paths with the highest conductivity, so that $\sigma = \sigma_0 \exp(-2\alpha R_{max} - \Delta E_{max}/kT)$, with $R_{max}^4 = 9/8\pi\alpha kT\ N(o)$ in Mott's theory, or, in Sheng and Abeles' theory $\sigma = \sigma_0 \exp(-2\alpha R_{max} - E_{cmax}/2kT)$ with $R_{max}^2 = K/4\alpha kT$, leading to the forms $\sigma = \sigma_0 \exp[-(T_0/T)^{1/n}]$ with $n = 4$ or 2 respectively. It should be noted that in one case activation is required because of disorder, in the other because of the Coulomb interaction. The Sheng-Abeles theory does not take into account that in small grains the electronic level spacing may be much greater than kT and so a further effect should come from the mismatch of the levels on adjacent grains if their sizes are slightly different. We might then expect a more complicated temperature dependence than either of the two fractional-exponent laws.

An illuminating alternative approach to Mott's hopping law, given by Ambegaokar, Halperin, and Langer[12], is worth discussing at this point since it is relevant to both the normal and superconducting phases of granular metals. Their discussion of hopping conduction treats the medium as a network of elementary resistors linking the sites on which electrons can be localized. The conductance between sites i and j, G_{ij}, is of the form $e^{-2\alpha R_{ij} - |\Delta E_{ij}|/kT}$. (For the exact definition of $|\Delta E_{ij}|$ see Ref. 12.) Suppose now that the elementary resistors are removed from the network in succession, starting with the smallest G_{ij} links and working towards the highest until, at the removal of some $G_{ij} = G_c$, the last percolation path from one end of the system to the other is broken. The key assumption in this approach is that the bulk conductivity of the system is proportional to G_c. The authors then go on to show, by an argument different from Mott's, that G_c is proportional to $\exp[-(T_0/T)^{1/4}]$. (They also discuss many reasons why the model can go wrong!). It is tempting to apply the same general approach to a granular metal and so to assume that the measured conductivity is dominated by the junctions between grains that break the percolation network when removed in order of increasing Josephson coupling energy. One would then expect the behavior in the tail of the resistive superconducting transition to be related to the normal state conductivity.

A completely different origin of the Sheng and Abeles half-power law has been suggested recently by Abrahams and Kulik.[7] Their exploration of the Hubbard model with attractive on-site correlations between electrons of opposite spin shows that when Debye screening is taken into account, the effective activation energy, E_a, is proportional to T^2, so that the factor $\exp[-(E_a/kT)]$ becomes $\exp(-const./T^2)$.

We now turn to the negative magnetoresistance which we reported in an earlier paper.[11] It is of importance in the present context because of the possibility that its detailed behavior may provide a means of telling whether or not the electron states are localized. A large negative magnetoresistance in granular metals was first observed in the Ni-SiO$_2$ system with 50 Å grains by

Gittleman, Goldstein, and Bozowski.[13] A theory based on the dependence of the charging energy on the exchange interactions within
the grains was developed by Helman and Abeles.[14] It implies,
however, that the effect should be absent if the grains are not
themselves ferromagnetic.

Negative magnetoresistance is well known in semiconductors
and various explanations have been given, some applying to small,
others to large impurity concentrations.[15] Although there are
general grounds for expecting that in metals the magnetoresistance
should be positive,[16] even in that case the effect can be negative
under special circumstances, for example if there are voids or
magnetic impurities. It seems more likely that the effect which we
observe is analogous to that of hopping conduction in semiconductors
for which a theory has recently been developed by Fukuyama and
Yosida.[17] The physical basis for their theory is that the decay
rate of the wavefunction, denoted earlier by α, is a function of
the Fermi energy. In the presence of a magnetic field electrons
with both spin orientations are in equilibrium and so their chemical potentials ζ are the same. The total energy of an electron
at the Fermi level is $E_F \pm \mu H$ so that the Fermi energies are
$E_{F\pm} = \zeta \mp \mu H$. Hence $\alpha = \alpha(E_F)$ becomes $\alpha_\pm = \alpha(\zeta \pm \mu H)$. It is then
assumed that the two electron-spin populations are equal but that
they contribute differently to the conductivity, i.e. $\sigma = \sigma_+ + \sigma_-$
where $\sigma_\pm = \frac{1}{2} \sigma(\alpha_\pm)$ and $\sigma(\alpha)$ is the conductivity in zero field. An
obvious difficulty of applying this theory to granular metals is
the assumption of equal populations. If the grains were large,
the fractional population difference would be of order $2\mu H/E_F$ and
the assumption would be a good approximation. However, Kubo[18] has
pointed out that if a grain is small enough so the level spacing at
the Fermi energy is large compared with kT, Fermi-Dirac statistics
no longer apply, and the fractional population difference on grains
with an even number of electrons is zero but on grains with an odd
number of electrons it is of order $\mu H/kT$. At 30kG and 2K, $\mu H/kT$ is
about equal to one, so that the temperature dependence of the
magnetoresistance is then different from that derived by Fukuyama
and Yosida.

Finally it should be mentioned that another mechanism proposed
to explain the negative magnetoresistance in semiconductors
involves field-dependent spin-flip scattering from magnetic
impurities or from the spins of single localized electrons.[15] This
explanation is meant to apply to cases where there are some states
that are not localized, for example, in semiconductors that are
heavily doped or when there are electrons above a mobility edge.
It does not appear to be relevant to the hopping case, where all
occupied states are localized. A further difficulty of this
explanation is that it seems to require the assumption of giant
magnetic moments (as large as 100 Bohr magnetons[19]) to fit the data.
In spite of much activity in this field for over a decade, there
is still a lack of consensus as to the basic origin of the
negative magnetoresistance.

EXPERIMENTAL RESULTS

The measurements were made on specimens similar to those which we have previously described.[11] Pure aluminum was evaporated from an electron-beam source under a small pressure of oxygen onto water-cooled glass substrates. It is well known that the metal then deposits in the form of grains surrounded by amorphous aluminum oxide. The grain size of our specimens is expected to be about 30 Å.[20]

Table I shows the characteristics of the specimens. We have no independent measure of the metal concentration, but we know that these specimens are in a very narrow range of concentration near the percolation threshold. Indirect evidence[21] suggests that the relation of room-temperature resistivity to concentration is the same as that reported for Al-SiO$_2$ by Abeles and Hanak.[22]

In this narrow region the room-temperature resistivity is extremely sensitive, not only to variations in the concentration, but also to details of the specimen preparation, such as the substrate temperature and the residual pressure. The absolute values of the resistivity in Table I are therefore to be regarded as nominal.

The listed room-temperature resistivities of the three super-conducting specimens (1, 2 and 5) are seen to vary by a factor of two, but the uncertainties are such that we can only say that all three are approximately the same.

Fig. 1 shows the temperature dependence of the measured resistance as a function of $T^{-\frac{1}{2}}$. A straight line on this graph indicates agreement with the Sheng-Abeles formula. It is seen that the two specimens in which we observe no superconducting transition (6 and 3) follow the formula but that the others do not.

To assess the disagreement of the superconducting specimens we have fitted the results to the empirical formula[11], $\sigma = \sigma_m + \sigma_0 \exp[-(T_0/T)^{\frac{1}{2}}]$. The parameters are shown in Table I. The table also shows the values of the temperature $T_{\frac{1}{2}}$ at which $\sigma = 2\sigma_m$. This parameter is independent of the absolute value of the conductivity and of our knowledge of the geometrical factor relating measured resistance to resistivity. It goes to zero when σ_m goes to zero, i.e. when the temperature dependence of the resistance follows the Sheng-Abeles formula.

Fig. 2 shows the superconducting transition temperature as a function of $T_{\frac{1}{2}}$. Since pure activation ($\sigma_m = 0$, $T_{\frac{1}{2}} = 0$) implies localization, the question of whether superconductivity is possible under these circumstances is the same as the question of where this graph meets the vertical axis.

Fig. 3a shows the magnetoresistance of specimen 6 at several temperatures. At 4.2K the field dependence is quadratic. At lower temperatures it begins quadratically but tends toward saturation at higher fields.

Fig. 3b shows the coefficient of the H^2-term as a function of temperature. The straight line is drawn with the slope which

TABLE I

Specimen #	ρ_{RT} (Ω cm)	$\rho_{4.2}$	σ_0 (Ω cm)$^{-1}$	σ_m	T_0 (K)	$T_{1/2}$	T_C	E_C (μeV)	E_J
1	(.04)	.16	11	4	8	6	1.9	30	3
2	(.02)	.12	15	3	5	4	1.8	20	5
5	(.02)	.1	38	1	9	1	1.2	40	7
6	(.05)	3	38	0	90	0	–	400	6
3	.3	32	6	0	120	0	–	500	1

Characteristics of the specimens. E_C is calculated from the relation[8] $E_C = T_0/4\alpha R$, with $\alpha = 1\text{Å}^{-1}$ and $R = 5\text{Å}$. E_J is calculated as described in Ref. 21, with $\rho_N = 1/\sigma_0$. For the non-superconducting specimens T_C was taken as 1K in order to obtain an upper limit for E_J.

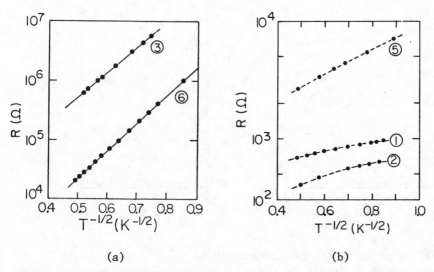

(a)   (b)

Fig. 1: Temperature dependence of the resistance, plotted as R against $T^{-\frac{1}{2}}$. A straight line corresponds to $\sigma = \sigma_0 [\exp -(T_0/T)^{\frac{1}{2}}]$. (a) The non-superconducting specimens, Nos. 3 and 6. (b) The superconducting specimens, Nos. 1, 2 and 5.

48

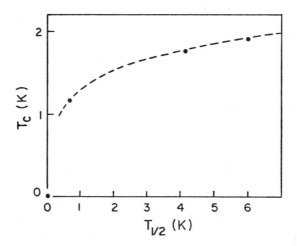

Fig. 2: Graph of T_c against $T_{\frac{1}{2}}$. $T_{\frac{1}{2}}$ is defined as the temperature at which $\sigma = 2\sigma_m$, where $\sigma = \sigma_m + \sigma_o^{\frac{1}{2}}\exp[-(T_o/T)^{\frac{1}{2}}]$. A value of zero for $T_{\frac{1}{2}}$ indicates that $\sigma_m = 0$ and agreement with the exponential form. A non-zero value of $T_{\frac{1}{2}}$ measures the departure from the exponential dependence.

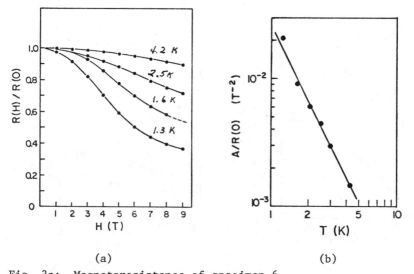

(a)   (b)

Fig. 3a: Magnetoresistance of specimen 6.

Fig. 3b: Log $[A/R(0)]$ plotted against log T, where A = $[R(0) - R(H)]/H^2$. The line has the slope of -2 which corresponds to a variation of $[R(0) - R(H)]$ proportional to H^2/T^2.

corresponds to the case where the initial parts of the curves on Fig. 3a are functions of H/T only.

This behavior is followed also by specimens 1 and 5. For specimen 3 the parabolic part is very small so that the uncertainty in the coefficient is large. Specimen 2 seems to depart from the behavior described here, especially at lower temperatures.

DISCUSSION

The results presented in Table 1 favor the view that super-conductivity exists in granular aluminum only when the electrons are not strongly localized. If agreement with the Sheng-Abeles formula $\sigma = \sigma_0 \exp[-(T_0/T)^{\frac{1}{2}}]$ is taken to indicate localization, we see that in such cases there is no observed superconducting transition. Nor is there any indication in the magnetoresistance measurements of fluctuation conductivity associated with a transition temperature several times smaller than our lowest accessible temperature. In the samples that are superconducting the Sheng-Abeles formula does not fit the data, as can be seen from the fact that the quantity σ_m is then non-zero. It should be noted that T_c decreases as the ratio σ_m/σ_0 decreases. (See also Fig. 2.) Whether T_c and σ_m/σ_0 continue to decrease smoothly as the volume fraction of metal is reduced or there is a discontinuous drop at some particular concentration is an interesting open question.

We wish to caution against attaching more significance to the formula $\sigma = \sigma_m + \sigma_0 \exp[-(T_0/T)^{\frac{1}{2}}]$ than that it merely indicates greater disorder in the system than is allowed for in the model of Sheng and Abeles. At first sight it implies that σ_m comes from metallic paths in parallel with the activated ones that give rise to $\sigma_0 \exp[-(T_0/T)^{\frac{1}{2}}]$, suggesting metallic threads running from one end of the sample to the other. There would then be no need to invoke Josephson tunnelling to explain the observed superconductivity! However, one can show by using an effective-medium approach[23] that disconnected short elongated metal regions immersed in a medium with conductivity proportional to $\exp[-(T_0/T)^{\frac{1}{2}}]$ can give rise to an effective-medium conductivity of the form $\sigma_{eff} = \sigma_m + \sigma_0 \exp[-(T_0/T)^{\frac{1}{2}}]$ providing that the temperature is not too low. At very low temperatures the real medium between the metal islands becomes an insulator thus cutting off connections between adjacent metal regions. Such elongated regions or threads may be a reasonable representation of the grain clusters that form just before the percolation threshold[24], since only the spines but not the side arms contribute to the conductivity.

Granular aluminum near its precolation threshold shows greater apparent disorder than other granular metals[6] that follow the Sheng-Abeles formula. This may be related to the fact that the percolation threshold in this system occurs at about 60% metal volume fraction as opposed to the 15-20% expected from classical models based on the random distribution of identical spheres[25].

(We recall that in a close-packed simple cubic array of spheres, the packing fraction is 52% and in the hexagonal close-packed case it is 74%.)

The strength of the localization was referred to at the beginning of this section in relation to the occurrence of superconductivity. Because the systems studied here would be estimated by most criteria to be three-dimensional and not two-dimensional, they might not be expected to reflect any of the interesting general results concerning localization obtained recently by Abrahams et al.[26] However, when the data shown in Fig. 1 are plotted on a graph showing R against log T it is seen that for specimens 1 and 2 which appear to be the least strongly localized but have negative temperature coefficients of resistance, they follow straight lines. This is not true for the other specimens which appear to be more strongly localized. This suggests that the logarithmic dependence recently found[27] for two-dimensional systems may be more generally applicable. This question will be discussed in a forthcoming publication[28].

We now turn to the negative magnetoresistance. The results shown in Fig. 3 are surprisingly similar to the theoretical results given in Fig. 2 of the paper by Fukuyama and Yosida, thus raising the expectation that there is an intimate connection between the hopping conduction and granular metal cases. On closer inspection there are two major obstacles. First of all the magnetoresistance can be large in this theory only when $E_c - E_F$, the energy difference between the mobility edge and the Fermi level, is comparable to μH, where μ is the magnetic moment associated with the electron spin. The quantity in the granular system analogous to $E_c - E_F$ is the work function of the metal-to-insulator interface. The work function of aluminum to vacuum is about 4 eV and, even if this has to be modified to allow for the effect of neighboring grains, it is unlikely that it can be reduced to be comparable with μH, even at 100kG. Secondly, although the observed temperature dependence agrees qualitatively with the theory, in quantitative detail it agrees with neither the original theory nor our modified version allowing for the breakdown of Fermi-Dirac statistics in very small particles. For these reasons it is not possible to link the experiment with the most promising of theories explicitly dealing with localization.

A possible clue to the origin of the negative magnetoresistance is that in most of our specimens the resistance for a given sample follows approximately the general law $R(H,T)/R(0,T) = f(H/T)$, where $f(x)$ is proportional to x^2 for small x. This suggests that the effect arises from a Boltzmann factor $\exp(-\mu H/kT)$.

ACKNOWLEDGEMENTS

We have profited greatly from the continued collaboration of G. Deutscher. We acknowledge illuminating conversations with E. Abrahams. G. Hughes provided technical assistance. The research was supported by the National Science Foundation, under grant

DMR 78-24213, and by the Rutgers University Research Council.
Helium gas was supplied by the Office of Naval Research.

REFERENCES

1. G. Deutscher, Y. Imry, and L. Gunther, Phys. Rev. B 10, 4598 (1974).
2. See J. Rosenblatt, Revue de Physique Appliquée 9, 15 (1974) and early references cited therein.
3. B. Abeles, Phys. Rev. B 15, 2828 (1977).
4. W. L. McLean and M. J. Stephen, Phys. Rev. B 19, 5925 (1979).
5. P. W. Anderson, in Lectures on the Many-Body Problem, edited by E. R. Caianiello (Academic Press, New York, 1964) Vol. 2, p. 127.
6. B. Abeles, Ping Sheng, M. D. Coutts, and Y. Arie, Advances in Phys. 24, 407 (1975).
7. E. Abrahams and I. O. Kulik, preprint.
8. P. Sheng, B. Abeles, and Y. Arie, Phys. Rev. Lett. 31, 44 (1973).
9. J. J. Hauser, Phys. Rev. B 7, 4099 (1973). A similar disparity of temperature dependences is found in discontinuous metal films. See for example, R. C. Dynes, J. P. Garno, and J. M. Rowell, Phys. Rev. Lett. 40, 479 (1978).
10. N. F. Mott, Phil. Mag. 19, 835 (1969).
11. W. L. McLean, P. Lindenfeld, and T. Worthington, A.I.P. Conf. Proc. 40, 403 (1977).
12. V. Ambegaokar, B. I. Halperin, and J. S. Langer, Phys. Rev. B 4, 2612 (1971).
13. J. I. Gittleman, Y. Goldstein, and S. Bozowski, Phys. Rev. B 5, 3609 (1972).
14. J. S. Helman and B. Abeles, Phys. Rev. Lett. 37, 1429 (1976).
15. For a recent set of references, see B. Sernelius and K.-F. Berggren, Phys. Rev. B 19, 6390 (1979).
16. A. B. Pippard, Dynamics of Conduction Electrons, Gordon and Breach, New York (1965).
17. H. Fukuyama and K. Yosida, Journ. Phys. Soc. Japan 46 102 (1979).
18. R. Kubo, Journ. Phys. Soc. Japan 17, 975 (1962).
19. Y. Goldstein and Y. Grinshpan, Phys. Rev. Lett. 39, 953 (1977); Y. Goldstein, Y. Grinshpan, and A. Many, Phys. Rev. 19, 2256 (1979).
20. G. Deutscher, H. Fenichel, M. Gershenson, E. Grünbaum, and Z. Ovadyahu, Journ. Low Temp. Phys. 10, 231 (1973).
21. T. Worthington, P. Lindenfeld, and G. Deutscher, Phys. Rev. Lett. 41, 316 (1978); R. L. Filler, P. Lindenfeld, T. Worthington, and G. Deutscher, to be published.
22. B. Abeles and J. J. Hanak, Physics Letters 34 A, 165 (1971).
23. W. L. McLean, to be published.
24. S. Kirkpatrick, A.I.P. Conf. Proc. 40, 99 (1978).
25. S. Kirkpatrick, Rev. Mod. Phys. 45, 570 (1973).
26. E. Abrahams, P. W. Anderson, D. C. Licciardello, and T. V. Ramakrishman, Phys. Rev. Lett. 42, 673 (1979).

27. P. W. Anderson, E. Abrahams, and T. V. Ramakrishnan, Phys.
     Rev. Lett. 43, 718 (1979); G. J. Dolan and D. D. Osheroff,
     Phys. Rev. Lett. 43, 721 (1979); N. Giordano, W. Gilson, and
     D. E. Prober, Phys. Rev. Lett. 43, 725 (1979).
28. G. Deutscher, B. Bandyopadhyay, T. Chui, P. Lindenfeld,
     W. L. McLean, and T. Worthington, to be published.

TRANSPORT PROPERTIES OF COMPOSITE SUPERCONDUCTORS

R.S. Newrock
University of Cincinnati, Cincinnati, Ohio

and

D.J. Resnick and J.C. Garland
Ohio State University, Columbus, Ohio

ABSTRACT

We report on the transport properties of normal metal–super-conductor small-particle composites. We have measured the electrical resistivity of NbTi/In and Nb/In composites from 3.4k to 12k, in magnetic fields to 6T and over a range of volume fraction of super-conductor from o to 35%. Several effects, possibly due to intergrain coupling, were observed and are discussed. In particular, specimens with volume fraction of superconductor near the critical percolation threshold exhibit "tails" in their R–T curves and a "double" superconducting transition.

In this paper we present the preliminary results of a series of investigations into the transport properties of superconductor-normal metal (S/N) composites. We have studied two nearly identical systems: niobium–titanium grains embedded in an indium matrix and pure niobium grains in the same matrix. In these systems indium is considered to be the normal metal. We have examined the electrical transport properties of these materials over a temperature range from 3.4K (the transition temperature of indium) to 12K, in magnetic fields from zero to 6 Tesla and over a range of volume fraction, p, of superconductor from 0 to 35%. This range of volume fraction takes us from below the critical percolation threshold, P_c to well above it.(1)

For $p \lll p_c$, no superconductivity is observed. The transport properties of such composites, both in and out of strong magnetic fields, are now very well understood in terms of current distortion effects and effective medium theory, and are discussed elsewhere in this volume. For $p > p_c$ the specimen becomes a superconductor at the transition temperature of the individual grains, T_{cg}, with critical currents that are well below the bulk values. For $p \lesssim p_c$ a transition to the superconducting state is observed but it occurs below T_{cg} and the critical currents are much lower. For $p < p_c$ the specimens are not superconducting ($T > 3.4K$) but significant changes in the resistivity vs. temperature curves are observed.

It is believed on theoretical grounds[2] that, depending on the intergrain barrier resistance and the temperature, long-range

Josephson or proximity coupling between grains may be possible.
Thus, a three-dimensional random array of grains may, depending on
the temperature, be simply a collection of isolated superconducting
islands or, if the order parameters of the various grain align, be a
"bulk" three-dimensional superconductor. Such an alignment of the
order parameters of the individual grains may have already been
observed in superconductor-insulator composites[3]; the data we report
here may be evidence for similar effects in random small-particle
S/N composites.

The specimens used in this work were prepared in the following
manner: The required quantity of niobium or niobium-titanium powder
was mixed thoroughly with indium powder. The two powders were mixed
in a vortex mixer for 40 minutes to ensure a uniform distribution of
the superconducting grains. The mixture was then pressed, in a
vacuum, into a pellet which was then rolled into a 1.5mm thick sheet.
This sheet was sliced into specimens with dimensions
1.5mm x 3mm x 20mm. Before each experiment each specimen was
annealed for one hour at 95°C.

The indium powder, when melted and formed into a specimen, had
a residual resistivity ratio of over 8000; however, specimens formed
by compressing the indium powder into a solid had residual
resistivity ratios of 400-500. The niobium-titanium grains were
irregularly shaped and had sizes ranging from 25 to 125μm in their
long dimensions, with a mean diameter of about 75μm. The indium
grains had a mean diameter of 20μm. For these specimens the average
diameter of the superconducting grains is much greater than the
coherence length ($D \gg \xi \approx 50 \text{\AA}$). The grains themselves are therefore
three-dimensional superconductors. In addition $D \gg \lambda_e$ the electron
mean free-path in the normal metal ($\approx 10\mu$m). The measurements were
performed using standard four-probe techniques, with an RF squid
serving as a null detector.

The data are displayed in Figures 1-3. Figure 1 shows the
behavior of the resistivity as a function of the temperature for an
indium specimen and for two composites with superconducting fractions
(Nb-Ti) of 25 and $27\frac{1}{2}$%. As may be seen from the figure the
homogeneous indium specimen behaves as expected; that is the
resistance decreases with temperature until the critical temperature
of indium is reached whereupon it decreases suddenly to zero. On
this scale there is essentially no width to the transition. The
behavior of the 25% composite is significantly different and the
effects of the presence of the superconducting grains are apparent.
The most obvious effect is the strong rounding of the resistive
transition near the indium critical temperature. This rounding is
probably due to proximity effects, which increase in strength as the
critical temperature of indium is approached and the indium coherence
length diverges. In this specimen we also observed that the normal
state temperature dependence of the resistivity was roughly T^5. The
coefficient of this term changed abruptly at T_{co}, that is, when the individual grains became superconductors. The volume fraction of the last
specimen shown,

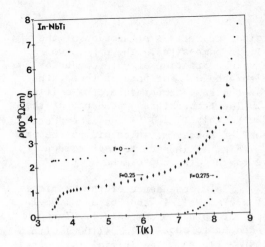

Fig. 1. Resistance vs.
temperature for an indium
specimen and two S/N
composites.

$27\frac{1}{2}\%$, is very close to the percolation threshold for this system.
The resistance of this specimen is seen to decrease rapidly at the
grain transition temperature. The resistivity does not, however,
decrease to zero but has a "tail" which slowly decreases to zero
resistance at $T_{ci} \approx 7.2K$. Such "tails" (and "feet") are often
observed in R vs. T plots for superconductor-insulator composites[3]
and have come to be associated with intergrain coupling and a
"double" superconducting transition. (We note that the actual value
of T_{ci} is difficult to determine exactly; it is very sensitive to
magnitude to the measuring currents employed).

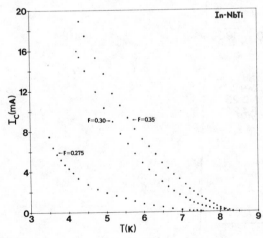

Fig. 2. Critical current
as a function of temperature
for these composite specimens.

Figure 2 displays the critical current as a function of the temperature for a number of NbTi/In composites. The upper two curves are for specimens whose volume fraction of superconductor is above the critical percolation threshold. For both of these, the critical currents become zero at the same temperature, the critical temperature of the grains, T_{cg}. The temperature dependence of the critical current was found to be roughly $(T-T_c)^{3/2}$ as is expected for a bulk superconductor. The $27\frac{1}{2}\%$ specimen, which did not become a superconductor until $T_{cj} < T_{cg}$ (Fig. 1) is seen to have a much lower critical current relative to the other specimens.

Figure 3 shows the magnetic field dependence of the critical current for two specimens: 3a) a $27\frac{1}{2}\%$ NbTi-In and 3b) a 23% Nb-In specimen (This latter is near p_c for NbIn S/N composite). In both cases I_c is extremely field dependent to about 10^{-2} T(100G) with a small but steady decrease in higher fields. The initial fall-off is most likely due to magnetic field effects on the intergrain coupling and on proximity effects.

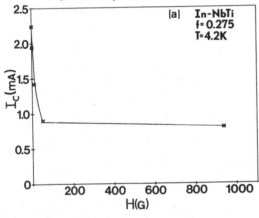

Fig. 3. Critical current as magnetic field for two composite specimens.

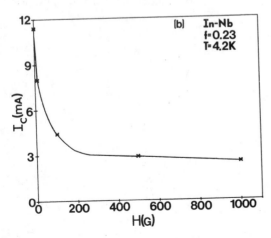

This work was supported by N.S.F. grant, DMR-78-09428.

REFERENCES

1. It should be noted that, because of proximity effects, it is difficult to determine precisely the critical percolation threshold for superconductivity.
2. See for example: B. Giovannini and L. Weiss, Sol. St. Comm. 27, 1005, (1978); G. Deutscher, Y. Imry, and L. Gunther, Phys. articles in this volume.
3. See for example: S. Wolf and W. H. Lowery, Phys. Rev. Lett. 39, 1038 (1977); G. Deutscher and M.L. Rappaport, J.Phys. C6, C6-581, (1978); T. Worthington, P. Lindenfeld, and G. Deutscher, Phys. Rev. Lett. 41, 316 (1978) and N.A.H.K. Rao, E.D. Dahlberg, A.M. Goldman and L.E. Toth, to be publishd. See also references listed in these articles and elsewhere in this volume.1.
4. D.J. Resnick, J.C. Garland and R.S. Newrck, Phys. Rev. Lett. 41, 818 (1978).

Hg-Xe Films Deposited at Low Temperatures:

A Model System for the Study of the Interplay

Between Disorder and Superconductivity*

K. Epstein, A.M. Goldman, E.D. Dahlberg, and R. Mikkelson**
University of Minnesota
Minneapolis, MN   55455

ABSTRACT

Random gaseous mixtures of Hg and Xe effusing from a molecular beam oven have been condensed onto substrates held at 4.2 K. The resultant films appear to be model systems for the study of the interplay between superconductivity and disorder brought about by increasing dilution of metallic Hg with Xe. A metal-nonmetal transition as a function of composition is observed near a volume fraction of metal close to that expected for random percolation. The increase of the resistivity near this transition is accompanied by a substantial drop in the superconducting transition temperature as determined resistively. At low Hg concentrations film resistances increase with decreasing temperature in a manner typical of disordered systems.

INTRODUCTION

The technique of preparing thin films by evaporation onto surfaces cooled to helium temperatures has been used to form amorphous metallic phases which would otherwise not be stable at higher temperatures,[1] or crystalline phases which are essentially structural modifications which would only be produced by the application of high pressure.[2] If metal vapor is simultaneously condensed onto a substrate with various other gases, the resultant films can be used to systematically study the local disorder brought about by increasing the dilution of the metal with a solid gaseous matrix. For the examples of the alkali metals mixed with rare gas atoms, metal-nonmetal transitions have been observed with increasing dilution. These transitions have been termed paridigms of the microscopic percolation transition.[3] The work we shall describe here has been concerned with the investigation of the electrical conductivity of the Hg-Xe system[4] where studies have been carried out at sufficiently low temperatures to permit the observation of the effects of the dilution and resultant disordering of the Hg atoms by Xe on the electrical conductivity in the normal state and

---

*Supported in part by the DOE under contract EY-76-S-02-1569-A002
**Permanent address: Macalaster College, St. Paul, Minn.

on the character and location of the superconducting transition. In particular, the normal state resistance at T = 4.2 K as a function of composition appears to undergo a metal-nonmetal transition which is consistent with percolation theory. Beyond the percolation threshold the conduction exhibits the negative temperature coefficient of resistance that characterizes disordered systems. The superconducting transition does not drop significantly until the normal-state resistance begins to increase substantially. High resistivity superconducting films exhibit a long tail in their resistive transitions.

Some of the effects revealed by these investigations are qualitatively similar to phenomena reported for other systems. The physical observations appear to depend on the character of the local order, which has not yet been determined quantitatively using electron microscopy or diffraction.

EXPERIMENTAL

Despite the existence of a long history in the study of the properties of thin films deposited onto cold substrates, little attention has been paid to the effects on the character of the films of the total energy incident on their surfaces during growth. This includes contributions from both the kinetic energy and the condensation energy of the particles in the vapor stream and from the thermal radiation emanating from the vapor source. The work of Tsymbalenko and Shal'nikov[5] on pure Hg films prepared on cold surfaces was the first study in which serious efforts to limit heating of the surfaces were undertaken.

In the present work this problem has been addressed by using a molecular beam oven as a vapor source. With this oven, which, except for its orifice, is surrounded by a liquid nitrogen shield at 77 K, it has been possible to deposit films which are subject to an energy flux of less than 10^{-4} W/cm^2 during their preparation.

The apparatus is different from that conventionally employed in the preparation and study of films condensed onto helium temperature substrates. Details of its overall construction have been given elsewhere.[6] For this experiment, the source of vapor is a copper-clad stainless steel molecular beam oven which is a true Knudsen source. The oven is suspended from a flange inside a 1" dia. stainless steel tube whose walls are kept at 4.2 K. The vapor stream from the orifice is projected vertically downward onto the substrate. The section of the vacuum system containing the oven and that containing the substrate are separated by a radiation shield which is cooled to 4.2 K. A second orifice allows the vapor stream to enter the chamber containing the substrate. The oven is itself surrounded by a vacuum jacket which in turn is surrounded by a liquid nitrogen cooled jacket. As a result of the various shields and jackets, the substrate is shielded from all radiation originating in the oven except for that emanating from its orifice.

The substrates, which are 2.54 cm x 2.54 cm glazed alumina squares, are mounted on a copper block connected by a controlled thermal link to the liquid helium bath. A mechanical feedthrough from the top of the apparatus allows for the positioning of a mask in any of six positions. Thus six films can be fabricated during one cool-down of the apparatus. A second mechanical feedthrough operates a shutter which can be used to interrupt the molecular beam.

Compositions of the vapor are calculated from the geometrical parameters of the oven using the Xe-gas pressure measured with an MKS capacitance manometer. The Hg pressure in the oven is determined from the vapor pressure-temperature curve with the oven temperature measured using a platinum resistance thermometer. An MKS automatic pressure controller and a Brooks electrically operated valve were used for pressure control and a Linear Research temperature controller was used to control temperature. Films were prepared with the oven held at a temperature of 340 K with an atomic flux of 10^{18} atoms/cm^2 sec.

Because of the possibility of small changes in geometry from run to run, one film out of each batch of six was prepared with a nominal 60 MPM composition. The resistance of this film was then used as a check on the run-to-run composition variation.

Compositions,determined to ±1 MPM,were calculated from the vapor fluxes taking the sticking coefficients of Hg and Xe to be unity, an assumption which is supported experimentally at substrate temperatures and vapor fluxes used here.[7] The conductances of films as measured during their formation were found to increase linearly with time at fixed deposition rates indicating that perhaps with the exception of the first several atomic layers, where the resistance was unmeasurable, the films are homogeneous across their thicknesses.

EXPERIMENTAL RESULTS

In Fig. 1 we plot the logarithm of the normal state resistivity measured at 4.2 K and the superconducting transition temperature T_c, of 2,000-5,000 Å thick films as a function of the atomic concentration of Hg in mole percent metal (MPM). The dashed line near X = 100 MPM represents the expected variation of the resistivity with concentration assuming linear dilution. The solid line associated with $\log_{10}\rho_N$ corresponds to a least squares fit to $\rho_N \sim (X-X_c)^\alpha$ with the exponent α forced to be 1.7, a value appropriate to three dimensional percolation.[8] The fit, which was carried out for compositions between 58 and 75 MPM, resulted in $X_c = 55 \pm 4$ MPM. The range of the fit was chosen so as to exclude films exhibiting negative temperature coefficients of resistance (TCR). All films with compositions to the right of the line, exhibit negative TCR's.

It should be noted that the critical concentration of 55 MPM corresponds to a critical volume fraction of about 13%. This result is obtained by assuming a packing fraction of 0.45 corresponding to a liquid of spheres of radii 1.49 Å and 2.17 Å which are appropriate to Hg and Xe respectively. It would thus seem that the composition variation of the resistivities of films when they are dominated by

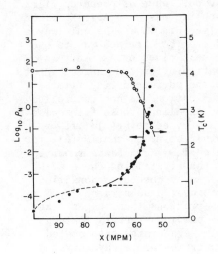

Fig. 1. Transition temperatures (open circles) and logarithms of normal state resistivity (closed circles) at 4.2 K vs. nominal composition X in mole-percent metal (MPM) for 1500-3000 Å thick Hg(Xe) films 0.5 mm wide and 0.4 cm long. Compositions are accurate to better than ± 1 MPM.

metallic conduction is consistent with random percolation theory.

Because of the unknown character of the crossover from percolation to the linear behavior at high metal concentrations and to conduction with a negative TCR at lower concentrations, a systematic least squares analysis of the data for metal concentrations outside the limited range of the fit would not be meaningful. Thus the present results must be considered to be suggestive rather than proof of the applicability of microscopic random percolation.

For each of the films, the corresponding superconducting transition temperatures are also plotted in Fig. 1. T_c has been arbitrarily chosen to be the temperature at which $R = 0.9\ R_N$ where R_N was the resistance at 4.2 K. For both metallic films of pure Hg and those containing substantial Xe, $T_c = 4.06$ K, close to the value reported for Hg films less than 100 Å thick in Ref. 5 where a molecular beam technique was also used.

In Fig. 2 we show representative normalized R(T) curves for as-prepared films. Exhibited are results characteristic of: a) films with a high metal concentration, b) films exhibiting tails in R(T), c) films with higher Xe concentrations, tails in R(T), and negative TCR's near T_c, and d) films which exhibit a metal-insulator transition with decreasing temperature rather than a superconducting transition.

For pure Hg films, the unusual transition temperature at 4.06 K raises the question that the as-prepared pure Hg films may be an amorphous, crystalline or microcrystalline phase different from Hg(α) or Hg(β) known previously.[9] First, crystalline Hg(β) with a T_c of 3.95 K was never produced when

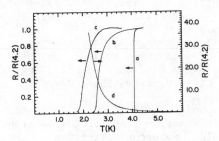

Fig. 2. Representative curves of R(T) for films (a), (b), (c) and (d) with X=100 MPM, 44 MPM, 54 MPM and 52 MPM, respectively. Lines have been drawn through discrete data points for clarity.

62

the liquid nitrogen shielded oven was used. When as-prepared films were annealed, T_c first dropped and then increased to 4.18 K which is close to the value for Hg(α) (see Fig. 3). The only way a pure Hg film with a T_c of 3.95 K could ever be obtained was to use an unshielded oven. In this configuration the thermal input to the surface during film fabrication was not controlled. On annealing, these films also transformed to Hg(α). It should be noted that Hg(β), for which T_c = 3.95 K was reported as the crystalline phase of Hg formed by quench condensation onto cooled substrates.[11] Our observations thus suggest that the previous reports that Hg films evaporated onto cooled substrates are always crystal- line Hg(β) may not be true if the thermal input to the surface is limited.

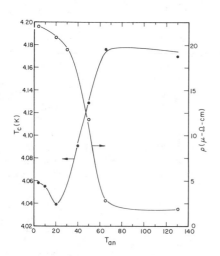

Fig. 3. Resistivities ρ_N and transition temperatures T_c of a pure Hg film prepared at 4.2 K and annealed for 1/4 hour at various temperatures T_{an}.

In the absence of electron or X-ray diffraction data a definitive statement as to structure cannot be made. It is interesting to note that the as-prepared normal state re- sistivities of pure Hg were equal to the resistivity of solid Hg rather than liquid at the melting temperature. The latter is the usual case for amorphous metals.[1] The measured resistivities were, on the other hand, equal to the calculated resistivity of liquid Hg at melting.[10]

Although low resistance Hg-Xe films exhibited sharp resistive transitions, when the film resistivities were greater than 10^{-3} Ω-cm, tails were observed in the superconducting transition. For films of resistivities the order of 5 x 10^{-2} Ω-cm such tails could typically be fit with three adjustable parameters to R = A(T-T_c)$^{3.7\pm0.5}$ over two decades of resistance (see Fig. 4). Although the exponent is the same as that found for anodized NbN films, the scaling analysis of Wolf, Gubser, and Imry[12] could not be carried out. Similar long tails were observed in thin Hg films of thicknesses the order of 200 Å.

Films with negative temperature coefficients of resistance and superconductivity were found only over a narrow range of composition very close to the percolation threshold. Superconductivity as measured resistively was not observed above T = 1.8 K in films with resistivities greater than 0.5 Ω-cm. A theory of the behavior of such systems may require a generalization of the BCS theory which takes into account electronic localization.

For as-prepared films such as film d in Fig. 2 no simple be- havior of log R vs $T^{-\lambda}$ with λ = 1/2, 1/3, or 1/4 was found. However,

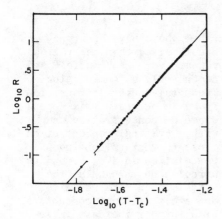

Fig. 4. $\log_{10} R$ vs $\log_{10}(T-T_c)$ plotted for data in the tail of the resistive transition of a film with a 60 MPM nominal composition such as that labeled b in Fig. 2. $R_N = 380 \ \Omega$, $T_c = 3.63$ K and the slope is 3.43.

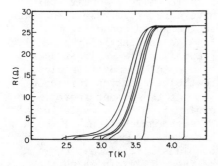

Fig. 5. Magnetic field dependence of a film with 85 MPM Hg exhibiting a tail. The leftmost curve was obtained in a perpendicular field of 7.2 kG. Subsequent curves to the right correspond to fields of 6.3 kG, 5 kG, 4.5 kG, 4 kG, 2 kG and zero field which is the righmost curve.

after annealing to 20 K, $\log R \sim T^{-1/4}$ was found. These films did not exhibit superconductivity as measured resistively down to the lowest temperatures attainable (T $\sim$ 1.8 K). A detailed study of the temperature dependence of the resistivities of films of this type may shed light on the behavior of 3-D localized systems.

The magnetic field dependence of R(T) for a 85 MPM film exhibiting a tail is shown in Fig. 5. The remarkable effect is that the tail seen in zero magnetic field is transformed to a foot as the field increases. The foot-shaped features are similar to those observed in Hg-Xe films prepared using an unshielded oven or prepared using a shielded oven and heated in an uncontrolled way above 20 K. For the latter, R(T) was typically found to fall to zero as $(T-T_c)^{0.7\pm0.5}$ over one decade of resistance in the best samples (see Fig. 6). The exponent is that predicted for 3D percolation in a random resistor lattice of superconducting and normal links.[13] Similar behavior and a similar exponent have been reported for granular Al(Ge) films by the Tel Aviv group.[14]

In the resistor lattice problem, the resistance $R \sim (X-X_c)^\alpha$ where X and X_c are respectively the concentration and critical concentration of superconducting links. If X, which is temperature dependent, can be expanded in a power series in $T-T_c$, where T_c is the temperature at which $X = X_c$ then a variation with $(X-X_c)^\alpha$ near X_c would map onto a variation with $(T-T_c)^\alpha$. The present results may not be definitive evidence for the applicatility of a percolation model to these samples.

DISCUSSION

Although some of the results described above have been presented in qualitative terms, it must be emphasized that the various features obtained using the shielded oven are very reproducible and depend only on composition. The metal-nonmetal transition in Hg-Xe occurs with a dependence on concentration and with a critical concentration close to that of continuous percolation in 3D. Beyond the percolation threshold, the systems acquire a negative TCR but are still superconductors. With further increase in Xe concentration, a regime in which the conductivity takes on a character usually associated with disordered systems is entered. It should be further emphasized that in contrast with other random superconducting systems the Hg-Xe system is one in which the insulating matrix appears to have a relatively small effect on the superconducting transition temperature of the metal trapped in it, at least down to a metal composition close to the percolation threshold.

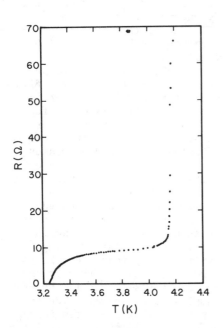

Fig. 6. R(T) for a film prepared using an unshielded oven. The resistance of the "foot" is proportional to $(T-T_c)^{0.75\pm0.05}$ when measured at a current density of 100 A/cm^2. Here T_c = 3.24 K and R_N = 70 Ω. The exponent appears to be current dependent dropping to .55 $\pm$ .15 at a current density of 1 A/cm^2.

At the moment there is no explanation of the variation of T_c with composition, although a variety of explanations may be plausible. If a picture of these films in which they consist of randomly packed spheres of Hg and Xe were correct, the fact that T_c does not change initially with Xe concentration might be a consequence of the existence of a connected network of domains or grains of a characteristic size on the average greater than the superconducting coherence length. The fall of T_c with dilution of the Hg by Xe could be a consequence of thermal fluctuations or noise, or both, disrupting the coupling between metallic domains or grains which would be weakening with increasing dilution.

Alternatively with decreasing Hg concentration, the electron concentration could be dropping in a way which would lead to a falling T_c. When the temperature coefficient of resistance becomes negative, there may be hopping between localized states. Cooper pairs associated with such states might lead to superconductivity with a T_c reduced relative to that obtained when the states are extended.

Another possibility is a reduction of T_c from a coupling of order parameter fluctuations to electromagnetic field fluctuations which may be important in high sheet resistance films.[15] In this instance the superconducting transition would be postponed until the condensation energy could in effect expel the black-body radiation of the environment. Such a model also predicts that all Type-I superconductors have transitions which are weakly first-order.[16] A fourth possibility is a lowering of T_c by a modification of the phonon spectrum of Hg by intimate contact with Xe atoms. Near the percolation threshold there is a large Hg surface-to-volume ratio and such an effect could be much larger than that reported in an adsorbed layer geometry.[17]

The tails in the resistive transitions of high-resistance films may be a manifestation of critical behavior or they may be a signature of the phase-locking transformation of Ref. 12. The fact that the ambient field in the present apparatus is the order of 1/2 G has prevented a truly quantitative study of this effect from being carried out.

The disappearance of superconductivity at temperatures above 1.8 K as determined resistively in films with resistivities greater than 0.5 Ω-cm may be a consequence of a lack of connectedness of metallic domains in these samples. In such an event a nontransport measurement would reveal the existence of superconductivity in such systems. Another possibility is that Cooper paired electrons which are localized are not superconducting in the sense of being able to carry current with zero resistance. Further experimental and theoretical work is required to clarify this issue.

REFERENCES

1. G. Bergman, Physics Reports 27, 159 (1976).
2. B. G. Lazarev, E. E. Semenenko, V. I. Tutov, and A. A. Chupikov, Fiz. Nizk. Temp. 4, 957 (1978) [Sov. J. Low Temp. Phys. 4, 451 (1978)].
3. D. J. Phelps and C. P. Flynn, Phys. Rev. B14, 5279 (1976) and references therein.
4. O. Chesnovski, U. Even, and J. Jortner, Solid State Commun. 22, 745 (1977) and references therein.
5. V. L. Tsymbalenko and A. I. Shal'nikov, Zh. Eksp. Teor. Fiz. 2068 (1973) [Soviet Physics JETP 38, 1943 (19740].
6. N. A. McNeal and A. M. Goldman, J. Low Temp. Phys. 31, 863 (1978).
7. L. L. Levenson, Nuovo Cimento Suppl. 5, 321 (1967).
8. K. S. Shante and S. Kirkpatrick, Adv. Phys. 20, 325 (1971).
9. J. E. Scherfer and C. A. Swenson, Phys. Rev. Lett. 2, 296, 296 (1969); Phys. Rev. 123, 1115 (1961).

66

10. T. E. Faber, Introduction to the Theory of Liquid Metals (Cambridge University Press, 1972).
11. H. Bülow and W. Buckel, Z. Physik 145, 141 (1956).
12. S. A. Wolf, D. U. Gubser, and Y. Imry, Phys. Rev. Lett. 42, 324 (1979).
13. J. P. Straley, Phys. Rev. B15, 5733 (1977).
14. G. Deutscher and M. L. Rappaport, Journal de Physique Colloque 6 39, C-581 (1978).
15. I. O. Kulik, Zh. Eksp. Teor. Fiz. Pis. Red. 14, 341 (1971) [Soviet Physics Letters 14, 228 (1971)].
16. B. I. Halperin, T. C. Lubensky, and Shang-Keng Ma, Phys. Rev. Lett. 32, 292 (1974).
17. D. G. Naugle, J. W. Baken, and R. E. Allen, Phys. Rev. B7, 3028 (1973).

HIGH-TRANSITION-TEMPERATURE SUPERCONDUCTING

PARTICLES IN AN INSULATING MATRIX

C.C. Tsuei and J.T.C. Yeh

IBM Thomas J. Watson Research Center

Yorktown Heights, N.Y. 10598

ABSTRACT

A number of new bulk granular superconductors consisting of high transition-temperature (T_{co}) superconducting particles of V_3Si, NbN or $Mo_5Pb_1S_8$ embbeded in a variety of resins have been prepared. The resistive superconducting transition temperature T_c for these composite conductors is, in general, less than half of T_{co}. In samples containing V_3Si powder ($\sim 20\mu m$ in average particle size), T_c as high as 7.5K has been achieved. The superconducting properties, electrical and magnetic, can be understood if these materials can be considered as 3-dimensional arrays of Josephson junctions. Potential applications for these bulk granular superconductors are discussed.

INTRODUCTION

In recent years, considerable interest has been expressed in the experimental and theoretical studies of granular superconductors.[1-6] These superconducting materials essentially consist of an assembly of superconducting grains (s) embedded in an insulating matrix (i). Previous work in this field concentrates mostly on systems of very small superconducting grains (~ 10-100Å) separated by their native oxides. Granular superconductors of this sort are characterized by the following features:

1) The superconducting transition temperature of the grains, T_{co}, is usually low (for example, T_{co} for granular Al is about 1.2 to 4K depending on the grain size). As a result, the zero-resistance transition temperature of the s+i composite materials, T_c, is also, in general, very low ($<<4.2K$).

2) The granular samples are generally prepared in the form of ultra thin films (thickness typically of the order of 100Å). The nature of the 2-or lower dimensionality of the these samples can be significant in interpreting the experimental results.

3) The small size of grains can lead to complications such as grain-size dependent T_{co}, charging effects[7], discreteness of the energy levels within grains.[8]

In this paper, we shall report some properties of several new granular superconducting systems which are composed of high T_{co} particles randomly distributed in an insulating matrix. The average size of the superconducting grains is of the order of microns or larger so that the size effects mentioned in 3) are insignificant. After a brief description of sample preparation, the superconducting as well as the normal-state properties of these inhomogeneous superconductors will be discussed in terms of the Josephson coupling between superconducting grains. Potential applications of these new materials will be also explored.

SAMPLE PREPARATION

The new granular superconductors prepared in this investigation are essentially a mixture of a high T_{co} superconducting powder and an insulating resin. The superconducting powders used include V_3Si (T_{co} ~ 15-17K), NbN (T_{co} ~ 15-18K), $Mo_5 Pb_1 S_8$ (T_{co} ~ 15K). The relatively high T_{co} and the unusual brittleness of these compounds make them the ideal superconducting constituents in the new granular superconductors. The size of the superconducting particles approximately falls in one of the following ranges: (1) 0.5-5μm, (2) 5-25μm, (3) 25-125μm. The insulating component of the new materials comes from a variety of resins which include a) Acryloid B66 dissolved in amyl acetate, b) Epon 820 and c) Stycast 1266. It should be pointed out that the superconducting particles are all to some extent coated with a thin insulating layer of native oxide(s) which should be considered as part of the insulating matrix.

The new granular superconductors are prepared simply by mixing appropriate amounts of the superconducting powder with one of the resins mentioned above while it is in the liquid state. It usually takes an hour or so for the mixture to set. The weight ratio of the metal to insulator, (s/i), varies depending on the superconducting and normal state properties of the composite material required. To achieve a relatively high value of T_c (>4.2K, for example), a relatively large s/i ratio is needed. In the case of V_3Si and Acryloid B66 (e.g. 2g of solid Acryloid B66 dissolved in 10 cc of amyl acetate), the ratio of s/i is about 30. In the case of V_3Si and Epon 820 or Stycast 1266 a s/i ratio of about 6 is necessary. The size of the samples for electrical measurements is about 0.2 mm^2 in cross section and 0.5 to 1 cm in length.

RESULTS AND DISCUSSION

To characterize the granular superconductors prepared in this study, the following measurements have been carried out: 1. electrical resistance R, 2. current-voltgage characteristics and critical current I_c, 3. microwave response, 4. magnetization σ, 5. inductance change ΔL near the superconducting transition temperature. Results of these experiments will be briefly described as follows:

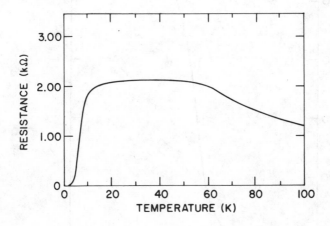

Fig.1   Electrical resistance as a function of temperature for a V_3Si granular superconductor.   s=V_3Si powder (0.5-5μm), i=Acryloid B66, and s/i ~ 15.

The temperature dependence of the resistance of the granular superconductors has been measured as a function of particle size and s to i
weight ratio. It is found that the value of T_c, the normal-state resistance
as well as its temperature coefficient are greatly determined by the
concentration of the superconducting particles. The effect of particle
size is minimal in the range studied. For example, the resistance as a
function of temperature for a sample of V_3Si powder (0.5-5μm) in
Acryloid B66 (weight ratio s/i $\sim$ 15) is shown in Fig. 1. Resistance
increases with decreasing temperature for T>40K and is essentially a
constant of temperature for 20$\leq$T $\leq$40K. This sample exhibits a broad
superconducting transition with onset at~20K and completion (R=0) at
2.4K (T_c). It should be mentioned the temperature coefficient of thermal expansion for resins is, in general, an order of magnitude larger than
that of metal. The effect of differential contraction between s and i on
the temperature dependence of resistance may be important, especially at

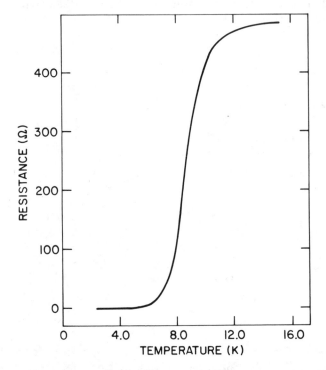

Fig.2   Electrical resistance as a function of temperature for a V_3Si
granular superconductor.   s=V_3Si powder (0.5-5μm),
i=Acryloid B66, and s/i $\sim$ 30.

relatively high temperatures. In Fig. 2, resistance versus temperature for a similar sample (V_3Si powder in Acryloid B66) with s/i ~ 30 is shown. The sample starts becoming superconducting at about 16K and completes the transition around 6K (T_c). It is noted that the normal-state resistance value at T ~20K is about an order of magnitude smaller than that of the previous sample (Fig. 1). The temperature coefficient of resistance is positive (resistance decreases a factor of ~10 from 300 to 20K) The critical current, I_c, as measured from I-V curves, is shown in Fig. 3 for the temperature range 1.8-6K.

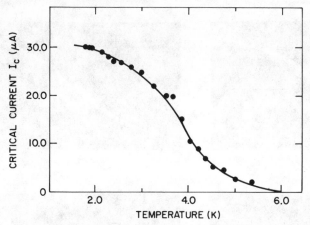

Fig.3   Critical current as a function of temperature for the same sample used in Fig. 2.

The critical current increases with decreasing temperature. There is some leveling-off of I_c at very low temperatures. This behavior is similar to that of a single tunnel junction. The temperature dependence of I_c near T_c must reflect the strength of Josephson coupling between the superconducting grains as a function of temperature.

The microwave response of the new materials is studied by monitoring the I-V characteristics, with or without microwave radiation on the samples. Typical results of such an experiment, as shown in Fig. 4, indicate that:

a)   Samples, such as those used in this microwave experiment, with relatively large normal state resistance (~$10^4\Omega$ for a 0.2 mm^2 x 1 cm sample) yield a very small critical current ($\leq 0.2\mu A$) even at very low temperatures. The I-V curves without microwave radiation on the sample bear a close resemblance to that of a weak-link.

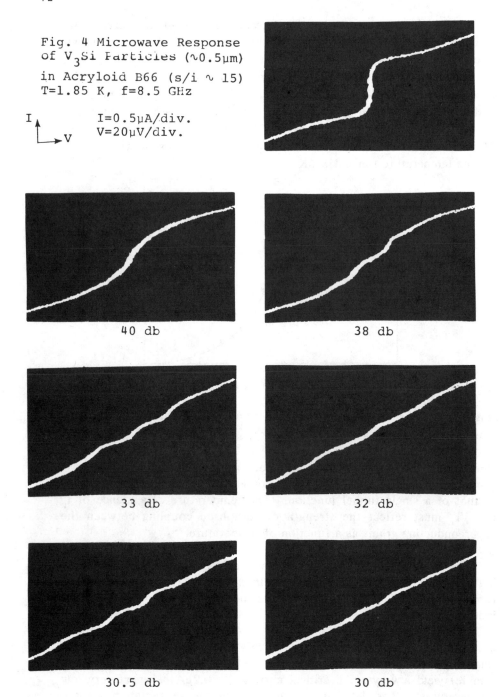

Fig. 4 Microwave Response
of V_3Si Particles (∿0.5μm)
in Acryloid B66 (s/i ∿ 15)
T=1.85 K, f=8.5 GHz

I=0.5μA/div.
V=20μV/div.

40 db

38 db

33 db

32 db

30.5 db

30 db

b) As shown by Fig. 4, the critical current and the I-V curve can be modulated by varying the power of the microwave incident on the sample. This finding strongly suggests that Josephson coupling between the superconducting particles through the oxide(s) or the resin is the main mechanism for electrical conduction for $T < T_{co}$.

c) In particular, it should be noted that the microwave induced current steps were observed at Josephson voltages corresponding to one weak link. This observation is interesting because the sample is presumably an assembly of many randomly packed Josephson weak links or tunnel junctions. This behavior is different from that reported by Yu and Sexena[9] on Sn granular superconducting systems with relatively higher critical currents than that of the sample in Fig.4. This difference in microwave response could be due to difference in coupling strength among particles.

To gain a better understanding of the coupling between the superconducting particles, the study of electrical properties was complemented by magnetic measurements under various experimental conditions. The results will be presented as follows:

The samples studied were a mixture of V_3Si powder ($\sim 0.5 - 25\mu m$ in size) and Stycast 1266 with a s/i ratio of about 6. The electrical resistance and critical current of such samples at zero magnetic field are plotted as a function of temperature in Fig. 5a. At about 17 K, the resistance starts to decrease with decreasing temperature and drops sharply between T~10K and T_c (R=0) =7K. The critical current, I_c increases rapidly with decreasing temperature. The magnetization of these samples at different magnetic fields and temperatures is shown in Figs. 5 (b) and 5 (c). The samples were cooled at nominally zero field to 4.2K and were then subjected to a surge of magnetic field up to ~1000 Oe, when the magnet was turned on. The magnetization was measured with a standard force-balance magnetometer as a function of temperature and field. The data as shown in Figs. 5 (b) and (c) are very interesting in the sense that there is a minimum in the σ vs T curves and that the temperature at which the σ minimum occurs (T_{min}) moves to lower temperatures as the external magnetic field increases. To understand the origin of the $\sigma(T)$ minimum, the inductance change ΔL (T) of (1) a V_3Si granular superconductor (2) V_3Si powder, and (3) a bulk piece of V_3Si was measured separately with a standard ac bridge

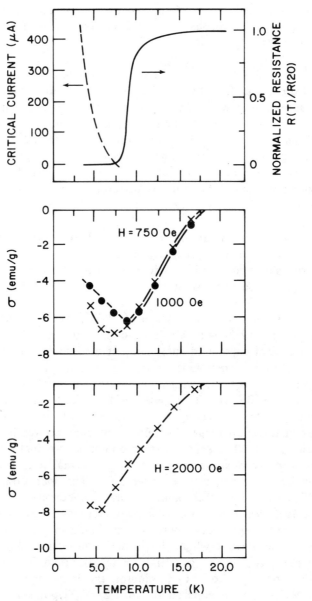

Fig.5   Electrical and Magnetic properties of a V_3Si granular superconductor as a function of temperature. s=V_3Si powder (0.5-25μm), i=Stycast 1266, and s/i ~ 6.

operated at a few hundreds Hz. The results of these measurements are shown in Fig. 6. It should be pointed out that the inductance change as detected by an ac bridge technique is a measure of the magnetization of the samples at low magnetic field (~1 Oe.) and low frequency (~100Hz). The results as shown in Fig. 6 suggest that: a. The superconducting transition of the bulk V_3Si (the solid curve) is sharp ($T_{co} \sim$ 16K). b. The powder V_3Si and the V_3Si granular superconductor show an identical temperature dependence of ΔL and a relatively broad transition (the dotted line) finished at T $\cong$ 12K. c. Most significantly, there is no change in ΔL (T) for T< 12K (The resistive superconducting transition temperature, T_c for the V_3Si granular superconductor is about 6K). From these results, it is clear that the σ increases with increasing temperature (for $T_{min} \lesssim T < T_{co}$) is a manifestation of the Meissner effect arising from the superconducting transition of the V_3Si particles. The increase in σ with decreasing temperature for $T < T_{min}$ has to do with the way that σ was measured. It is probable that a large amount of magnetic flux was trapped in the sample when the field was turned on at 4.2K. As the sample temperature increases the critical current I_c decreases sharply (Fig. 5 a). As a result of this rapid decrease in I_c, the number of superconducting loops connecting the V_3Si particles greatly decreases. This effect leads to a reduction of flux-trapping and consequently a

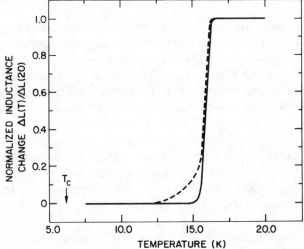

Fig.6   Normalized inductance change, $\Delta L(T)/\Delta L(20)$,

(1)   a V_3Si granular superconductor and
(2) V_3Si powder
(3)   bulk V_3Si.

decrease in σ. When the temperature reaches T_c (R=0) for a given field, all trapped flux should be released from the sample and the temperature dependence of σ should reflect only the Meissner effect. This is in fact what was observed (Figs. 5b, 5c and 6). This is also consistent with the fact that T_{min} decreases with increasing magnetic fields because both I_c and T_c are expected to be suppressed by magnetic fields.

It should be mentioned that the results described so far are limited to granular systems containing V_3Si particles. We have prepared similar materials with $Mo_5Pb_1S_8$ or NbN powder embbeded in various resins. Preliminary results on T_c, and I_c are very similar to those for V_3Si granular superconductors and will not be presented here.

SUMMARY AND CONCLUSIONS

A number of new bulk granular superconductors containing high-T_{co} superconducting particles in various resins have been prepared. The electrical and magnetic properties of these materials in the superconducting state can be understood if they can be viewed as arrays (3-dimensional) of Josephson junctions.

These new superconductors are characterized by the following properties:

1) The normal-state resistivity for these granular materials can be of the order of 0.01 -1 Ω cm depending on the size and the concentration of the superconducting particles. The temperature coefficient of resistance can be positive or negative and can be controlled by the amount of the metallic conductor in the sample. Materials with a large superconductor to insulator ratio become superconducting at T_c which is, in general, less than half of T_{co} (i.e. $T_c < \frac{1}{2} T_{co}$).

2) The critical current I_c is extremely low and is also a function of the particle size and concentration of the superconducting powder (critical current density $J_c \sim 0.001 - 0.3$ A/cm^2). For comparison, it should be noted that J_c for granular Al is about 10^2-10^4A/cm^2.

3) The critical current and the I-V curve can be modulated by varying the power of the microwave. Microwave induced current steps at Josephson voltages can also be modulated in amplitude by the microwave power.

While the properties of the new high-T_c granular superconductors are interesting from a fundamental point of view, they should find some useful practical applications in the future. In the following, a few examples for potential applications will be given:

1.   SQUIDs: One of the constraints in designing a SQUID is $L\,I_c \cong \Phi_o$, where L is SQUID inductance and Φ_o the flux quantum. Deutcher and Rosenbaum[10] have made use of relatively low I_c of granular Al to make rf-SQUIDs with weak-link configuration as wide as 40μm. The unusually low values and the wide range of the I_c of the high-T_c granular superconductors should be valuable in constructing an optimum SQUID.

2.   Radiation Detectors: The properties associated with the Josephson coupling between the superconducting particles should be very useful in millimeter and sub-millimeter wave detection. There are already some experimental results for this type of application.[11]

3.   A superconductive glue and paint: With a relatively high T_c, the new composite materials can be used also as a superconductive epoxy to patch up cryogenic electronic circuits or as a conducting line to reduce the dissipative path for heat and signal. They can be used as a superconducting coating as a shield for magnetic field.

ACKNOWLEDGEMENTS

The authors wish to thank A. Davidson for helpful discussions and W. Kateley and H. Lilienthal for their skillful technical assistance.

REFERENCES

1. G. Pellam, G. Dousselin, H. Cortes and J. Rosenblatt, Solid State Commun. *11*, 427 (1972).

2. J. Rosenblatt, Rev. de Phys. Appl. *9*, 217 (1974).

3. G. Dentscher, Y. Imry and L. Gunther, Phys. Rev. *B10*, 4598 (1974).

4. E. Simanek and S. Cremer, Solid State Commun. *23*, 887 (1977).

5. D.Abraham, S. Alterovitz and R. Rosenbaum, IEEE Trans. Magn. *MAG*-13. 866 (1977).

6. S.A. Wolf, D.U. Gubser and Y. Imry, Phys. Rev. Lett. *42*, 324 (1979).

7. B. Abelis, Phys. Rev. *B15*, 2828 (1977).

8. P.W. Anderson, J. Phys. Chem. Solids, *11*, 26 (1959).

9. M. L. Yu and A. M. Saxena, IEEE Trans. on Magnetics, *MAG-11*, 674 (1975).

10 G. Deutscher and R. Rosenbaum, Appl. Phys. Lett. *27*, 366 (1975).

11. A.L. Solovev, E.V. Khristenko, and V.M. Dmitriev, Fiz. Nizk. Temp. (USSR) *4*, 152 (1978).

Percolation Thresholds in Granular Films —
Non-Universality and Critical Current

Scott Kirkpatrick

IBM Research Center, Yorktown Heights, N.Y. 10598

SUMMARY

Three results are reported which should be applicable to the percolation threshold seen in the low temperature properties of inhomogeneous super-conductors as the fraction of superconducting material is varied. First, we introduce a simplified model for the deposition of granular films, with an interaction energy favoring the formation of metal clumps. The percolation problem defined on random samples prepared by this process is non-universal: critical exponents are continuous functions of the interaction strength and differ from the conventional values. Second, we treat the critical current, using the network model introduced recently by Deutscher and Rappaport[1], and by Huse and Guyer[2], neglecting the effects of structural correlation. Results are presented for 2D and 3D networks. In the course of these calculations, we have obtained a measure of the "tortuousity" of percolation paths close to threshold. Both results are conveniently expressed in terms of the percolation coherence length, ξ_p. The critical current density, I_c, is found to be $\propto \xi_p^{1-d}$. The ratio of the shortest path length across a random network to the linear dimensions of the network is $\propto \ln \xi_p$ in 2D and $\propto \xi_p^{\delta/\nu}$ in 3D, with $\delta \approx .35$.

METASTABLE STRUCTURES AND UNIVERSALITY

It might be useful to begin by describing the domain of validity of the calculations presented here. Fig. 1 is a sketch of the phase diagram of a typical inhomogeneous superconductor. The results of percolation theory have been applied by other speakers at this conference to describe the behavior of their systems as the temperature is lowered. As long as the dominant physical effect is the formation of finite clusters of material linked by couplings which are stronger than average, such calculations should give correct results (and that seems to be the case). However, sufficiently close to the phase boundary, whether it is approached at fixed concentration (a), as in cermets [1,3], or (b) with the concentration increasing through prox-imity effect as the temperature is decreased [4], the critical properties will be those of the pure system. Renormalization group arguments show that only at $T = 0$ will the percolation critical properties remain applicable all the way to the phase boundary. Otherwise some sort of crossover, sketched as a dashed line in Fig. 1, will occur. Thus our results are for the zero-

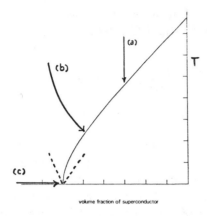

1. Phase diagram for a dilute inhomogeneous superconductor. Arrows represent the directions by which the transition is approached under various experimental and theoretical circumstances.

temperature trajectory (c) in Fig. 1, and should be mapped into other situations only with appropriate caution.

Almost all discussions of percolation thresholds in real materials [5] employ results of model calculations of the connectivity properties of sites or bonds randomly arranged on regular lattices. In such models, the probability that a given site (or bond) is present or absent is independent of whatever happens on the surrounding sites (or bonds). This simplification is a great convenience, and is usually justified by appeal to the universality of critical phenemona. Since properties of the idealized models can be extracted from the partition function of a Potts lattice gas [6,7], our present understanding of equilibrium statistical mechanics suggests that these critical properties are independent of lattice type and valid for random as well as regular lattices. Connectivity properties in the more general case when the site occupation properties are locally correlated have only recently received attention [8].

We consider here a model which goes beyond the work in [8]. To model deposition we take a lattice of sites, intially empty, and allow atoms to impinge on it. The sticking probability will vary from site to site, depending on the number of occupied neighboring sites to which the incoming atom may bind. Thus if the adsorption energy per bond is E, and site i has z_i out of its z neighboring sites occupied,

$$p_i^{(d)} = \exp[-E(z - z_i)/kT = \alpha^{z - z_i} ,$$ (1)

where

$$\alpha \equiv \exp(-E/kT)$$ (2)

When α is sufficiently small, the first few atoms deposited act as seeds, and a strongly clumped arrangement evolves, as seen in Fig. 2. This gives a reasonable resemblance to electron micrographs of some inhomogeneous films of experimental interest [1,3].

2. Arrangement of material in the correlated deposition model with $\alpha = 0.25$. In this 120×120 site sample, .56 of the sites have been occupied (white regions), .51 lie in the largest cluster, and complete paths cross the sample in both horizontal and vertical directions.

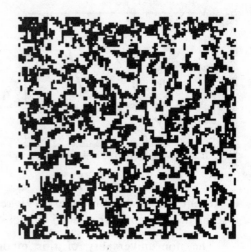

One can also imagine an evaporation process which is the reverse of (1), with the evaporation probability per unit time for an atom given by

$$p_i^{(e)} = \exp(-z_i E/kT) = \alpha^{z_i} \tag{3}$$

A film in equilibrium with a vapor would experience both processes, with their relative rates fixed by conditions of detailed balance. But that is not the typical preparation condition. Here we shall study the two processes separately.

Fig. 3 shows that the two processes are not inverses, by comparing the fraction of samples resulting from each process which are connected at a given coverage. The percolation threshold, estimated as the concentration where half of the samples are conducting, requires 7 per cent greater coverage in the deposited samples than in the evaporated ones. Thus this system is not time reversal invariant, and has no Hamiltonian description.

More important, the correlations (here $\alpha = 0.25$) have shifted the position of the percolation threshold and broadened the range of concentrations in which the correlation length associated with the percolation threshold exceeds the sample size. This can be seen by comparing curves (a) and (b) in Fig. 3, and taking the "critical region" for an $L \times L$ sample, $\Delta x(L)$, to be the range of concentrations during which the fraction of conducting samples passes from nearly zero to nearly unity. By study of the narrowing of $\Delta x(L)$ as L increases we can extract the critical exponent, ν, for the diverging correlation length $\xi_p(x) \propto (x - x_c)^{-\nu}$ [See the lectures in Ref. 4 for a discussion of this sort of analysis.] Analysis of this size dependence shows that ν is increased by ≈ 25 per cent when $\alpha = 0.5$ in 2D. The larger exponent is consistent with a broadened critical regime. Both the sign and the magnitude of the change are comparable to the discrepancies observed

82

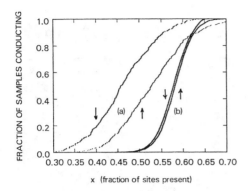

FRACTION OF SAMPLES CONDUCTING

x (fraction of sites present)

3. Fraction of 30×30 samples which were conducting at a given fractional occupancy under pure deposition (↑) and evaporation (↓), with correlation factors of (a) $\alpha = 0.25$ and (b) $\alpha = 1.0$, which produces no correlation.

in recent experimental papers [9] reporting values of the conductivity threshold exponents for quench condensed films.

The non-universality of this model should not come as a surprise. Coniglio, Stanley and co-workers [8] have found in equilibrium correlated percolation models that the percolation exponents were unchanged if the correlations were sufficiently weak, but that first-order transitions could occur for strongly correlated systems, i.e., those which phase separate and never form regions in which the concentration takes the value needed for a continuous onset of percolation. In our model, the sites do not rearrange after deposition, so phase separation cannot occur and the transition must be continuous. Apparently, this departure from equilibrium produces non-universal critical connectivity properties.

CRITICAL CURRENT AT THRESHOLD

Two recent papers have proposed a simple starting point for considering the concentration dependence of the critical current density near a percolation threshold in any superfluid, be it helium or superconductor. The essential idea is that the supercurrent is limited by the cross sectional area of the narrowest point through which it flows. If we model a granular superconductor as a random network of superconducting points (the grains) interacting by nearest neighbor bonds, this minimum cross section is given by the number of distinct paths which can be constructed to cross the network simultaneously. Since there are efficient algorithms for solving this problem on specific networks [10], we have determined this quantity for the most commonly studied 3D and 2D percolation network models.

Huse and Guyer [2] calculate $I_c(x)$ approximately and predict that in 2D $I_c(x) \propto (x - x_c)/|\ln(x - x_c)|$. They comment that this suggests that $I_c(x) \propto \sigma(x)$, the conductivity, in 2D. However, I do not find their approximations very compelling, and these predictions disagree with experiment [1] and with the numerical results to be reported here. Deutscher and Rappaport [1] find that $I_c(x)$ has a larger critical exponent than $\sigma(x)$ in Pb-Ge films, which are presumed to be 2D, while $I_c(x) \propto \sigma(x)$ in thicker (3D) Al-Ge films. Both cases are consistent with

$$I_c(x) \propto (x - x_c)^{(d-1)\nu} \propto \xi_p^{1-d} \,, \tag{4}$$

a prediction which follows from the "nodes and links" picture of the current flow close to a percolation threshold [11].

Our numerical results support Deutscher and Rappaport's observations. The conductivity in the 2D bond percolation model is very nearly linear in $(x - 0.5)$, departing significantly only close to threshold, as shown in Fig. 4. The critical current, on the other hand, droops well below the conductivity data. Similar behavior is displayed for I_c in both site and bond percolation in 2D, as Fig. 4 shows. In 3D, however, $\sigma(x)$ and $I_c(x)$ are practically indistinguishable (Fig. 5).

To obtain a more quantitative prediction of the behavior of $I_c(x)$ near the percolation threshold we make use of the dependence of this quantity on sample size in finite samples, again using insights gained from real-space

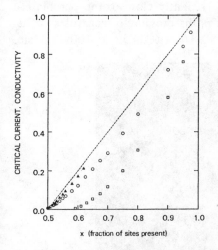
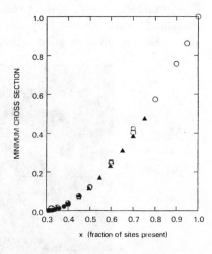

4. Critical current density as a function of concentration, for 2D bond (circles) and site (squares) percolation, in 100×100 site samples. For contrast, the conductivity of the bond percolation model is also shown (solid points), as well as the effective medium theory prediction (dashed line).

5. Critical current vs. concentration for 3D site percolation, with sample dimensions of L = 30 (squares) and L = 10 (circles). The solid data points indicate the relative conductivity, $\sigma(x)$, for samples with L = 20 (dots) and L = 10 (triangles).

renormalization group calculations. Away from x_c, the number of parallel paths which can be constructed in a sample is proportional to the cross sectional area of the sample, L^{d-1}. Close to x_c this number is observed to vary as some other power of L, say L^y. This is an example of an "anomalous dimension" or "fractal dimensionality" [12], but here we shall simply demonstrate that this behavior is equivalent to the expected power-law dependence at threshold.

For any value of x, we can approximate the minimum cross sectional area of an infinite system by breaking the system into many sufficiently large cells, and averaging the properties of those cells. The smallest cells which will give a reasonable approximation are those with $L \approx \xi_p(x)$. Therefore, sufficiently close to threshold, the current density per unit cross sectional area will be given by

$$I_c \propto \xi_p^{y+1-d} \quad , \tag{5}$$

and the threshold exponent can be identified as $\nu(d-1-y)$.

Direct examination of the "backbone" region [12], the multiply-connected component of a percolation network through which a current may flow, indicates the surprising result that sufficiently close to the percolation threshold, a sample has only one or a few paths crossing it, regardless of its size. Fig. 6 gives a good example of this, for it shows a 400x400 site

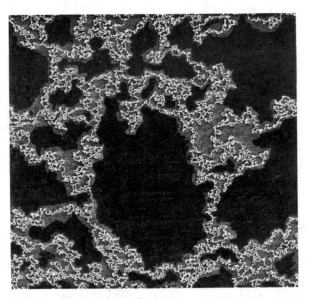

6. Backbone (largest biconnected component) of a 400×400 site sample with x = .596 $\approx x_c$, in the 2D site percolation model.

system close to x_c, and no more than two distinct paths can be constructed to cross the sample in either direction, vertical or horizontal. We studied populations of several hundred to 10,000 samples of networks at x_c with L ranging from 4 to 400 (for 2D site and bond percolation), and from 4 to 50 (3D site percolation). In each case, the mean number of distinct paths crossing a conducting sample is 1.2 $\pm$ .1, and insensitive to sample size. Thus y = 0 to a fairly good accuracy, and (4) is a correct result.

Several authors have speculated recently about the twistedness or tortuousity of the paths for current flow near threshold. This characteristic has implications for the critical exponents [5,11,12], and for the smoothing out of anisotropies close to x_c [13]. The algorithm we employed to find the minimal cross section of a network constructs the shortest possible paths first for the sake of efficiency. Thus one piece of information obtained in the process is the length, L_{min}, of the shortest path through a dilute network L sites on a side. L_{min} increases with decreasing concentration, with the most dramatic enhancements occurring just above x_c. If we study $L_{min}(x,L)$ at fixed x, with L varying, we find that L_{min} is proportional to L sufficiently far from threshold, but increases more rapidly at x_c. This shows evidence of an anomalous dimensionality, hence critical behavior.

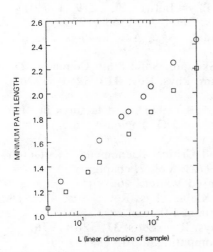 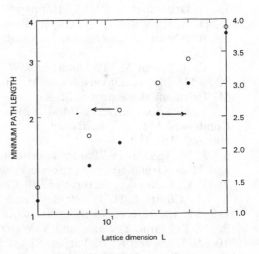

7. Semilog plot of the normalized minimum path length, L_{min}/L, to cross a connected sample with x = x_c in 2D bond (circles) and site (squares) percolation, as functions of L.

8. Minimum path length, L_{min}/L, for 3D site percolation at threshold. Solid data points give a semilog plot, open data points a log-log plot, from which the critical exponent δ was determined.

Figs. 7 and 8 show L_{min}/L as a function of L at x_c for 2d site and bond percolation (Fig. 7), and for 3D site percolation (Fig. 8). 2D, $L_{min}/L \propto \ln$ (L), while in 3D it seems more likely that $L_{min}/L \propto L^{.41}$, since the points fall on a straight line in a log-log plot (open data points), but are curved on a semilog plot (solid data points in Fig. 8). If we define a tortuousity exponent, δ, by

$$L_{min}(x)/L \propto (x - x_c)^{-\delta} \quad , \tag{6}$$

where L must be $>> \xi_p$ for the expression to hold, then $\delta \approx .35$ in 3D, and $= 0$ in 2D, but with logarithmic corrections in the latter case. This difference between 2D and 3D is consistent with recent calculations by Sarachev and Vinogradoff [13]. They find that an initially anisotropic system becomes isotropic as $x \rightarrow x_c^+$ in 3D, but that in 2D, the anisotropy is only strongly reduced. Since the logarithmic increase in tortuousity we find in 2D is rather weak, analysis of the size dependence of numerical results will probably be necessary to determine whether conduction processes at a percolation threshold become isotropic in 2D as well. The expectation is that they should.

REFERENCES

1. G. Deutscher and M. L. Rappaport, J. Phys. Lettres **40**, L219 (1979).
2. D. A. Huse and R. A. Guyer, Phys. Rev. Letts. **43**, 1163 (1979).
3. B. Abeles, P. Sheng, M. D. Coutts and Y. Arie, Adv. in Phys. **24**, 407 (1975).
4. C. J. Lobb, M. Tinkham, and W. J. Skocpol, Solid State Commun. **27**, 1273 (1978); A. Davidson and M. Tinkham, Phys. Rev. **B13**, 3261 (1976); M. Tinkham, these proceedings.
5. S. Kirkpatrick, Revs. Mod. Phys. **45**, 570 (1973), and lectures in "Ill-Condensed Matter," R. Balian, R. Maynard, and G. Toulouse, eds., (North-Holland, 1979).
6. J. W. Essam, in "Phase Transitions and Critical Phenomena," C. Domb and M. S. Green eds., (Academic Press, 1972), Vol. 2, chapter 6.
7. T. C. Lubensky, lectures in "Ill-Condensed Matter," loc. cit.
8. A. Coniglio, H. E. Stanley, and W. Klein, Phys. Rev. Letts. **42**, 518 (1979), and references to earlier work contained therein.
9. N. T. Liang, Y. Shan, and S. Wang, Phys. Rev. Letts. **37**, 526 (1976).
10. S. Even and R. E. Tarjan, SIAM J. Computing **4**, 507 (1975).
11. A. Skal and B. I. Shklovskii, Sov. Phys. Semicond. **8**, 1029 (1975); D. Stauffer, Z. Phys. **B22**, 161 (1975); P.-G. de Gennes, Lettres au J. de Phys. **37**, L1 (1976).
12. S. Kirkpatrick, A. I. P. Conf. Proc. **40**, 99 (1977).
13. A. K. Sarychev and A. P. Vinogradoff, J. Phys. **C12**, L681 (1979).

TOPOLOGICAL EXCITATIONS IN THIN SUPERCONDUCTING FILMS: a review.

B.A. Huberman
Xerox Palo Alto Research Center, Palo Alto, CA 94304

S. Doniach
Department of Applied Physics, Stanford University, Stanford CA 94305

I. INTRODUCTION

Over the past few years we have witnessed a surge of interest in a new class of phase transitions that are likely to occur in nearly two-dimensional systems. In contrast to the extended elementary excitations that have been thoroughly studied for many years, the objects responsible for this new type of critical behavior in two dimensions are topological in character. A topological excitation consists of a metastable localized region in which the order parameter goes to zero and such that this state is a local minimum in the free energy of the system. Examples of this kind of excitation in two dimensional systems are quantum vortices in superfluids (liquid helium and superconductors) and crystal lattice dislocations and disclinations as they occur in solids such as epitaxial films and smectic liquid crystals.

In 1972, Berezinskii,[1] Popov,[2] and Kosterlitz and Thouless[3] predicted that in neutral superfluids a thermodynamic instability would occur at a non-zero temperature, T_{2D}, in which vortex-antivortex pairs would spontaneously start dissociating into free vortices. Furthermore, it was shown by several authors[3,4,5] that while the positional correlation functions decay exponentially with distance above T_{2D}, they exhibit power law behavior below this temperature, a fact that implies the existence of a line of critical points in the temperature range $0 < T < T_{2D}$. The value of T_{2D} has been conveniently expressed by Kosterlitz[6] in terms of the effective dielectric constant of this vortex gas $\varepsilon(r,T)$. If the "charge" of the vortex is denoted by q, the critical temperature is then given by

$$k_B T_{2D} = \frac{q^2}{2\varepsilon(\infty, T_{2D})} \qquad (1)$$

with $\varepsilon(\infty, T_{2D})$ of order unity. Moreover, it was shown that at T_{2D} the superfluid density undergoes a universal jump[6,7] which was recently confirmed for helium films by several groups.[8,9,10]

The experimental impetus to these ideas was provided by the observation of vortex depairing in He^4 films using several techniques. In particular, Bishop and Reppy[9] and Telschow and Hallock[10] have observed an increase in dissipation of the superflow as T_{2D} is approached from below; a fact that may be accounted for by the vortex depairing picture once the dynamics are incorporated into the theory.[11,12]

0094-243X/80/580087-08$1.50 Copyright 1980 American Institute of Physics

Recently it was suggested that dirty thin film superconductors could display the same type of topological phase transition that is observed in neutral superfluids.[13, 14, 15, 16] The key idea is the observation[13] that in small thin superconducting samples with impurities, the effective London penetration depth of magnetic flux lines could be made larger than the sample size. In that limit, vortices interact through logarithmic interactions and the superconductor exhibits the same type of topological behavior as He[4] films. Moreover, we showed[14, 17] that the effects of an internal magnetic field on vortex crystallization and depairing dissipation can be quite non-linear, leading to a rich phase diagram which is just beginning to be explored experimentally.

II. IN THE ABSENCE OF AN EXTERNAL MAGNETIC FIELD

As was first shown by Pearl,[18] vortex pairs in thin superconducting films have a logarithmic interaction energy out to a characteristic distance $\lambda_\perp = \lambda^2/d$, with λ the London penetration length and d the thickness of the film. Beyond this distance, the interaction energy crosses over to a $1/r$ dependence. Experimentally $\lambda_\perp$ can be made of the order of cms. Therefore, if we ignore the finite size effects, for sample sizes such that $\lambda_\perp \gg R$, vortex pair dissociation will start taking place at a temperature T_{2D} which is given by Eq.(1). Since the effective charge for the vortices is given by $q = (\phi_0/4\pi)\lambda_\perp^{-\frac{1}{2}}$, and $\varepsilon(\infty, T_{2D}) \cong 1$, Eq.(1) can be written as:

$$T_{2D} = \left(\frac{\phi_0}{4\pi}\right)^2 \frac{1}{\lambda_\perp (T)} \tag{2}$$

Using the expression for the temperature dependence of $\lambda_\perp$ in the dirty limit,[19] T_{2D} can be expressed in terms of the sheet resistance of the film in a form which may be approximated by[13]

$$\frac{T_{2D}}{T_{BCS}} = \frac{1}{1 + .173 \, R_\square/R_c} \tag{3}$$

with $R_c = \hbar/e^2$, a value which corresponds to a sheet resistance of $4.12\text{k}\Omega/\square$. As can be seen from these equations, the larger $R_\square$ the longer $\lambda_\perp$ and hence the lower the transition temperature T_{2D} when compared to T_{BCS}.

The presence of a vortex plasma above T_{2D} implies that free vortices will be swept across the sample by an infinitesimal current, giving rise to a finite resistivity for $T_{2D} < T < T_{BCS}$, decreasing to zero as $T \to T_{2D}^+$. A comparison between the observed broadening in the resistive transition of high-sheet-resistance films and Eq. (3) has been carried out by Beasley et al.[13] Although the detailed behavior of the resistivity near T_{2D} has not yet been compared with the theoretical predictions of Section IV, it appears that the observed resistive broadening is consistent with the vortex depairing phase transition. For $T < T_{2D}$, the analogy with the Helium film case suggests that the presence of a finite current will stimulate the unbinding of vortex pairs leading to a non-ohmic resistive behavior $R(T) \propto j^{\beta(T)}$. This kind of behavior has been observed by Wolf et al.,[27] although their interpretation of it is different.

III. H-T PHASE DIAGRAM OF A 2-D SUPERCONDUCTOR

In the presence of an external magnetic field the effective Hamiltonian of a system of vortices in a superconducting film can be written as [14]

$$H = N\mu_0 + U_0 \left| \sum_i \text{sgn} (q_i) \right|^2 + \frac{1}{2} \sum_{i \neq j} U_{ij} + H \sum_i m_i \qquad (4)$$

where N is the total number of vortices, μ_0 is the chemical potential associated with the vortex core ($\mu_0 = d\xi^2 H_c^2/8$ with ξ the core radius and H_c the thermodynamic critical field), U_0 is the magnetic energy associated with an excess of vortices of a given sign, which is given by

$$U_0 = q^2 \ln (R/\xi) \qquad (5)$$

and m_i is the paramagnetic moment of the ith vortex, $m_i = m \, \text{sgn}(q_i)$ with

$$m = \frac{\phi_0}{16\pi} \frac{R^2}{\lambda_\perp} . \qquad (6)$$

At $T = 0$ the field H_c, for which the film becomes unstable to the nucleation of a single vortex is given by the ratio $(\mu_0 + U_0)/m$. Using Eqs. (5) and (6) Pearl[18] obtained the size dependent value $H_{c_1} \cong 4\phi_0 R^{-2} \ln (R/\xi)$ which is extremely small for reasonable sample sizes ($H_{c_1} \cong 10^{-5}$ Gauss for $R \sim 1$ cm and $\xi = 20$ Å). For $0 < T < T_{2D}$ the nucleation energy for a single vortex will be lowered because of the finite polarizability of the gas of bound thermally excited vortex pairs, which interact with the nucleated vortex leading to a critical field $\tilde{H}_{c1} = H_{c1} \epsilon^{-1}(\infty, T)$, with $\epsilon^{-1}(\infty, T)$ the long distance dielectric constant of the vortex gas. If the effects of the finite sample size on the dielectric behavior predicted for the infinite system are ignored $\tilde{H}_{c1}/H_{c1}$ ($T = 0$) will display the same universal behavior near T_{2D} predicted for the superfluid density jump in He^4 films.[7,8]

At T = 0 and for magnetic fields such that $H_{c_1} < H < H_{c_2}$, with H_{c_2} the depairing field, the magnetic flux lines will rearrange themselves into a triangular lattice. This is directly analogous to the vortex lattice, now rotating with the sample, which is induced by the rotation of a thin film of superfluid He[4] about an axis normal to the film plane. In the superconducting case the vortex lattice is stabilized by a counter-rotating diamagnetic shielding current induced in the finite sample by the external field, so remains static. The question which can be posed is: could this vortex lattice melt by a process in which the topological excitations of a two dimensional solid, i.e., dislocations, undergo an unbinding process similar to the one we have just discussed for vortices? The answer is yes,[17] and the melting temperature is given, in the limit where we do not assume a large renormalization of the rigidity modulus by the dislocation pairs,[20] by

$$k_B T_M = (\frac{\phi_0}{4\pi})^2 \frac{1}{4\pi\sqrt{3} \ \lambda_\perp (T)} \quad . \tag{7}$$

In the low temperature, very thin limit, where $\lambda_\perp$ becomes independent of temperature, a comparison of this equation with Eq. (2) gives a simple numerical scaling relation, i.e.,

$$\frac{T_M}{T_{2D}} = \frac{1}{4\pi\sqrt{3}} \quad . \tag{8}$$

As the film thickness is increased however, the ratio of T_M to T_{2D} will change and we will obtain the behavior shown in Fig. 1.

Above the melting temperature of the vortex lattice, there may or may not exist an additional "hexatic" phase, in which although the positional correlation function of the vortex lattice decays exponentially the correlation function for orientational order of the lattice persists at large distances.[21] In particular, Halperin and Nelson have shown[22] that the hexatic phase can itself "melt" by dissociation of disclination pairs, with a transition temperature T_H given by

$$k_B T_H = k_A (T_H)/72 \tag{9}$$

with $k_A(T_H)$ the renormalized value of the Franck constant. Our present lack of knowledge of k_A for a vortex lattice means that we do not know whether this phase exists or not in 2-D superconductors.

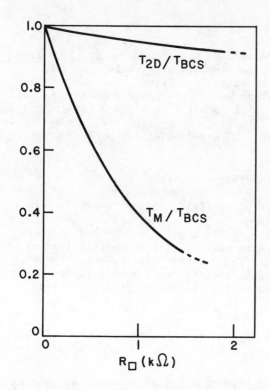

Figure 1.

Initial dependence of vortex lattice melting temperature T_M and vortex plasma transition temperature T_{2D}, on $R_\square$. For large values of $R_\square$ the asymptotic ratio (8) is reached.

In order to obtain a complete phase diagram for a 2-D superconductor, we need to know the behavior of the rigidity modulus of the vortex lattice at very high fields, near H_{c_2}. Conen and Schmid have shown[23] that this decreases quadratically[2] with the applied magnetic field, so that both T_M and T_H will go to zero as $H \to H_{c_2}$. Thus, we are led to the following phase diagram for the two-dimensional superconductor in the magnetic field-temperature plane.[28]

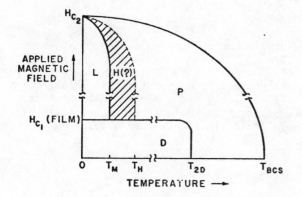

Figure 2

Phase diagram of a thin film superconductor : L denotes the rigid vortex lattice phase, D the weakly diamagnetic Meissner phase with no vortices present, and P the vortex plasma. The shaded area H indicates a possible hexatic phase.

In closing, we should mention that although the H_{c_2} boundary has been drawn with the traditional solid line, this does not imply the existence of a sharp phase transition. Just as in the three-dimensional bulk situation where the presence of a magnetic field renders the superconducting-normal transition a one-dimensional problem,[24,25] in the thin film case the applied field transforms the Ginzburg-Landau theory into a zero-dimensional situation, which can be computed exactly.

IV. THE RESISTIVE TRANSITION

As mentioned above, for applied fields larger than $\tilde{H}_{c_1}$, with $T < T_{2D}$ or in all finite fields at $T > T_{2D}$, the superconducting film will always have a finite density of unbound vortices $n_+(T,H)$ with paramagnetic moments parallel (+) or antiparallel (−) to the field respectively. These free vortices will be swept towards the film boundaries by a current, thereby leading to a finite resistivity $\rho(T,H)$ which may be written in the absence of pinning effect as

$$\frac{\rho(T,H)}{\rho_n(T,H)} = 2\pi\xi^2(n_+ + n_-) \tag{10}$$

In ref. 14, we proposed a semi-phenomenological scaling law leading to a calculation of the temperature and field dependent density of unbound vortices. Using arguments similar to those of Kosterlitz and Thouless, we proposed that for $T > T_{2D}$ the density of free vortices $[(n_+ + n_-) = n_{free}]$ is given by the solutions of a pair of self consistent equations. If $M = \pi R^2(n_+ - n_-)$ measures the vortex imbalance, we can write these equations as

$$M = \pi R^2 n_{free} \sinh \beta (mH - m_B M) \tag{11}$$

$$n_{free} = 2\xi^{-2}[\exp(-\beta\tilde{\mu}_0) \cosh\beta(mH - m_B M)]^\nu \tag{12}$$

with $\tilde{\mu}_0$ a renormalized chemical potential, $m_B = \frac{1}{2}(3q^2) \ln R/\xi)$, and $\nu(T) = 1/(t + xt^{\frac{1}{2}})$ with $t = [(T/T_{2D}) - 1]$ and x a numerical constant.

In order to study the behavior of the solutions of Eqs. (11) and (12), we first look at the zero field limit. We then obtain

$$\frac{\rho(T)}{\rho_n} = 4\pi[\exp(-\beta\tilde{\mu}_0)]^{\nu(T)} \tag{13}$$

which implies an essential singularity at $T = T_{2D}$ of a form which continuously crosses from Kosterlitz scaling to Zittartz scaling for $t \gtrsim x^{2}$ [24]. As the temperature approaches T_{BCS} Eq. (13) is no longer valid. In this regime, Halperin and Nelson[25] have suggested an interpolation scheme which smoothly joins the behavior of $\rho(T)$ at $T = T_{2D}^{+}$ with the results of the Aslamazov-Larkin theory valid for $T \gtrsim T_{BCS}$.

For a very small applied field, $H \lesssim H_{c_1}(0)$, Eqs. (11) and (12) give rise to very interesting non-linear effects. Since for $T > T_{2D}$, $H_{c_1} = 0$, it follows that an external magnetic field, however small, will always inject vortices of one sign into the film. Moreover, the effects of this vortex imbalance are by no means linear.

As the applied field is increased, the injection of vortices of one sign leads to a change in the total vortex density, which, in turn, via a reduction in the Debye screening length of the vortex plasma, leads to a field stimulated unbinding of vortex pairs at a given temperature. Following the scheme proposed in ref. 14, this leads for $H \gg H_{c_1}(0)$ to an equation for the total number of free vortices,

$$\bar{n}_f = \bar{n}_0^{\frac{\nu}{1+\nu}} \bar{n}_f^{\frac{\nu}{1+\nu}} + \bar{n}_H \qquad (14)$$

where $\bar{n}$ denotes $n\xi^2$, n_0 is the zero field vortex density and n_H is the density of vortices injected by the applied field $= 2[H/H_{c_1}(0)]/\pi R^2$. Solution of this implicit equation leads to a characteristic peeling off of the resistivity from the zero field essential singularity as a function of field and temperature, in qualitative agreement with observations made 10 years ago by Masker et al.[26] This qualitative evidence for field induced vortex unbinding provides strong support for the existence of a population of bound vortex pairs in thin film superconductors.

VI. REFERENCES

1. V.L. Berezinskii, Sov. Phys. JETP **34**, 6101 (1972).
2. V.N. Popov, Teor. Matem. Fiz. **11**, 354 (1972) and Soviet Phys. JETP **37**, 341 (1973).
3. J.M. Kosterlitz and D.M. Thouless, J. Phys. **C6**, 1181 (1973).
4. J. Zittartz, Z. Phys. **23**, 55 (1976).
5. J. Jose, L.P. Kadanoff, D.R. Nelson, and S. Kirkpatrick, Phys. Rev. **B16**, 1217 (1977).
6. J.M. Kosterlitz, J. Phys. **C7**, 1046 (1974).
7. D. Nelson and J.M. Kosterlitz, Phys. Rev. Lett. **39**,1201 (1977).
8. I. Rudnick, Phys. Rev. Lett. **40**, 1453 (1978).
9. D.J. Bishop and J.D. Reppy, Phys. Rev. Lett. **40**, 1727 (1978).
10. K.L. Telschow and R.B. Hallock, Phys. Rev. Lett. 37, 1484 (1976).
11. B.A. Huberman, R.J. Meyerson, and S. Doniach, Phys. Rev. Lett. **40**, 780 (1978).
12. V. Ambegaokar, B.I. Halperin, D.R. Nelson, and E.D. Siggia, Phys. Rev. Lett. 40, 783 (1978) and preprint (1979). See also V. Ambegaokar and S. Teitel, Phys. Rev. **B19**, 1667 (1979).
13. M.R. Beasley, J.E. Mooij, and T.P. Orlando, Phys. Rev. Lett., 42, 1165 (1979).
14. S. Doniach and B. Huberman, Phys. Rev. Lett. **42**, 1169 (1979).
15. B.I. Halperin and D.R. Nelson, J. Low Temp. Phys. **36**, 599 (1979).
16. L.A. Turkevich, J. Phys. C. **12**, 385 (1979).
17. B.A. Huberman and S. Doniach, Phys. Rev. Lett. 43, 950 (1979).
18. J. Pearl, L. Temp. Physics –LT9, Ed. J.G. Daunt, D.O. Edwards, F.J. Milford, and M. Yagub (Plenum, NY, (965) 566.
19. M. Tinkham, "Introduction to Superconductivity", (McGraw-Hill, NY 1975).
20. As shown by R.H. Morf, Phys. Rev. Lett. **43**, 931 (1979), in the case of 2-D solids there is a large decrease in the rigidity modulus as $T \rightarrow T_M$. It is not clear however, how severe this effect will be in vortex lattices.
21. D. Mermin, Phys. Rev. **176**, 250 (1968).
22. B.I. Halperin and D.R. Nelson, Phys. Rev. Lett. **41**, 131 (1978) and D.R. Nelson and B.I. Halperin, Phys. Rev. **B19**, 2457 (1979).
23. E. Conen and A. Schmid, J. Low Temp. Phys. **17** 331 (1974).
24. P.A. Lee and S.R. Shenoy, Phys. Rev. Lett. **28**, 1025 (1972).
25. D.J. Thouless, Phys. Rev. Lett. **34**, 946 (1975) and S.P. Farrant and C.E. Gough, Phys. Rev. Lett. **34**, 943 (1975).
26. W.E. Masker, S. Marcelja, and R.D. Parks, Phys. Rev. **188**, 745 (1969).
27. S.A. Wolf, D.U. Gubser, and Y. Imry, Phys. Rev. Lett. **42**, 324 (1979).

28. As D. S. Fisher (private communication) points out, very near H_{c2}, this argument implies T_m is concave rather than convex as depicted in Fig.2.

FLUX LATTICE MELTING IN
THIN FILM SUPERCONDUCTORS

Daniel S. Fisher
Bell Laboratories
Murray Hill, NJ 07974

ABSTRACT

Melting of flux-lattices in thin film type II superconductors is analyzed and the phase diagram at a function of magnetic field is discussed. Several experimental consequences are explored, in particular the possibilities for observing flux lattice melting.

INTRODUCTION AND PHASE DIAGRAM

It has been clear for some time that the equilibrium state of a type II superconductor in a magnetic field $B > H_{c1}$ consists of a triangular lattice of vortex lines each containing one quantum of flux (Φ_0). In this paper we discuss the melting of flux lattices in thin films due to thermal fluctuations and investigate some of the experimental consequences.[1,2]

In a film geometry it is impossible to exclude flux in any non-zero magnetic field perpendicular to the film, and hence H_{c1} vanishes. In any field there will thus be vortices present with areal density, $n = B/\Phi_0$. At low temperatures these vortices will form a lattice with a well-defined shear modulus, μ. However, as first pointed out by Kosterlitz and Thouless,[3] any two-dimensional solid becomes unstable to the presence of free dislocations at temperatures above a melting temperature, T_M, given approximately by

$$\frac{\mu(T_M)}{n\, T_M} = 2\pi\sqrt{3} \quad . \tag{1}$$

At T_M there will be a second order transition from the flux lattice phase to a vortex fluid phase in which the long wavelength shear modulus will vanish due to the presence of free dislocations.

Using Eq. (1) and calculated values for μ,[4] we can estimate the melting temperature of a flux-lattice in a thin superconducting film of thickness d. We note that this melting transition will take the place of the transition at $H_{c2}(T)$ in a bulk (or thin film) superconductor. There are two regimes of experimental interest:

1. Large Magnetic Fields

In high magnetic fields, $B \lesssim H_{c2}(T)$, the flux-lattice melting temperature will depend on B and we find in particular that

$$T_M \propto (H_{c2}(0)-B)^2 \tag{2}$$

for low temperatures.

2. Small Magnetic Fields

For magnetic fields, $B \ll H_{c2}(T)$ (except for extremely small fields $B \lesssim d\Phi_0/\lambda^2(T)$ where λ is the bulk Ginzburg Landau penetration depth), we find, on the other hand, that the flux lattice melting temperature is <u>independent</u> of B and is implicitly determined by

$$T_M = \frac{A_2}{128\sqrt{3}\pi^3} \frac{d\Phi_0{}^2}{\lambda^2(T_M)} \tag{3}$$

where A_2 is a constant which comes from renormalizations of the low temperature shear modulus of the flux-lattice due to nonlinear thermal vibrations and dislocation pairs.[5] This constant is probably in the range[1]

$$.4 \leq A_2 \leq .75 \tag{4}$$

It is useful to express the flux lattice melting temperature in the low field regime in terms of experimentally measurable quantities, in particular the normal state sheet resistance R_n and the bulk transition temperature T_{c0}. As R_n increases (i.e., as the film gets thinner), T_M decreases continuously from T_{c0}. In the dirty limit,[6] and for R_n not too large,

$$\frac{T_M}{T_{c0}} \simeq \frac{1}{1 + \frac{3.8}{A_2} \frac{R_n}{R_c}} \tag{5}$$

independent of B where $R_c = \hbar/e^2 = 4.12 k\Omega/\square$. We can compare this result with the resistive transition in <u>zero</u> field in thin films which, as several authors[6,7] have recently pointed out, occurs not at the bulk transition temperature T_{c0} but at a temperature given by

$$\frac{T_c}{T_{c0}} \simeq \frac{1}{1 + .17 \frac{R_n}{R_c}} \tag{6}$$

which we note is of the same form as Eq. (5) but T_c is considerably closer to T_{c0} than T_M is. For temperatures above T_c there will be thermally activated vortices of <u>both</u> signs present in the film which give rise to a finite resistance even for B=0. However, for T < T_C and nonzero magnetic field (the regime of interest here), almost all the vortices will be of one sign and we will ignore thermal excitation of vortex pairs.

The flux-lattice melting curve is sketched in the figure as a function of B and T along with the bulk $H_{C2}(T)$ which we emphasize is <u>not</u> a phase boundary in thin films. [In addition to the flux lattice and fluid phases, there may also be an intermediate anisotropic "hexatic" phase with a phase boundary (shown dashed in the figure) roughly parallel to the melting curve. This hexatic phase will be hard to distinguish experimentally from the isotropic fluid and we will ignore it henceforth.]

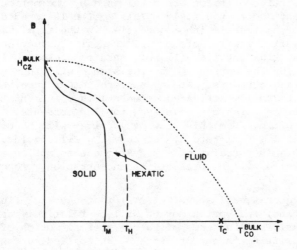

Figure 1. The phase diagram of a thin film superconductor is sketched showing vortex solid, hexatic and fluid phases. The solid line is the flux-lattice melting curve (T_M) and the dashed line the hexatic-isotropic fluid phase boundary (T_H). The zero magnetic field resistive transition temperature, T_c, is marked by an X. For comparison the <u>bulk</u> upper critical field $H_{c2}(T)$ is shown as a dotted line.

EXPERIMENTAL CONSEQUENCES

It will be very difficult to observe a sharp phase transition in thin films at T_M due largely to the existence of solid-like order of the vortices on scales smaller than a rapidly diverging correlation length, ξ_V, above the melting temperature:

$$\xi_v(T) \propto e^{\dfrac{b}{(T-T_M)^{\overline{v}}}} \qquad (7)$$

where $\overline{v} \approx .43$ and b is a non-universal constant.[3] However several measurable quantities will show interesting changes in behavior as the system is cooled from the vortex fluid phase to the flux-lattice phase. We consider here only two: flux flow resistance and the flux-lattice shear modulus.

1. Flux-Flow Resistance

In a magnetic field and at temperatures below T_c, the resistive properties of films are determined by the motion of the vortices present due to the field. This motion is impeded by pinning due to small scale inhomogeneities in the film. At temperatures well below T_M, effects of thermal fluctuations can be ignored and the flux lattice will be pinned completely below some critical value of the current. The resistance will thus vanish for small applied currents. At any nonzero temperature, however, there will be thermally activated defects (e.g., interstitials) in the vortex lattice which can move even for low currents. The resistance resulting from this flow of vortices will be continuous through the melting temperature, and above T_M will include flow of parts of the highly correlated flux system due to motion of free dislocations which will be present in concentrations proportional to $\xi_v^{-2}(T)$ for $T \gtrsim T_M$.

At temperatures well above $T_M (T \lesssim T_c)$ in the vortex-fluid phase, on the other hand, the vortex motion will be relatively uncorrelated and can be considered in terms of random thermal motion of individual vortices drifting in the presence of an applied current. The resistance in this region will be determined by the ratio of a typical pinning energy $\tilde{U}_p$ to the temperature. For strong pinning, $\tilde{U}_p(T_c) \sim T_c$, there will be a range of temperatures with thermally activated flow of individual vortices and

$$R \approx R_f \, e^{-\tilde{U}_p(T)/T} \qquad (8)$$

where R_f is the flux flow resistance in the absence of pinning.

For materials with only weak inhomogeneity which is on scales small compared to the Ginzburg-Landau coherence length $\xi(T)$ (e.g., granular aluminum films) $U_p(T)/T$ will be small at temperatures above melting and the pinning will not significantly alter the flux flow resistance until the vortex fluid becomes strongly correlated. In this limit there should be a relatively sharp cross-over from unpinned, individual vortex behavior to pinned, lattice-like behavior at a temperature, T, above T_M where

$$n\xi_v^2(T)\ \frac{U_p(T)}{T}\sim 1 \tag{9}$$

Thus the weaker the pinning, the sharper will be the cross-over from fluid-like to lattice-like behavior. For this reason, it may be desirable experimentally to use (relatively) thick, high resistivity films (where the relative pinning energy may be smaller) rather than extremely thin films of lower resistivity material.

2. Measurement of the Shear Modulus

If a flux lattice is driven through a random pinning potential by a transport current greater than the critical current, dissipative fluctuations of the vortex lattice will be excited.[8,9] In an ingenious experiment, Fiory[8] was able to couple to these fluctuations with an rf current and extract the shear modulus from the width of steps observed in the I-V characteristics.

The Kosterlitz-Thouless melting theory[3] predicts that the infinite wavelength shear modulus will jump to zero at the melting temperature, with a discontinuity given approximately by Eq. (1). Ideally, it should be possible to measure this jump, however there are difficulties. At any finite wavelength, L (or finite frequency), the vortex system above T_M will support shear as long as $L < \xi_v(T)$ and the measured shear modulus will be continuous through the melting temperature and drop gradually when $\xi_v(T)\sim L$.

In Fiory's experiment at low temperatures,[9] the results are sensitive to very long wavelength lattice distortions and hence to the long wavelength shear modulus.[8,9] However, for $T \lesssim T_M$, a detailed analysis following Schmid and Hauger[9] shows that the experiment is sensitive to rather short wavelengths ($L \sim 10$ vortex-lattice spacings) and hence the extracted shear modulus should only show a continuous decrease to zero at temperatures somewhat above T_M.

While Fiory's method will thus not be useful for measuring the desired long wavelength shear modulus near T_M, other more direct measurements may be possible. In particular, as suggested by Kramers, if the flux-lattice in one part of a film is strongly pinned and a shear (via a transport current) is applied to the lattice in another part of the film, it may be possible to extract the shear modulus from the resulting response of the system. This and other possible experiments will be investigated in the future.

CONCLUSIONS AND ACKNOWLEDGMENTS

While it may be difficult to verify experimentally some of the quantitative predictions of the Kosterlitz-Thouless melting theory for the vortex system (e.g., the detailed form of $\xi_v(T)$, many of the general features should be observable. In particular, by studying systems with a variety of R_n and pinning strengths, it should be possible to observe the high temperature vortex fluid-like behavior and the strong cross-over to lattice-like behavior.

Some quantitative measurements of the shear modulus should also be possible. In addition, other experimental probes may be sensitive to the different regimes of vortex behavior; these will be left for future consideration.

The author wishes to thank P. C. Hohenberg and W. F. Brinkman for stimulating theoretical discussions and A. F. Hebard and A. T. Fiory for many fruitful interactions concerning experiments and experimental possibilities.

REFERENCES

1. This paper is a brief summary of some of the results contained in a longer preprint by this author to be submitted to Phys. Rev. B.

2. B. A. Huberman and S. Doniach, Phys. Rev. Lett. $\underline{43}$, 950 (1979), have recently discussed the phase diagram of a thin super-conducting film in a magnetic field. Discussion of the discrepancies between their results and those of this author is contained in Ref. 1.

3. J. M. Kosterlitz and D. J. Thouless, J. Phys. $\underline{C6}$, 1181 (1973); B. I. Halperin and D. R. Nelson, Phys. Rev. Lett. $\underline{41}$, 121 (1978), $\underline{E41}$, 519 (1978) and Phys. Rev. $\underline{B19}$, 2457 (1979); A. P. Young, Phys. Rev. $\underline{B19}$, 1855 (1979).

4. E. Conen and A. Schmid, J. Low-Temp Phys. $\underline{17}$, 331 (1974).

5. D. S. Fisher, unpublished.

6. M. R. Beasley, J. E. Mooij, T. P. Orlando, Phys. Rev. Lett. $\underline{42}$, 1165 (1979).

7. B. I. Halperin and D. R. Nelson, J. Low-Temp. Phys. $\underline{36}$, 599 (1979); S. Doniach and B. A. Huberman, Phys. Rev. Lett. $\underline{42}$, 1169 (1979).

8. A. T. Fiory, Phys. Rev. $\underline{B8}$, 5039 (1973).

9. A. Schmid and W. Hauger, J. Low-Temp. Phys. $\underline{11}$, 667 (1973).

TWO-DIMENSIONAL SUPERCONDUCTING TRANSITION
IN FILMS WITH MINIMIZED INHOMOGENEITY,
THE KOSTERLITZ-THOULESS TRANSITION

R. E. Glover, III and Ming K. Chien*
Department of Physics and Astronomy,
University of Maryland, College Park, Maryland 20742

ABSTRACT

Measurements of the width of the resistive transition of 39 superconducting amorphous bismuth films with thicknesses between 150
and 2800 Å are compared with theoretical predictions based on the
existence of a Kosterlitz-Thouless vortex-antivortex dissociation
transition. The superconducting transition region is found to
broaden with increased residual resistance of the films as expected.
The observed width is less than predicted.

INTRODUCTION

Beasley, Mooij, and Orlando[1] have recently proposed that a Kosterlitz-Thouless type transition should occur in superconducting
thin films and that it should be observable in the resistive transition of these samples. The "unbinding" transition from a lower
temperature state in which current vortices of opposite circulation
are bound in pairs to a higher temperature one consisting of a free
vortex plasma is expected to occur at a temperature T_c^{KT} lying below the BCS transition temperature by an amount depending on the residual resistance per square, $R_{o\square}$, of the sample. The quantitative
prediction, assuming $(T_c^{BCS} - T_c^{KT})/T_c^{BCS} \ll 1$, is

$$\frac{T_c^{KT}}{T_c^{BCS}} = \frac{1}{1 + \dfrac{R_{o\square}}{23,800\Omega}} \tag{1}$$

The constant is given[2] by $[\pi^4/14\zeta(3)][\hbar/e^2] = 23,800\Omega$. Associated
problems are discussed in several recent publications.[3,4] How to
obtain precise values of critical temperatures involved from film
measurements is not clear. Beasley et al.[1] point out that the presence above T_c^{KT} of vortices free to move across the film in the
presence of a transport current would result in resistance and propose that the temperature at which easily measured resistance disappears is a reasonable approximation to T_c^{KT}. T_c^{BCS} is presumably
the temperature at which the film resistance would become zero if
the effect of the vortices could be removed. Unfortunately this

*Present address: Computer Science Corporation, Silver Spring,
                   Maryland 20910

would require theory which is not available. Experimentally measuring T_c^{BSC} is complicated by the fact that the initial reduction of resistance with decreasing temperature is a fluctuation effect and does not directly signal the phase transition. Beasley et al. propose that T_c^{BCS} corresponds approximately to the point of maximum slope in the R vs T transition curves. The spirit of the approach is to take the width of the region where resistance is dropping rapidly as a measure of the separation between T_c^{KT} and T_c^{BCS}

In testing Eq. 1 it would seem attractive to have large values of the residual sheet resistance, $R_{0\square}$, since they correspond to large predicted ratios of T_c^{KT} to T_c^{BCS}. Transition width measurements are available[1] in the literature for films having residual resistances on the order of $10^4\Omega$ per square. It is clear however that these samples cannot in any reasonable approximation be viewed as homogeneous metallic films of uniform cross section.[5] This complicates interpretation and makes spurious distortions of the transition region difficult to rule out. Beasley et al.[1] have compared existing transition width data for high residual resistance films with Eq. 1. A general increase in transition width with $R_{0\square}$ is found as suggested by the formula. Quantitative agreement is lacking.

We have taken an oppositely directed approach. Sample inhomogeneity, as far as possible, is reduced even though this leads to reduced sheet resistance, $R_{0\square}$. Fortunately the good temperature resolution available in the liquid helium range makes possible a detailed study of the resulting narrow superconducting transition region. As reported previously[6] a measure of the transition region width for superconducting amorphous bismuth films has the form given by Eq. 1. The purpose of this paper is to present a quantitative comparison of the experimental results with the predictions based on the assumed presence of a Kosterlitz-Thouless transition.

EXPERIMENT

We have measured the dc electrical resistance in the superconducting transition region of 39 amorphous, metallic bismuth films formed by vacuum evaporation onto substrates held at liquid helium temperatures.[7] Three atomic % Tl was added to the Bi to help stabilize the amorphous structure. Film thicknesses ranged from 150 to 2800 Å corresponding to residual resistance per square values between 5 and 100 ohms. Measurements of resistance vs temperature for a 500 Å film are indicated by the dots in Figure 1.

Factors that have been shown to distort or shift the resistive transition of thin films are strain, thickness, contamination by impurities from the vacuum, presence of magnetic fields, and surface roughness of the substrate. Amorphous bismuth is an intrinsically favorable material with respect to some of these factors. Considerable experimental work was required to reduce the effects of others. A favorable property of amorphous Bi films is that experiments have shown that the level of strains present is much lower than for polycrystalline films deposited at low temperature.[8] A feature that has both favorable and unfavorable consequences is the strong dependence

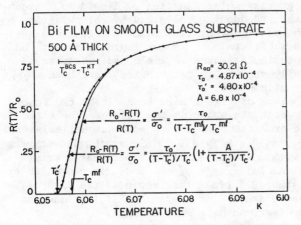

Fig. 1. Normalized resistance of an amorphous bismuth film. Points indicate measured values. R_o, $R_{o\square}$ and σ_o are respectively the residual normal-state resistance, the residual resistance per square, and the residual conductivity of the film. σ' is the superconductivity related fluctuation conductivity $\sigma' \equiv \sigma(T) - \sigma_o$. Values of the parameters T_c^{mf}, T_c', τ_o, τ_o', and A are obtained from curve fitting. The indicated $T_c^{BCS} - T_c^{KT}$ interval is that predicted for the film by Eq. (1) of the text.

of the superconducting transition temperature on residual resistance per square or alternately on thickness.[9] For the range of residual sheet resistance, $R_{o\square}$, covered by the present work,[7] this dependence has been shown to be well represented by

$$\frac{T_c'}{T_c'^{\infty}} = \frac{1}{1 + \frac{R_{o\square}}{1700\Omega}} \quad . \tag{2}$$

T_c' is the transition temperature (see Fig. 1) for a film of residual sheet resistance $R_{o\square}$ and $T_c'^{\infty}$ is the corresponding transition temperature for a thick sample $[R_{o\square} \to 0]$. Decreasing film thickness (increasing $R_{o\square}$) results in a lowering of the transition temperature. Because of this the thin regions along the film edges are not expected to contribute appreciably to the resistance measured in the transition region, very different from the situation that would pertain if the transition temperature increased with decreasing thickness as is found for Al. Evaporation geometry was chosen to hold thickness variation along the length of the films below the level at which the shape of the transition curve would be appreciably affected. With a 30 cm vapor source to substrate distance tests showed that macroscopic thickness variations were less than 0.5%. The vacuum at the film location was good enough to prevent contamination which could appreciably alter the transition region as shown by the constancy of the measurements with time. Perpendicular magnetic fields seen by the films were on the order of 10^{-2} gauss. Remaining magnetic field related resistance was smaller than can be resolved on the scale of Fig. 1. Finally, substrate roughness was shown[6] to be a main contributor to the "resistance tail" at temperatures just below T_c' (see Fig. 1). This tail was more pronounced for films made on optically polished single crystal quartz substrates than on specially smooth glass made by a process in which

104

the glass is leveled by gravity while floating on liquid Sn. A confirming observation is that roughening the glass by polishing increases resistance in the tail region. The film of Fig. 1 was deposited on a float glass substrate. It is our impression that the combined effects of perpendicular magnetic field and substrate roughness which principally show up in tail region, have been largely but not entirely eliminated.

The measured data points of Fig. 1 have been fit by two functions, the formulas for which are shown in the figure. The solid line to the right is the prediction of the two-dimensional Aslamazov-Larkin mean-field theory,[10] For $R(T) \geq 0.75 R_0$ agreement with the experimental points is within the 0.15% of R_0 experimental error, This agrement holds for the full range of the measurements which extends to the right a distance 25 times that shown in the figure. The mean-field transition temperature T_c^{mf} where the fitting function crosses the abscissa is experimentally well defined.

The solid curve to the left in Fig. 1 is seen to fit the data to very much lower $R(T)/R_0$ values. The expanded view in Fig. 2

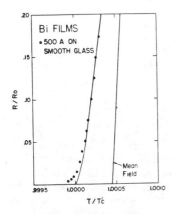

Fig. 2. Expanded view of the lower left-hand region of Fig. 1.

shows reasonable agreement for $R(T)/R_0 > 0.05$. T_c', defined by the interception of the curve with the abscissa is seen to lie a little above the temperature at which the measured resistance tends toward zero. The formula for the imperical fitting function used is shown in the figure. The important point for the present consideration is that fitting the experimental data to the indicated functions results in the determination of two experimentally well defined temperatures T_c^{mf} and T_c' whose difference gives a measure of the width of the transition. The points in Fig. 3 show this transition region width in units of T_c' plotted against residual resistance for the 39 films. The line is a least-squares fit and can be represented by $(T_c^{mf} - T_c')/T_c' = R_{0\square}/73,000\Omega$

or equivalently

$$\frac{T_c'}{T_c^{mf}} = \frac{1}{1 + \dfrac{R_{o\square}}{73,000\Omega}} . \tag{3}$$

DISCUSSION

A reasonable assumption on the basis of the vortex picture discussed in the introduction is that T_c' which is close to the temperature at which the film resistance tends toward zero can be identified with the Korterlitz-Thouless transition temperature T_c^{KT} below which vortices are supposedly bound. As a first guess T_c^{BCS} might be associated with the mean-field transition temperature T_c^{mf} which is experimentally determined at temperatures above those at which the vortex plasma would be expected to be important in determining the observed resistance. It is interesting that the experimentally found dependence of T_c'/T_c^{mf} on $R_{0\square}$ given in Eq. (3) is of the same form as that proposed by Beasley et al. for T_c^{KT}/T_c^{BCS} in Eq. (1). However the constants are rather different, the width of the transition region suggested by Eq. 1 being about three times that actually found. The situation is shown in Fig. 1 for a 500 Å film where the appropriate value of $T_c^{BCS} - T_c^{KT}$ has been inserted for comparison

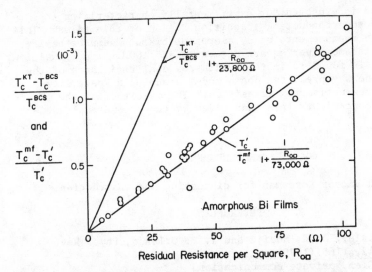

Fig. 3. Dependence of the width of the superconducting transition region on residual resistance of amorphous bismuth films. Circles are experimental values. The lines through them is a least-squares fit. T_c' and T_c^{mf} are shown for a 500 Å thick film in Fig. 1. T_c^{KT} and T_c^{BCS} are described in the text. The upper line is the theoretically proposed dependence of $(T_c^{KT} - T_c^{BCS})/T_c^{BCS}$ on residual resistance per square $R_{0\square}$.

with the $T_c^{mf} - T_c'$ measure of the transition width. The dependence on $R_{0\square}$ of T_c^{KT}/T_c^{BCS} predicted by Eq. (1) has been included in Fig. 3 for comparison with the measured T_c'/T_c^{mf} ratios.

The identification of T_c' and T_c^{mf} with T_c^{KT} and T_c^{BCS} respectively is of course crude. As seen in Fig. 2 the film resistance remains finite at temperatures slightly below T_c' so presumably this somewhat over-estimates T_c^{KT}. Probably an appreciably larger error is intorduced by identifying T_c^{mf} with the thermodynamic phase transition temperature T_c^{BCS}. While T_c^{mf} does include the effect of independent fluctuation it ignores interactions which become important where the resistance approaches zero. Including effects of the

106

$|\psi|^4$ term in the Ginzburg-Landau free energy expression, Korenman[11] and Van Vechten[12] have been able to fit the R vs T measurements for the Bi films to considerably lower $R(T)/R_0$ values than is possible when only mean-field effects are considered. Their conclusion is that at least half the $T_c' - T_c^{mf}$ transition width, seen for example in Fig. 1, is explainable in terms of the $|\psi|^4$ term contributions. This in turn reduces by half the width which can be interpreted in terms of the vortex plasma picture.

CONCLUSIONS

A method is proposed for experimentally characterizing the width of the superconducting transition region of thin films. This is applied to measurements on 39 amorphous bismuth samples having residual resistances per square between 5 and 100Ω. The transition region width is found to increase with residual resistance of the samples in the way predicted[1] on a model assuming a Kosterlitz-Thouless vortex-antivortex transition. The magnitude of the observed width is appreciably less than given by the theoretical estimate.

ACKNOWLEDGMENT

We thank Victor Korenman for discussion and instruction.

REFERENCES

1. M. R. Beasley, J. E. Mooij, and T. P. Orlando, Phys. Rev. Letters 42, 1165 (1979).
2. John R. Clem, private communication.
3. S. Doniach and B. A. Huberman, Phys. Rev. Letters 42, 1169 (1979) and preprint.
4. B. I. Halperin and D. R. Nelson, J. Low Temp. Phys. 36, 599 (1979).
5. Assuming (unfairly) that $D = \rho/R_{0\square}$ for a film having a residual resistance of $R_{0\square} = 10^4\Omega$, leads for amorphous Bi to a thickness of 1.6 Å, about half an atomic layer. The appropriate value of the resistivity ρ (which corresponds to an electron mean-free path on the order of the atomic separation) is $1.6\times10^{-4}\Omega$cm.
6. M. K. Chien and R. E. Glover, III, in Low Temp. Physics LT-13, K. D. Timmerhaus, W. J. O'Sullivan, and E. F. Hammel editors, Plenum Press, New York, 1974, Vol. 3, p. 649.
7. Ming K. Chien, Thesis, University of Maryland, College Park, Md., 1972.
8. W. Buckel, J. Vacuum Sci. Tech. 6, 606 (1969).
9. D. G. Naugle, W. Moorman, and R. E. Glover, III, published Proc. Int. Conf. on Science of Superconductivity, Stanford, 1969, North Holland, Amsterdam, 1971, p. 250.

10. L. G. Aslamazov and A. I. Larkin, Fiz. Tverd. Tela <u>10</u>, 1104 (1968); English translation, Soviet Phys.-Solid State <u>10</u>, 875 (1968).
11. Victor Korenman, private communication.
12. Deborah Van Vechten, Thesis, Univ. of Maryland, College Park, Md. 1979.

EXPERIMENTAL INVESTIGATION OF THE RESISTANCE IN THIN

SUPERCONDUCTING FILMS OF NIOBIUM-GERMANIUM[*]

N.A.H.K. Rao[**], E.D. Dahlberg, and A.M. Goldman
School of Physics and Astronomy
University of Minnesota

and

L.E. Toth and C. Umbach
School of Chemical Engineering and Materials Science
University of Minnesota
Minneapolis, MN   55455

ABSTRACT

We discuss the resistance of thin superconducting films of amorphous niobium-germanium below the BCS thermodynamic transition temperature as determined by measurements of the heat capacity. This resistance is shown to be consistent with a model in which the dissociation of thermally excited vortex pairs gives rise to a flux flow resistivity. The magnetic field dependence of the resistance has been investigated though only qualitatively.

I.   INTRODUCTION

In 1935 Peierls[1] argued one should not observe long range order in two dimensional (2-D) solids. Mermin and Wagner[2] showed the same to be true in 2-D magnets and Hohenberg[3] in 2-D superfluids. It is generally believed that long range order as customarily defined by the properties of the two-point correlation functions of an order parameter does not occur in 2-D systems at a finite temperature. Recently, however, the necessity of long range order for the production of the characteristic singular behavior of response functions that distinguish between the ordered and disordered phases has been questioned in the work of Kosterlitz and Thouless[4] (K-T) and independently in the work of Berezinskii.[5] The K-T theory defines a 2-D phase transition not in terms of long range order of a correlation function but in terms of the response of the system to applied stimuli. The transition from the liquid to the solid state in 2-D is not determined by changes in the correlation function or the structure factor but by the change from a viscous to an elastic response to shearing stress.

---

* Supported in part by NSF Grant DMR-78-08513
**Present address: Dept. of Physics, Ohio State University.

Since its inception, the K-T transition is believed to be relevant to an increasing number of problems both inside and outside the realm of condensed matter physics.[6] Because of the fundamental nature of this theory, model systems which might exhibit this type of 2-D phase transition are of great importance. Helium films have thus far been the main source of experimental information on the K-T transition.[7,8] In this example there is believed to be a Bose condensation which leads to a local order parameter. For $T > T_{KT}$, the Kosterlitz-Thouless transition temperature, isolated single vortex excitations lead to dissipative flow. At T_{KT} the system undergoes a change from viscous to nondissipative response since the singly excited vortices become bound in vortex-antivortex pairs. This transition has been modeled in terms of a discontinuity in the superfluid density at T_{KT}. This interpretation has not gone uncontested, however, because of the question of the influence of the substrate on which the films are collected.[9] In their original work K-T stated this type of toplogical phase transition would not occur in charged superfluids or superconductors. As in superfluid helium, this order-disorder transition would involve vortex-antivortex pairs dissociating at some temperature (T_{KT}) but whereas in superfluid helium the energy to create a single vortex is very large, in a superconductor this energy is much smaller and thus there would always be a background of free vortices and at large separations the vortex-antivortex interaction energy was not logarithmic in separation. These arguments would seem to preclude a topological phase transition in superconductors.

Recently several authors[10,11,12,13] have suggested that these arguments are not sufficiently compelling as to negate the possibility of this type of phase transition in superconductors. This opens up the possibility of studying 2-D phase transitions in a different system, in particular one which may not leave an open question as to the role of the substrate. The theories of a Kosterlitz-Thouless transition in superconductors are based on the premise that the 2-D melting of vortex-antivortex pairs would be manifested in the resistance of thin superconducting films. Below T_{K-T} the vortex-antivortex pairs would be bound and thus not contribute to the measured resistivity. Above T_{K-T} the pairs are dissociated and therefore swept across the film and generate a voltage in the manner of flux flow resistance but in this case without an externally applied magnetic field. In all of the theories, four material and sample dependent parameters are necessary to describe the temperature dependent voltage. These are the normal state resistivity (ρ_N), the film thickness (d), the bulk magnetic field penetration depth (λ) and the bulk superconducting transition temperature (T_{BCS}). In two of the theories[11,12] λ is related to ρ_N and d in a fashion which reduces the number of parameters to three.

We have measured the relative specific heat and the resistance of amorphous niobium-germanium (a-Nb$_3$Ge) as a function of temperature for films of different thicknesses. In previous measurements[14] on granular aluminum films the resistance was always found to fall to zero prior to any thermodynamic signature in the heat capacity. Our films, however, exhibit the opposite behavior in that the thermodynamic transition temperature (T_{BCS}) occurs when the sample is still resistive. A possible resolution of this discrepancy is that in amorphous films of high sheet resistance the resistance below T_{BCS} is due to thermally excited vortex pairs which yield a flux flow resistance as one would imagine in the K-T model of vortex-antivortex unbinding. The work on granular aluminum was carried out on low sheet resistance films of very high resistivity in which this phenomenon might not take place.

In Section II we describe the sample preparation along with the specific heat apparatus and data. In this section we also include the resistive transition data in relation to T_{BCS}. Section III contains the relevant equations for the temperature dependent resistance and a comparison of the data and with a theory of Turkevich[10] which has been modified in a manner which takes into account the temperature dependence of the penetration depth. The theory with this modification describes the data over five decades in resistance below T_{BCS}. Data obtained in a magnetic field applied perpendicular to the films in qualitative agreement with the theory of Doniach and Huberman[12] will also be shown. Our conclusion will be detailed in Section IV.

II. EXPERIMENTAL DETAILS AND RESULTS

The films are cryogetter d.c. sputtered from a target of $Nb_{2.75}Ge$. The substrates are nominally 0.0025 cm thick aligned single crystal sapphire. Prior to sputtering, the base pressure for the system was 10^{-9} to 10^{-10} Torr. It was then backfilled with 0.25 Torr of research grade argon. The thicknesses of the films were determined by sputtering time and checked by optical interferometry. Electron diffraction pictures of the films show three diffuse rings (see Fig. 1), while a typical brightfield transmission electron microscope picture from a cracked film is shown in Fig. 2. Both the electron diffraction and electron microscopy results are reasonably consistent with what would be expected of a binary amorphous material.[15] The structure which is observed in Fig. 2 is typical of that observed in amorphous materials.[15] The darkfield transmission electron microscopy and scanning electron microscopy were carried out and the results assured us that the films were homogeneous.

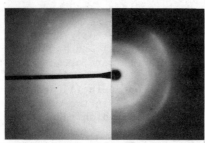

Fig. 1. Electron diffraction photographs of two of the films investigated here. One photograph is overexposed to enhance the outer ring.

The heat capacity measurements were performed in a manner similar to those of Sullivan and Seidel[16] using technology developed by Viswanathan and Varmazis.[17] Even though the heat capacity of the films comprised only a few percent of the total heat capacity of the calorimeter, high resolution measurements (one part in 10^4) gave enough accuracy to fit the heat capacity of the film to the BCS theory. An example of the raw data is exhibited in Fig. 3a. An important point in this

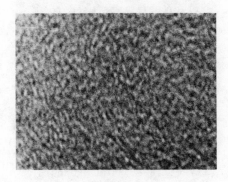

H—H
100 Å

Fig. 2. Brightfield transmission electron micrograph of an edge cracked from one of the films.

figure is that above T_{BCS}, the total heat capacity (sample and calorimeter) can be completely fitted with only linear and cubic temperature terms of the form $C_V = \gamma_T T + \beta_T T^3$ where γ_T is the total (film + calorimeter) electronic contribution to the heat capacity and β_T is the total phonon contribution. For temperatures less than T_{BCS} ($T < .8\ T_{BCS}$) the data were fitted to a form $C_V = (\gamma_T - \gamma_F)T + \beta_T T^3 + C_{BCS}(\gamma_F)$ where γ_F is the electronic contribution to the heat capacity of the film and C_{BCS} is the weak coupled BCS superconducting heat capacity.[18] The applicability of weak coupled theory to a-Nb_3Ge was demonstrated in an analysis of specific heat measurements on thick a-Nb_3Ge films by Tsuei and co-workers.[19] The fitting procedure we have used allows us to uniquely determine the BCS transition temperature of the films investigated. The BCS transition temperature of the films are given in Table I. The measured resistivities of the films are also given in Table I and although at first they might appear large, it should be noted that the films are disordered and that the measured resistivities are not greater than the maximum metallic resistivity.[20]

In cooling the films from liquid nitrogen temperature to 4.2 K, the resistivity increases slightly ($\approx 2.5\%$). The specific heat measurements and the temperature dependent resistance measurements were acquired in a background magnetic field less than 1 mOe unless otherwise noted. Fig. 4 shows an expanded plot of the excess heat capacity for two of the films over a range of temperatures starting at a temperature slightly greater than T_{BCS} and extending down to 1.1 K. We should point out that the low temperature fitting procedure is extremely sensitive to the value of T_{BCS}. If T_{BCS} is shifted to a lower temperature by only 0.03 K for the film shown in Fig. 2a, then the heat capacity calculated using this value gives a resultant square error between the measured and calculated heat capacities increased by nearly 20% over the same quantity computed using the fitted value of T_{BCS}. In this figure the resistive transition for these films is also plotted. In both Figs. 4a and 4b there is measurable resistance in the films for temperatures less than T_{BCS}. It is the nature of this resistance in the superconducting state which we wish to discuss. Four terminal resistance measurements were taken after the specific heat data were accumulated. The measurements were carried out in the calorimeter using the same thermometry as was used in the specific heat work.

112

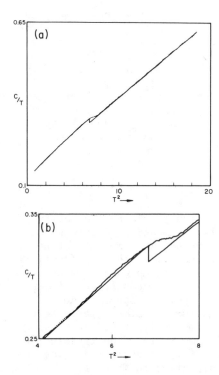

Silver paint was used to form leads on the sample. The current density in the films was maintained at 1 A/cm^2 for all the temperature dependent measurements. The region between the voltage leads was a rectangle of dimensions roughly 1.0 cm x 0.8 cm. Figure 5 shows data from the film Nb$_3$-Ge-6 in the vicinity of T_{BCS}. The expanded Y-axis scale (.7 Ω) shows that resistance is still present in the film for temperatures more than 0.1 K below T_{BCS}. This is well outside the error in the estimate of the T_{BCS} as determined by the fitting procedure. The resistance of the films was also measured in the presence of magnetic fields applied perpendicular to the plane of the films in fields up to 20 Oe.

Fig. 3. Raw data of the specific heat/temperature vs. (temperature)^2 for the film labeled Nb$_3$Ge-6. Note that the measured specific heat is explained by terms linear and cubic in temperature only.

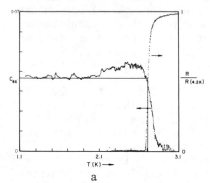
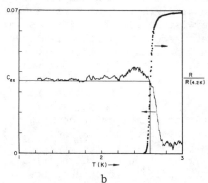

Fig. 4. Expanded plot of the excess heat where capacity vs. temperature, the solid line is the fitted BCS result. In this figure is also the resistive transition as a function of temperature.
a) Nb$_3$Ge-4, b) Nb$_3$Ge-6.

III. THEORY AND COMPARISON WITH EXPERIMENTAL RESULTS

At the present time there are three theoretical papers which indicate one should anticipate resistance in thin superconducting films at temperatures less than T_{BCS}. The explanation for this phenomena is based on the K-T theory which has been expanded to include charged superfluids (superconductors). The film characteristic which is most important for this effect is that the temperature dependent penetration depth, $\lambda(T)$, be much greater than the film thickness. Thus in our case although the films are thicker than the temperature-dependent coherence length ($\xi(T) = 50 \, \overset{o}{A} \left[\frac{T_c - T}{T_c} \right]^{-1/2}$ for all temperatures except in a region of 5 mK around T_{BCS}, they are 2-D at all temperatures in a magnetic sense since the zero temperature penetration depth, $\lambda(0)$, is much larger than the thickness of the films ($\lambda(0) \approx 30,000 \, \overset{o}{A}$). One would therefore expect 2-D behavior in terms of the magnetic properties of the system. All three of the above mentioned papers consider films which are 2-D in terms of $\lambda(T)$ and predict a flux flow resistance due to thermal unbinding of vortex-antivortex pairs at temperatures $T < T_{BCS}$. Following the original K-T line of thought, it was felt that the vortex pair excitations would be bound at low temperatures and then dissociate at T_{K-T}. In all three papers T_{KT} is less than T_{BCS} and is defined as follows:

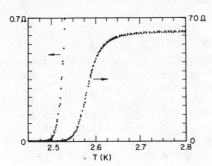

Fig. 5. Expanded view of the resistance vs. temperature in the vicinity of T_{BCS} (= 2.6) for Nb$_3$Ge-6. Note that even at temperatures well below T_{BCS} there is still resistance present.

$$ k_B T_{KT} = \frac{\phi_o^2}{32\pi^2} \frac{d}{2\lambda^2} . \tag{1} $$

Here ϕ_o is the flux quantum, d is the film thickness and λ is again the penetration depth of the film. Since λ is a temperature dependent quantity, T_{KT} must be determined self-consistently from Eq. 1. as outlined in Ref. 11. Based on the K-T theory of vortex-antivortex unbinding, the equations relevant to the resistivity in zero field presented in the three theoretical papers are

$$ R = 4\pi R_N \exp[-2(T_{KT}/T)^2] \tag{2} $$

$$R = 4 R_N \exp\left\{ \left(-\frac{1}{k_B} \frac{\phi_o}{32\pi^2} \frac{d}{2\lambda^2} \right) \frac{T_{KT}}{T(T-T_{KT})} \right\} \qquad (3)$$

$$R = 2.7b\, R_N \sinh^{-2} \left[b\left(\frac{T_{BCS}-T_{KT}}{T-T_{KT}} \right) \right]^{1/2} \qquad (4)$$

where Eqs. 2, 3, and 4 are given in Refs. 10, 12 and 13 respectively. In these equations R_N is the normal state resistance and d, λ, and T_{KT} and T_{BCS} are as defined previously. For our films, R_N, d and T_{BCS} are measured quantities and from Ref. 11, T_{KT} and λ are related to R_N. Thus <u>all</u> the variables in the theories are experimentally determined quantities and one (hopefully) could explain the measured resistivities for $T < T_{BCS}$. Unfortunately this was not the case. Because we have measured the resistance over range of 10^{-5} $R(T=T_{BCS})$ < R(T) < $R(T=T_{BCS})$, our data require a precise theory for fitting. Because of the possibility of a grain-grain coupling transition,[21] we also tried to fit the data to a power law of the form

$$R = R_o (T-T_T)^\mu \qquad (5)$$

where T_T would be the phase locking transition temperature. Equation 5 also could not fit our data. However, with a certain modification, L. Turkevich's theory (our Eq. 2) did in fact fit the data over the entire range of resistances investigated. In deriving his equation for the resistivity Turkevich implicitly assumes $T \ll T_{BCS}$ and thus the temperature depndence of λ is removed and $\frac{\phi_o}{32\pi^2} \frac{d}{2\lambda^2(T=0)} = T_{KT}$. In our case, however, such a condition is not

satisfied as $T \lesssim T_{BCS}$ and λ is a rapidly varying function of temperature. We therefore modified his equation by retaining the explicit temperature dependence of λ and obtained:

$$R = 4\pi R_N \exp\left[-2\left(\frac{\phi_o^2}{k_B 32\pi^2} \frac{d}{2\lambda^2(T=0)} \right) \left(\frac{T_{BCS}-T}{T\, T_{BCS}} \right)^2 \right] \qquad (6)$$

In fitting to this equation we fixed $4\pi R_N = R(T=T_{BCS})$, and allowed $\lambda(0)$ to be the only adjustable parameter. As shown in Fig. 6, the solid line is Eq. 6 with $\lambda(0) = 30,000$ Å. The open circles in this figure are the experimental data points. Since a-Nb_3Ge is a BCS superconductor, one can use the BCS value of $\lambda(0)$ to calculate the zero temperature coherence length $\xi(0)$ which gives $\xi(0) \approx 50$ Å, a reasonable value for an amorphous superconductor. The other curve in this figure is the resistance of the film measured with a 20 Oe field applied perpendicular to the plane. Other data were taken on the films in as many as seven different fields from less than

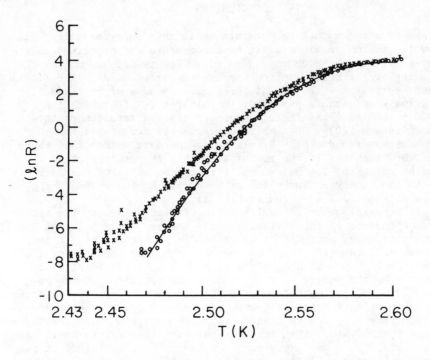

Fig. 6. ln R vs. T for Nb$_3$Ge-6. The (O)'s are zero magnetic field data with the solid line being a fit to Turkevich's modified theory (see text) with λ = 30,000 Å. The (X)'s are data accumulated in a 20 G magnetic field applied perpendicular to the plane of the film.

0.001 Oe to 20 Oe. Qualitatively the effect of an externally applied magnetic field agrees with that predicted in the inset of Fig. 1 of Ref. 12 even though the detailed theory of Ref. 12 for the applied field equal to zero did not fit the data. With the value of $\lambda(0)$ experimentally determined, one can calculate T_{KT} self-consistently from Eq. 1. For the data shown in Figs. 5 and 6, T_{KT} would be 2.54 K. Reference 11 calculates T_{KT} self-consistently by relating $\lambda(0)$ to the normal state sheet resistance ($R_\square$) of the films. Following this procedure we find T_{KT} = 2.59. The reason for the difference between the two estimates of T_{KT} might lie in the fact that the theory of Ref. 11 employs the nearly free electron model to calculate T_{KT} from R_N whereas the value determined from R(T) depends on a model of the vortex flux flow resistance. However, with either temperature, scrutiny of the data reveals no dramatic effect in the resistivity in this temperature range (2.54 → 2.59). Nevertheless, the temperature dependence of the resistivity can be explained by flux flow resistance due to vortex-antivortex pair dissociation.

IV. CONCLUSIONS

We have shown that the resistance in thin superconducting films below the thermodynamic transition temperature can be fitted to the model of Turkevich which considers flux flow resistance due to the unbinding of thermally excited vortex-antivortex pairs. The fit is in good agreement with the data over five decades of resistance. The primary adjustable parameter in this fit is $\lambda(0)$ which is 30,000 ± 1000 Å. This fitted parameter gives a zero temperature coherence length $\xi(0) \approx 50$ Å which is certainly reasonable for an amorphous superconductor. By examining the data we see that there is no abrupt change in the resistivity in a temperature range spanning values of T_{KT} determined either from a fit of the data for $R(T)$ to the theory of Turkevich or by a calculation based on the free electron model as given in Ref. 11.

In explaining these results one possibility is that the temperature dependence of the resistivity may not be a good probe of 2-D vortex-antivortex unbinding transitions in superconducting films. Alternatively the effect may be suppressed by the presence of the ambient field which although less than 10^{-3} G is not identically zero. Given the uncertainty as to both the magnitude of the ambient field and the magnitude of H_{c1}, this must be considered to be an open question insofar as these measurements are concerned.[22]

Nevertheless, the resistance vanishes at a temperature well below the thermodynamic transition temperature in a fairly small magnetic field. This may imply that further theoretical study of the vortex-antivortex unbinding transition, taking into account the possible renormalization of the transition temperature by the vortex-antivortex plasma, is required for an understanding of these results.

REFERENCES

1.   R. E. Peierls, Ann. Inst. Henri Poincaré 5, 177 (1935).
2.   N. D. Mermin and H. Wagner, Phys. Rev. Lett. 22, 1133 (1966).
3.   P. C. Hohenberg, Phys. Rev. 158, 383 (1967).
4.   J. M. Kosterlitz and D. J. Thouless, J. Phys. C: Solid State Phys. 5, L124 (1972) and J. Phys. C: Solid State Phys. 6, 1181 (1973).
5.   V. L. Berezinskii, Sov. Phys.-JETP 32, 493 (1970) and Zh. Eksp. Teor. Fiz. 61, 1144 (1971).
6.   Physics Today, 17 (August 1978).
7.   D. J. Bishop and J. D. Reppy, Phys. Rev. Lett. 40, 1727 (1978).
8.   E. Webster, G. Webster, and M. Chester, Phys. Rev. Lett. 42, 243 (1979).
9.   J. G. Dash, Phys. Rev. Lett. 41, 1178 (1978).
10. L. A. Turkevich, J. Phys. C: Solid State Phys. 12, L385 (1979).
11. M. R. Beasley, J. E. Mooij, and T. P. Orlando. Phys. Rev. Lett. 42, 1165 (1979).
12. S. Doniach and B. A. Huberman, Phys. Rev. Lett. 42, 1169 (1979).
13. B. I. Halperin and D. R. Nelson, Jour. Low Temp. Phys. 36, 316 (1978).

14. T. Worthington, P. Lindenfeld, and G. Deutscher, Phys. Rev. Lett. 41, 316 (1978).
15. T. M. Donovan and K. Heinemann, Phys. Rev. Lett. 27, 1794 (1971).
16. P. F. Sullivan and G. Seidel, Phys. Rev. 173, 679 (1968).
17. R. Viswanathan and C. Varmazis, private communication.
18. B. Mühlschlegel, Z. Physik 155, 313 (1959).
19. C. C. Tsuei, S. von Molnar, and J. M. Coey, Phys. Rev. Lett. 41, 664 (1978).
20. N. F. Mott and E. A. Davis, Electronic Processes in Non-Crystalline Materials, 2nd Ed., Clarendon Press, Oxford (1979) p. 28.
21. S. A. Wolf, D. U. Gubser, and Y. Imry, Phys. Rev. Lett. 42, 324 (1979).
22. B. A. Huberman and S. Doniach, Phys. Rev. Lett. 43, 950 (1979).

Table I

Thickness	T_{BCS}	R_q	ρ_{Normal}	T_{K-T} from Ref. 11	T_{K-T} with fitted λ
1000 Å	2.59	75±15	750±150 $\mu\Omega$-cm	2.58	2.54
1500 Å	2.71	65±10	950±150 $\mu\Omega$-cm	2.7	
1200 Å	2.6	63±10	800±150 $\mu\Omega$-cm	2.59	2.54

RECENT EXPERIMENTS ON ANDERSON LOCALIZATION
IN ONE AND TWO DIMENSIONAL DISORDERED ELECTRONIC SYSTEMS

G. J. Dolan
Bell Laboratories, Murray Hill, New Jersey 07974

There are several experiments indicating anomalous temperature dependent rises in low temperature resistance for systems of reduced dimensionality. Dolan and Osheroff[1] studied discontinuous thin films of various widths and lengths and interpreted the behaviors they observed as characteristic of one or two dimensional systems based on rather complicated reasoning which I will try to describe at length below. Giordano, Gilson, and Prober[2] studied the resistance of continuous but very narrow films which exhibited one dimensional behavior and Chaudhari and Habermeier[3] have observed similar effects on narrow amorphous films of a different material. Bishop, Tsui and Dynes[4] have conducted an extensive investigation of the resistive properties of the inversion layer of Si-MOSFETs and corroborate the Dolan and Osheroff results on the two dimensional phenomena. All of the experiments have been interpreted in terms of what I shall call the scaling theory of localization. All were stimulated by Thouless' paper[5] predicting that electronic states in a long wire would be localized and that any wire having resistance greater than $2\hbar/e^2 \sim 8000\Omega$ would be an insulator at $T = 0$. I will try to summarize the results of the scaling theory as represented in several recent papers[5,6,7] with emphasis on the interpretation of the experiments in terms of the theory. I will also emphasize the problems with this interpretation and point out that a recent result by Lee[13] apparently provides an alternative, equally satisfactory explanation for some of the experimental observations.

Various theoretical considerations suggest a minimum metallic conductivity for a homogeneous system for mean free paths $\ell \sim a$, the interatomic spacing.[8] Expressed in terms of a resistivity one expects insulating behavior for any system with microscopic resistivity in excess of $\rho_m \sim 10^2$ to 10^3 $\mu\Omega$-cm depending on the assumptions made. This would imply for a thin film a maximum metallic sheet resistance $R_c \sim 3$–30 kΩ assuming the minimum film thickness of $t \sim a$. Numerical studies of the variation of conductance with sample size or scale have suggested a maximum metallic resistance $R_c \tilde{\sim} 8\, \hbar/e^2 \sim 30$ kΩ for any two dimensional system including inhomogeneous systems and quasi-two dimensional systems with $t > a$.[9,10] The implication of these studies was that there was a mobility edge defined by R_c. For sufficiently high resistivities the electronic states should be localized to regions $\ell \sim a$ in size in either three or two dimensions for a continuous system. In an inhomogeneous system, e.g., a cermet with particle size s, the localization size is s; this is conceptually somewhat different, I think, but the limits should still apply according to some interpretations of the theory.

It is a new idea that there might still be a long localization length for the electrons even in a relatively low resistivity system for which the electronic states appear extended on microscopic scales, e.g., ℓ, a, s. This idea first appeared in an explicit calculation in Thouless' paper on "one dimensional" wires although the idea was foreshadowed elsewhere. Thouless' result[5,11] for the resistance of a wire at $T = 0$ may be expressed:

$$R(L) = r_0\{\exp (L/L_\ell) -1\}$$

$$\cong (R(L_0)L/L_0) \ (1 - \frac{1}{2} L/L_\ell), \ L \ll L_\ell \qquad (1)$$

where $r_0 = 2\hbar/e^2$ and $L_\ell = r_0 L_0/R(L_0)$.

I have defined here a scale L_0 which is so small that localization effects are negligible. For example, in a low resistivity homogeneous system choose $L_0 \backsim \ell$ and $R(L_0)/L_0 = \rho(\ell)/A$ where A is the wire cross-sectional area. In a cermet one can define an effective free path from the measured resistivity or choose $L_0 = s$ with $R(L_0)$ the coupling resistance between conducting particles separated by the distance s. According to Eq. (1) the electronic states are always localized to lengths of the wire having resistance $2\hbar/e^2 \backsim 8000 \ \Omega$. Eq. (1) may not be precisely right but contains the essential features of Thouless' prediction. Thouless also considered the effects of finite temperature on observability of the phenomenon. At finite temperatures, inelastic processes, characterized by a time $\tau_i = cT^{-p}$, will break the coherence of a diffusing wave packet every τ_i on average. In this time the packet will have diffused a distance $L_T \cong (v_F \ell \tau_i)^{1/2} \backsim T^{-p/2}$. One criterion for observation of the length dependence R(L) is then $L < L_T$. But even if this is not true, so long as $L > L_\ell$, one would expect to see "insulating" behavior, with a strong temperature dependent increase in resistivity at temperatures so low that $L_T > L_\ell$. Assuming the electric field used is small, conduction will be activated by phonon assisted mechanisms. If the electric field is so high that eEL_ℓ is comparable to the energy

spacing of the localized states $(\Delta E \backsim (\frac{dn}{dE} L_\ell A)^{-1})$ field induced

effects will be important so it is desirable to use small fields in an experiment. Since L_ℓ may be very large, this requirement may be quite severe. When $L < L_\ell$ the exponential nature of Eq. (1) will not be apparent but even in this 'metallic regime' Thouless predicts still a length dependence in R/L; at finite temperatures a temperature dependence reflecting the small scale version of Eq. (1) can be predicted by substituting L_T for L in Eq. (1).

$$R(T) = R(L_T) = \{R(L_0) \ L/L_0\} \ \{1 - \frac{1}{2} L_T/L_\ell\}, \ \ L_T < L_\ell$$

$$= \{R(L_0) \ L/L_0\} \ \{1 - \frac{1}{2} (v_F \ c\ell)^{1/2} \ T^{-p/2}/L_\ell\} \qquad (2)$$

The substitution is based on the idea that L_T is effectively the scale of the measurement and the scale on which the structure of the electronic states is sampled in a measurement. The envelope of the wave functions for the states has an exponential shape ($\sim\exp(-L/L_\ell)$). At small L the contribution to conduction by the states is still less than would be obtained for extended states (a flat envelope). A wave packet formed at $T = 0$ and $X = 0$ will be formed predominantly of states centered at $X = 0$. It will be reformed on the average at a position $X = L_T$ at finite temperatures with the new packet being composed primarily of states centered at $X = L_T$. The resistance measured will be approximately $R(L_T) \cdot \dfrac{L}{L_T}$ if $L \gg L_T$ and $L_\ell \gg L_T$.

Although Thouless considered only ordinary electron–phonon ($p = 1$, 2, 3 or 4 depending on the phonon dimensionality and disorder) and electron–electron ($p = 2$) scattering, any process which will break the coherence of a diffusing wave packet will define a length L_T and the dominant mechanism will be that providing the shortest length.

On a similar basis, Abrahams, Anderson, Licciardello, and Ramakrishnan (AALR)[6] have predicted a long localization length and the absence of metallic behavior even for low resistivities in the two dimensional case. Their result for a two dimensional system is based on an intuitively constructed perturbation theory applicable to the low resistivity regime and arguments of continuity and regularity. Expressed in terms of a resistance their result in the "metallic" ($L \ll L_\ell$) regime is:

$$R(L) = R(L_0) \ \{1 + (R(L_0)/R_c) \ \ell n \ (L/L_0)\}$$

$$\text{with } R_c = \frac{\pi^2 \hbar}{\alpha e^2} \cong \frac{\pi^2 \hbar}{e^2} \gg R(L_0) \tag{3}$$

Equation (3) predicts a monotonic increase in the sheet resistance of a thin film with L so that for large enough L one always has $R(L) \sim R_c$. One can estimate the implied localization length for the electronic state using Eq. (3) and $R(L_\ell) = R_c$:

$$L_\ell \stackrel{\sim}{=} L_0 \ \{\exp \frac{R_c}{R(L_0)} - 1\} \tag{4}$$

L_ℓ is astronomical for $R(L_0)$ less than a few thousand ohms, microscopic for $R(L_0) \sim R_c$ and sweeps through experimentally accessible scales for intermediate resistances. In response to the measurements by Dolan and Osheroff, Anderson, Abrahams, and Ramakrishnan (AAR)[7] have noted that Eq. (3) implies a logarithmic temperature dependence for resistance if one substitutes L_T for L:

$$R(T) = R(L_T) = R(L_0) \ \{1 - \frac{p}{2} \ (R(L_0)/R_c) \ \ell n \ T + \text{const}\}$$

$$= R(T_0) \ \{1 - \frac{p}{2} \ (R(T_0)/R_c) \ \ell n \ T/T_0\} \tag{5}$$

where $R(T_0)$ and T_0 are defined self-consistently.

Besides assuming that L_T defines the scale of a finite temperature measurement when $L_T < L$, AAR and Dolan and Osheroff assume that the effective dimensionality of a system may also depend on L_T. For definiteness consider a system of dimensions $L \gg W \gg t \gg a$. In different regimes a system's characteristics and behavior may be one, two, or three dimensional. If $\rho > \rho_m$, the electronic states are localized with a three dimensional envelope $\sim \exp(-L/L_\ell)$ and $L_\ell \sim a < t$. For $\rho < \rho_m$, the states envelopes are approximately flat in the direction parallel to t but according to the scaling theory will be localized at some scale $L_\ell > t$ in the film plane. If L_ℓ from Eq. (4) is less than W, the states envelopes fall off in a two dimensional way until scales $\sim W$ are considered. If $L_\ell > W$, the states will be relatively flat across the strip but their small scale ($\sim W$) structure will still be determined by the two dimensional considerations. Equation (1) for a one dimensional system will define the localization length and $R(L)$. However, to take into account (approximately) the two dimensional, small scale structure of the electronic states one might choose $L_0 \sim W$ in Eq. (1) and calculate $R(W)$ using Eq. (3). An appropriate L_0 to choose for the two dimensional construction would be $L_0 \sim t$. Although our system is one dimensional at $T = 0$ and will be an insulator if $R(L) > 2\hbar/e^2$, the idea that L_T is an effective scale for finite temperature measurements means that we will observe one dimensional behavior (e.g., Eq. (2)) only when $L_T > W$. At high enough temperatures that $L_T < W$, the electronic states structure is being sampled at a scale where the structure of the electronic states is two dimensional and Eq. (5) will describe the temperature dependence. A crossover from one to two dimensional behavior should occur if one covers a sufficiently wide temperature range.

A system like a thick ($> s$) granular aluminum film is a suitable experimental system in this kind of picture except that it makes no physical sense to talk of scales smaller than the granule size. A thin discontinuous film, a two dimensional array of metallic islands on a substrate, is also suitable except that again scales smaller than the island size should not be considered (there is a lower cutoff on the effect of L_T). The system is intrinsically two dimensional since the conductivity in the t direction is large and the sheet resistance arises primarily from the coupling resistance between the islands. The triangular cross-section wires of Giordano et al., could be one or three dimensional in the sense of this discussion but not two dimensional. The inversion layer of a Si-MOSFET is a genuinely two dimensional system in the sense that $t \sim \lambda_F$ usually.

Figure 1 shows the I-V curve of an Au-Pd film with $L = 2$mm, $W = 20\mu$m, $t \sim 3$nm and $R \sim 16$ kΩ so that the sheet resistance is $R_\square \stackrel{\sim}{\sim} 160 \ \Omega/\square$. A constant resistance has been subtracted from the actual I-V curve so that what is shown is the exaggerated departure from linearity. Figure 2 shows schematically the circuit and the subtraction. Figure 3 is from Ref. 1 and shows for various temperatures the quantity $\Delta R = (V/I - R_0)/R_0$ vs. log V for a similar film

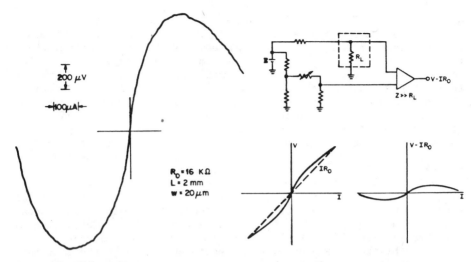

Fig. 1 "I-V curve" for an AuPd film with a sheet resistance $\sim160\Omega/\square$ after a constant resistance, R_O, is subtracted (see Fig. 2).

Fig. 2 Schematic of circuit used to exaggerate small non-linearity in I-V for low resistivity thin films.

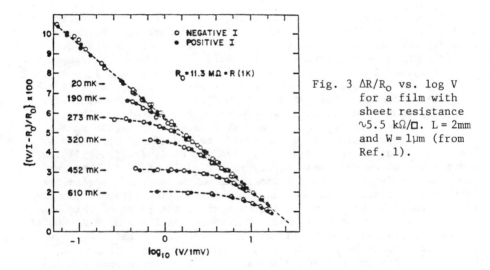

Fig. 3 $\Delta R/R_O$ vs. log V for a film with sheet resistance ~5.5 k$\Omega/\square$. L = 2mm and W = 1μm (from Ref. 1).

which is narrower (W $\sim$ 1 μm) and has $R_\square \sim 5$ k$\Omega/\square$. The data is taken from curves like that in Fig. 1. The curves are linear in log V at low T. At higher T plateau values, the "zero bias" values of $\Delta R(T)$

are approached at small V. R(T) was found to be logarithmic in T so
that the behavior of such films can be expressed

$$\lim_{E \to 0} R(T,E) = R(T_0,0) \{1 - S_T \ell n(T/T_0)\} \qquad (6a)$$

$$\lim_{T \to 0} R(T,E) = R(0,E_0) \{1 - S_V \ell n(E/E_0)\} \qquad (6b)$$

with T_0, E_0, $R(T_0,0)$ and $R(0,E_0)$ defined self-consistently and

$$S_T \sim \alpha_T R(T_0,0)/R_C$$

$$S_V \sim \alpha_V R(0,E_0)/R_C \qquad (7)$$

This behavior has subsequently been found to describe the
behavior of similar films of a Au-Cu alloy. In very beautiful
experiments of Bishop, Tsui, and Dynes on the inversion layer of
square Si-MOSFETs the same behavior is found. In these experiments
R can be varied continuously by varying the FET gate voltage. Figure 4 shows a plot of the quantities S_T and S_V from two devices and
includes thin film data for Au-Cu, and Au-Pd alloy films of various
widths (W = 1µm, 2µm, 20µm, 200µm, 1000µm in different cases).

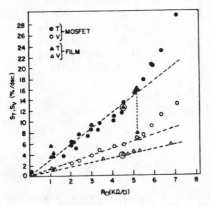

Fig. 4 Accumulated measurements of
logarithmic slopes S_T and S_V
(expressed as %/decade. Divide
by 2.3 for consistency with
Eq. (6)) defined by Eq. (6).
Data from two Si MOSFETs in
the experiments by Bishop,
Tsui, and Dynes (Ref. 4)
are included with thin film
data for Au-Cu and Au-Pd films
of various widths and thicknesses. Several of the thin
film points represent two
films with different widths.

The data supports the proportionality of the logarithmic slopes to
R and indicates that α_T/α_V is approximately constant. AAR have
pointed out that the electric field effect arises from joule heating
of the electrons and is simply another manifestation of the temperature effect. For low bath temperature the electron temperature is
related to the electric field by:

$$\pi k_B Te \stackrel{\sim}{=} 2e \, EL_{ep} \qquad (8)$$

where $L_{ep} = (\frac{1}{2} v_F \tau_{ep} \ell)^{1/2}$ and τ_{ep} is the usual electron-phonon scattering time. Equation (6b) is obtained from Eq. (6a) by replacing T by $T_e(E)$. If $\tau_{ep} \sim T^{-p\prime}$ then $\alpha_T/\alpha_v = \frac{2+p\prime}{2}$. For the MOSFET data $p\prime = 3$ which is appropriate for two dimensional phonons in a dirty system.[5,7] For the films both $p\prime = 3$ and more often $p\prime = 4$ have been observed. The latter power would require an interaction with the three dimensional phonons in the substrate. $R(T_e(E))$ can be obtained for any E from I-V and compared to the measured quantity $R(T,0)$; using Eq. (7) a direct measure of L_{ep} can be obtained. For example the plateau values in Fig. 2 give an equivalent temperature and electric field which gives $L_{ep} \alpha T^{-1.5}$ as shown in Fig. 5. It is apparent that $L_{ep} \gg W$ for the film over the entire temperature range. The equivalent electron-electron scattering length can be only estimated; it is smaller than L_{ep} but still $\gg W$ over the temperature range. The interpretation of the behavior Eq. (6) as a two dimensional effect is confirmed by the MOSFET experiments but is consistent with the scaling theory only if another mechanism, producing a shorter L_T, is responsible for the cutoff in the length dependence. AAR have suggested a shorter length determined by the collision broadening of the energy levels associated with the scattering. However, this

length is simply $\sqrt{R_\square/R_c} \, L_T$ and is not sufficiently small to remove the discrepancy.

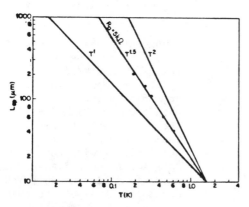

Fig. 5 The diffusion distance between electron-phonon collisions determined from Fig. 3 and Eq. (8).

It may be more sensible to look for an alternative explanation of the logarithmic effects. Lee[13] has recently shown that a detailed consideration of coulomb effects in the resistivity problem produces in two dimensions a correction to the resistivity of exactly the form Eq. (6a). The calculation is based on the earlier work by Altschuler and Aronov[14] on the effects of coulomb scattering for the three dimensional case. Lee's result agrees exactly with the AALR result for finite T if one sets $p = 1$ in Eq. (6a). Moreover, the characteristic length for the coulomb effect is $\sim(\hbar v_F \ell / k_B T)^{1/2}$. This length is in the range 10-100 nm for the various experiments. The Lee interpretation has apparently no relation to the localization problem and is at least as satisfactory in explaining the data on two dimensional systems of low resistivity. It may be considered by some to be more plausible than the localization theory result of AAR. However, it is clear, especially from the MOSFET experiments, that the "metal-insulator transition" at least appears to be a smooth crossover from an insulating regime characterized by exponential $R(T)$ to a pseudo-metallic, logarithmic regime. From the data in Fig. 4 one obtains $\alpha_T \sim .5$ which agrees with either explanation but requires $p = 1$ for the process which determines L_T in the AAR picture. Since p is not determined independently in the experiments the experiments cannot distinguish between the two phenomena.

Figure 6 shows the highly nonlinear I-V curves of an Au-Pd film with high temperature resistance $R_\square \sim 11$ kΩ/$\square$. The zero bias resistance was shown in Ref. 1 to be exponential in 1/T. Dolan and Osheroff interpreted this film as being localized as a two dimensional system although $W = 1$ μm $<< L$ because of the two dimensional behavior of the otherwise identical film with $R_\square$ only one-half as large.

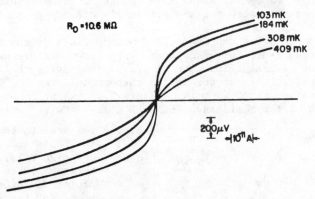

Fig. 6 I-V curves for an Au-Pd film with $W = 1$ μm but sheet resistance ~ 11 kΩ/$\square$ and total resistance ~ 11 MΩ at high temperatures. Curves for several temperatures are shown and R_O has been subtracted off (see Fig. 2).

Figure 7 shows data presented analogously to Fig. 3 for this high resistivity film and is shown to emphasize the importance of using sufficiently small electric fields in determining the "zero bias" resistance. This is relevant because some earlier experiments used fields so high (3-30 V/m) that the exponential character of this film would probably not have been recognized.[12] The earlier experiments apparently confirmed the existence of a mobility edge at $R_c \sim 30$ kΩ. However, in the thin film experiments and also the MOSFET experiments of Bishop et al., exponential behavior is observed for $R_\square$ in the range 10-15 kΩ. It is clear from the MOSFET experiments (see Fig. 4) that

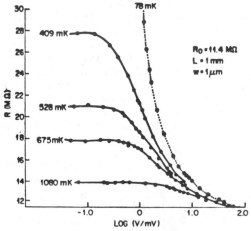

Fig. 7 R = V/I vs. log V for the film of Fig. 7.

the crossover is smooth although very rapid. The strict adherence to behavior Eq. (6) ceases above $R \sim 5$ kΩ and the temperature dependence becomes gradually stronger and eventually clearly exponential in the range 10-15 kΩ.

Although Dolan and Osheroff found no width dependence in their effect for $W \gtrsim 1$ μm, they did report larger temperature dependent effects for several films with $W \sim 0.1$ μm indicating that if L_T was really a relevant parameter in the phenomenon it was of this order in the temperature range $T > 0.1$K. Figure 8 shows the temperature dependence of the resistance for such a Au-Pd "wire" with $R_\square \sim 400\Omega$.

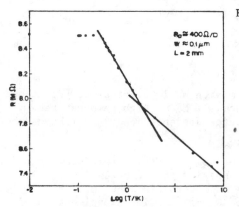

Fig. 8 Temperature dependence of the resistance of a narrower Au-Pd film. If the region between 0.3 to 2K is interpreted as logarithmic, the slope is approximately ten times too large to be included with the data for the wider films (Fig. 4).

The resistance increase (if interpreted as logarithmic) is small but too large by about 10 at low temperature to be consistent with the behavior of the wider wires. Also similar wires showed even bigger effects. A wire with $R_\square \sim 5$ kΩ and normal width 0.1 μm had a resistance exponential in $T^{-1/2}$ at low T. [1]

This is consistent with one dimensional variable range hopping; but the inconsistency of the results indicated long range variations in the wire widths. Giordano, Gilson, and Prober had much more precise control on their wire dimensions in their beautiful experiment on continuous Au-Pd films of triangular cross-section. They interpreted $R(T)$ to be logarithmic or possibly to vary as $T^{-1/2}$. Chaudhari and Habermeier[3] have observed similar but less well characterized phenomena in amorphous W - Re film strips with $W \sim 150 - 500$ nm. Most importantly, Giordano et al. determined that the resistance increment at constant temperatures was proportional to A^{-1} in agreement with the idea that the phenomenon was a one dimensional effect (Eqs. (1), (2)). The temperature range covered was inadequate to distinguish between $\Delta R \sim \log T$ or $\Delta R \sim T^{-1/2}$; if the latter behavior was observed the observations may represent the high temperature tail of an exponential in $T^{-1/2}$ implying a rather slowly varying L_T in the localization picture. Or it may be the one dimensional version of the coulomb effect interpretation. Although Lee does not discuss this it seems that his picture would yield $\Delta R \sim T^{-1/2}$ for a one dimensional system and the characteristic length for the coulomb effect seems to be of the right size approximately to be consistent with the data.

Summarizing the experimental picture, it seems that the cross-over from localized to metallic behavior in two dimensions at least appears to be a gradual one at finite temperature and that the "metallic" regime is characterized by logarithmically increasing resistance with decreasing temperature. The magnitude of the increase is within factors ~ 2 of that predicted by the AALR-AAR version of the scaling theory of localization but Lee has produced an alternative explanation at least as satisfactory in this regime. The larger effects seen for very narrow samples indicate that there is a one dimensional phonomenon which can be observed in experimental systems with dimensions in the range $W \sim 0.5$ μm and this may be Thouless' one dimensional localization. However, in this case as well further experimental information (unquestionably imminent) is needed and improved theoretical understanding of the resistivity problem at high resistivities is also required. The localization theory, if it is to hold up, must deal with the fact that the required length scale L_T is much smaller than originally believed. Theories such as Lee's which seem independent of localization must deal with the apparent continuous crossover to the localized regime.

The experiments so far are very limited - resistance measurements only - and further work on the effects of magnetic fields and finite frequencies as well as on dimensionality and on different systems should soon provide more information.

In our article (Ref. 1) we noted that the temperature dependent increases in the resistance of our samples always "saturated" i.e., ceased to increase with decreasing temperature for $T \sim 0.1K$. Such a saturation is clearly observed in Fig. 8. I have not mentioned this above because it is still not clear that the "saturation" is not an experimental problem. For example, one sees from Fig. 6 that

$L_{ep} \sim L$ at $T \sim 0.1K$ for that particular sample which means that the electrons are not in equilibrium with the lattice. It is not clear therefore that in our experiments the saturation effects observed were not simply a heating problem. However, we have not been able to consistently correlate the saturation temperature with $L_{ep} \sim L$ for example. Such saturations are also observed in the MOSFET experiments and are still being investigated.

I would like to acknowledge many conversations with my colleagues at Bell Laboratories and especially D. J. Bishop, D. C. Tsui and R. C. Dynes for access to their experimental results prior to publication.

REFERENCES

1. G. J. Dolan and D. D. Osheroff, Phys. Rev. Lett. <u>43</u>, 721 (1979).
2. N. Giordano, W. Gilson and D. E. Prober, Phys. Rev. Lett. <u>43</u>, 725 (1979).
3. P. Chaudhari and H-U Habermeier, preprint.
4. D. J. Bishop, D. C. Tsui and R. C. Dynes, to be published.
5. D. J. Thouless, Phys. Rev. Lett. <u>39</u>, 1167 (1977).
6. E. Abrahams, P. W. Anderson, D. C. Licciardello and T. V. Ramakrishnan, Phys. Rev. Lett. <u>42</u>, 673 (1979).
7. P. W. Anderson, E. Abrahams and T. V. Ramakrishnan, Phys. Rev. Lett. <u>43</u>, 718 (1979).
8. N. F. Mott, <u>Metal Insulator Transitions</u>, Taylor and Francis Ltd (London) pub. (1974).
9. J. T. Edwards and D. J. Thouless, J. Phys. <u>C5</u>, 807 (1977; D. C. Licciardello and D. J. Thouless, J. Phys. <u>C8</u>, 4157 (1975); and J. Phys. <u>C11</u>, 925 (1978); P. A. Lee, Phys. Rev. Lett. <u>42</u>, 1492 (1979); D. J. Thouless, Les Houches Lectures (unpublished 1978)
10. Experimental evidence for a mobility edge in two dimensional systems near $R_c \sim 30,000$ $\Omega/\square$ was provided by a large number of experiments on the inversion layers of IGFETs. Many of these experiments are discussed in a review article by C. J. Adkins, J. Phys. <u>C11</u>, 851 (1978). Also similar evidence for thin films was obtained by R. C. Dynes, J. P. Garno and J. M. Rowell, Phys. Rev. Lett. <u>40</u>, 479 (1978).
11. D. J. Thouless, preprint. Formula (1) is an interpolation formula suggested by P. W. Anderson to provide the correct behavior in the limits of large and small L/L_ℓ.
12. I do not consider the earlier experiments (see Ref. 10) to be in conflict with the present experiments for reasons such as this. Also in the theoretical perspective of the earlier experiments, the small effects we observe for $R < R_c$ would not have been considered significant or perhaps simply not noticed.
13. P. A. Lee, to be published and private communication.
14. B. L. Altschuler and A. G. Aronov, Solid State Comm. <u>30</u>, 115 (1979).

SYSTEMATICS OF THE RESISTIVE TRANSITION
IN 2D JOSEPHSON-COUPLED GRANULAR LEAD FILMS
NEAR THE MAXIMUM METALLIC RESISTIVITY

A. F. Hebard
Bell Laboratories, Murray Hill, New Jersey 07974

ABSTRACT

The resistive transition and current-voltage characteristics of two-dimensional Josephson-coupled granular lead films have been studied for films with the normal state resistance per square $R_\square^N$ near the maximum metallic resistivity of 30,000 Ω. The data implies that there is a distribution of coupling energies between grains in this inhomogeneous system which favors the formation of superconducting clusters. The deleterious effect of electrostatic charging energies on the Josephson coupling is moderated by the presence of these clusters and we can therefore attribute the absence of zero resistance transitions at $R_\square^N \simeq 30,000\Omega$ to the presence of localized electronic states. The appearance of these localized states is most probably responsible for the rapid onset of temperature broadening as a function of $R_\square^N$, and suggests that recent theories of thermodynamic instabilities predicting a gradual broadening should be modified to take these localization effects into account.

INTRODUCTION

The study of two-dimensional (2D) thin film superconductors with normal state resistance per square $R_\square^N$ approaching 30,000Ω has, for all practical purposes, been limited to inhomogeneous composites. This limitation exists primarily because the maximum bulk resistivity of homogeneous conductors, as determined by the Ioffe-Regel[1] condition, would require the technically difficult fabrication of continuous films less than 10 Å thick. Consequently most of the experimental effort to date has been concerned with metal-insulator or metal-island composites[2] in which the primary mechanism for charge transport is by low probability (high resistance) tunneling across the insulating regions surrounding the metallic component and/or by conduction along metallic threads embedded in the insulating matrix.

A feature common to nearly all of the existing data on these films is the broadening in the resistive transitions[3] as $R_\square^N$ approaches the maximum metallic resistivity[4] of 30,000Ω. There is a growing opinion that these rather broad resistive transitions into the zero resistance state are examples of phase transitions and a variety of suggestions have been made which include percolation effects,[5] thermodynamic fluctuations,[6,7] a paracoherent to coherent transition of the Josephson phase,[8] universal current scaling,[9] and the possibility of a Kosterlitz-Thouless[10] vortex-antivortex dissociation transition.[3,11] Notwithstanding these different interpretations, a characteristic common to all of the data on high sheet resistance 2D films, as confirmed by recent measurements on thin films of Pb, Sn and Aℓ[12] is that a transition to zero resistance will not occur if $R_\square^N$ is greater than 30,000Ω.

In this paper we present a study on the superconducting properties of granular lead films which have been prepared by reactive ion-beam sputter deposition in the presence of oxygen impurities.[13] The resulting films are inhomogeneous granular composites, primarily of Pb and PbO, in which the dominant mechanism for electron transport is by tunneling across the oxide barriers separating the metallic grains. This tunneling mechanism is uniquely demonstrated (Section III) by the appearance at low temperatures of hysteretic current-voltage characteristics on which there is superimposed a sequence of voltage steps equal in magnitude to twice the energy gap 2Δ of lead.[14] The appearance of these voltage steps is convincing evidence for the existence of superconducting tunneling between clusters[14-16] or aggregations of strongly coupled grains which can have a spatial extent equal to the film width. We argue that these clusters are a direct manifestation of the fact that in such granular systems the distribution of coupling energies between grains is such that superconductivity is maintained across macroscopic regions of strongly coupled grains which are separated from each other by more weakly coupled regions.

As $R_\square^N$ increases, and the strength of the coupling between grains is diminished, one would expect that electrostatic charging effects[17] should eventually become comparable to the Josephson coupling energy between grains and therefore prevent transitions to zero resistance. We show in Section IV however that these charging effects are not dominant in our granular lead films with $R_\square^N \approx$ 30,000Ω because the tunneling is between clusters with relatively large capacitance (and hence lower charging energy) rather than between single grains with correspondingly smaller capacitances. We therefore suggest that the absence of zero resistance transitions at $R_\square^N \approx$ 30,000 Ω is due to the appearance of localized electronic states.[14] We find it convenient to recast the previously published ideas on electrostatic charging[17] in terms of a maximum Josephson coupling resistivity $R_\square^J$ which is a materials dependent parameter. Localization effects are only expected to be observed when $R_\square^J >$ 30,000Ω, as is the case for our granular Pb films. Finally, in Section V, we discuss the experimentally observed rapid temperature broadening as a function of increasing $R_\square^N$ and relate our observations to predictions expected from applying the Kosterlitz-Thouless notions of thermodynamic instabilities in 2D superconductors[3,11] to Josephson coupled granular films.

THE RESISTIVE TRANSITION - EXPERIMENTAL DETAILS

The granular lead films are made by directing a 1.0 kV ($\sim$.5 mA/cm^2) beam of Argon ions onto a Pb target biased at -3.0 kV. The sputtered Pb and PbO[13] is deposited on a nearby oxidized silicon wafer at a rate of 1-2 Å/sec for total film thicknesses of 200-300 Å. By controlling the partial pressure of oxygen during the deposition, films with $R_\square^N$ of 100Ω to 10$^8\Omega$ were easily obtained. Nominal grain sizes of 100-200Å were determined by TEM analysis.[18]

In contrast to Pb films deposited on helium temperature substrates,[12,19] the ion-beam deposited granular lead films are mechanically and electrically stable with respect to temperature cycling. Also, in the presence of air at room temperature, the resistance of the high sheet resistance samples tends to decrease by typically less than 1%, rather than undergoing further oxidation and eventually becoming open circuits as is true for Pb evaporated from resistively heated sources in the presence of oxygen.[20] We find however that heating the film approximately 60°C will cause an irreversible increase in oxide thickness surrounding each grain which results in films with successively higher stable values of $R_\square^N$.

Using this technique of annealing the sample to higher $R_\square^N$ after each measurement, we were able to study the systematics of the resistive transitions for the same film as $R_\square^N$ was incrementally and irreversibly increased through 30,000Ω. Figure 1 represents a subset of such transitions for a 2mm long by 200 μm wide by 250 Å thick (ten squares) film with $R_\square^N = 16.3$ kΩ (squares) and $R_\square^N = 28.3$ kΩ (triangles). Two general features of these transitions which we wish to note at this point are: 1. There is a pronounced decrease ΔR in the resistance at a temperature $T_{\Delta R}$ which is slightly less than the bulk $T_c = 7.2$°K of Pb and is relatively insensitive to $R_\square^N$. 2. Below $T_{\Delta R}$ there is a broad transition towards the zero resistance state occurring at a projected temperature T_{2D} (see Section V) which rapidly decreases towards zero as $R_\square^N$ increases towards 30,000Ω.

Excitation currents as low as 10 nA rms at 25 Hz were used in a low noise configuration to insure that the resistance measurements were made in regions in which the voltage scaled linearly with current. We did not observe current dependent resistances reported, for example, in the critical current scaling results on thin granular NbN films.[9]

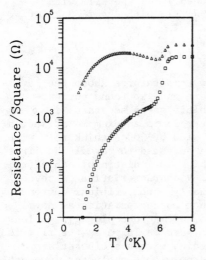

Fig. 1 Resistive transitions for a film 2 mm long by 200 μm wide by 250 Å thick with $R_\square^N = 16.3$ kΩ (squares) and $R_\square^N = 28.3$ kΩ (triangles).

132

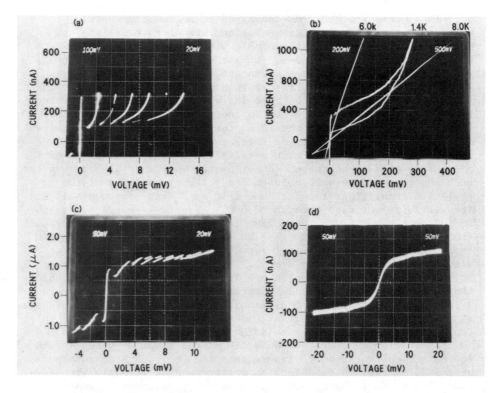

Fig. 2 Current-voltage I-V characteristics at 1.4 K corresponding
to: a) a film 2mm long by 20 μm wide by 300 Å thick with
$R_\square^N$ = 3.1 kΩ, b) the same film but with compressed current and
voltage scales. (The I-V characteristics at 6.0 K and 8.0 K,
the normal state, are superimposed.) c) The film with
$R_\square^N$ = 16.3 kΩ of Fig. 1 and d) the film with $R_\square^N$ = 28.3 kΩ of
Fig. 1.

THE CLUSTER INTERPRETATION

As the current is increased at low temperatures above the levels
at which the resistance measurements were made we found current-
voltage (I-V) characteristics which exhibit steps separated in voltage
by twice the energy gap 2Δ of Pb. Figure 2a is an example of such a
characteristic for a 2mm long by 20 μm wide by 300 Å thick film with
$R_\square^N$ = 3100 Ω. The current sweep has been adjusted to reveal the first
seven critical currents in a display which is indistinguishable from
that which would be expected from the I-V characteristics of seven
discrete Josephson junctions with nominally equal critical currents
connected in series.[21] We interpret such characteristics as novel
evidence for tunneling between clusters, or macroscopic aggregations
of grains, which in the case of Fig. 2a, are as large as the film is
wide. The critical currents between grains within a cluster are
sufficiently high so that the voltage drop within a cluster is close

to zero. Presumably the measuring current exceeds the critical currents of the more weakly coupled grains only at the boundaries between the clusters. The I-V characteristics are therefore a manifestation of the electronic tunneling (Pb-PbO-Pb) processes occurring at these boundaries.

Additional evidence for this cluster interpretation can be found by referring to the ΔR feature in the typical resistive transition of Fig. 1. Because the resistivity of isolated Pb grains is insignificant compared to the resistivity of the granular film, it can be argued that the sudden large change in resistance ΔR at $T_{\Delta R}$ occurs only when the grains become sufficiently well-coupled over large enough regions to short out a significant fraction of the sample. A similar interpretation has been made with respect to the resistive transitions observed for thin film AℓGe composites.[5] Because the temperature-dependent coupling has an observable effect on the resistance only when the coupling extends over sufficiently large regions of many grains, it is not surprising that $T_{\Delta R} < T_{cb}$, where $T_{cb} = 7.2°K$ is the bulk transition temperature of Pb. In fact, the grains themselves most likely have a transition temperature $T_{cg} < T_{cb}$ because of their small size.[19]

Figure 2b displays the I-V characteristics of Fig. 2a with a more compressed current and voltage axis on which is superimposed the I-V characteristics at 6.0°K and the normal state resistance at 8.0°K. We have been able to identify 108 critical currents for this one hundred square sample which implies approximately one cluster per square of film. It is interesting to note that the highest observed critical current at slightly greater than 1 μA occurs when the differential resistance is approximately equal to the resistance of the sample just below the ΔR feature. At this temperature of approximately 6.5°K the total resistance of the sample is 88 kΩ which for 108 series-connected clusters would imply an average tunneling resistance $<R>$ between clusters of 815 Ω. An estimate[22] $I_c(0) = \pi\Delta(0)/2<R> = 2.7$ μA of the zero temperature critical current is somewhat higher than the range of currents (.3 – 1.0 μA) actually observed. This is actually quite satisfactory agreement when one takes into account the rough approximations involved and also the possibility that the combination of thermal and extraneous noise could be suppressing the observed critical currents. This example of series-connected behavior reinforces the notion that clusters with reasonably well defined boundaries form at $T \lesssim T_{\Delta R}$ and that the principle contribution to the resistance at lower temperatures arises from the single particle tunneling between these clusters.

As $R_\square^N$ increases with increasing oxidation of the grains, one would expect the diminished superconducting coupling between grains to give rise to smaller clusters. This notion is confirmed in the plot of $\Delta R/R_\square^N$ vs $R_\square^N$ of Fig. 3. As $R_\square^N$ increases and the clusters shrink in size, a smaller percentage $\Delta R/R_\square^N$ of the sample is shorted out. We can envision two limits to this behavior: (1) The high $R_\square^N$ limit when a cluster becomes as small as a grain and $\Delta R \sim 0$ because the perturbation on the resistance due to the superconducting transitions of the grains is small, and (2) the low $R_\square^N$ limit in which a "giant cluster", larger than the area of the sample, forms and gives

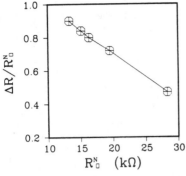

Fig. 3 Plot of $\Delta R/R_\square^N$ vs. $R_\square^N$ showing the decrease in cluster size with increasing $R_\square^N$. The data of Fig. 1 is a subset of the larger number of transitions used to obtain this plot.

rise to a zero resistance transition with $\Delta R = R_\square^N$ at $T_{\Delta R}$. This behavior is also confirmed in a qualitative manner by the appearance of the I-V characteristics which cross over from a series-connected like behavior of Fig. 2a and 2b (20 μm width film) to a series-parallel behavior[20] of Fig. 2c (200 μm width film) in which the voltage steps are diminished in magnitude and appear superimposed on a rising conductance background.

THE EFFECTS OF CHARGING AND LOCALIZATION

As $R_\square^N$ approaches 30,000 Ω the resistive transition becomes increasingly broad (see Fig. 1, triangles), the clusters decrease in size, the "critical currents" are diminished (compare Figs. 2c and 2d), and evidence of steps is barely discernible (Fig. 2d). In the over thirty samples we have measured, activated behavior has always been observed for samples with $R_\square^N > 30,000$ Ω. Such behavior is shown in the logarithmic plot of the resistance per square vs $1/T^{1/2}$ of Fig. 4 for a 2mm long × 200 μm wide by 200 Å thick film. The discontinuity in slope in the plot of Fig. 4 near the bulk transition temperature has also been observed in thin films of lead quench-condensed at helium temperature[12] and has been attributed to the development of a superconducting energy gap which decreases the probability of tunneling between grains. Similar behavior has also been noted in thin films of $(SN)_x$ and In.[23] The crucial implication of this data is that the isolated grains of insulating films with $R_\square^N > 30,000$ Ω retain their superconducting properties and that it is not the superconductivity of the grains but rather the superconducting coupling between the grains which disappears when $R_\square^N \stackrel{\sim}{\sim} 30,000$ Ω.

Abeles[17] has argued, using an analysis by Anderson,[24] that Josephson coupling between isolated grains in granular metals cannot be responsible for zero resistance transitions because the electrostatic charging energy can exceed the Josephson coupling energy by a large factor. The central implication of such an argument is that the observed superconductivity must be due to a connected network of superconducting filaments threading the material. For the granular lead films this cannot be the case because of the evidence that tunneling across insulating oxide barriers is the primary mechanism for conduction. It is for this reason that we now treat in more

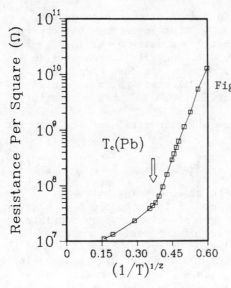

Fig. 4 Logarithmic plot of the
resistance per square vs.
$1/T^{1/2}$ for a 2 mm long by
200 μm wide by 200 A thick
film in the strongly activated regime. The arrow
marks the distinct change
in slope near the transi-
tion temperature T_{cg} of the
grains.

detail the effects of charging energy on the tunneling between
clusters rather than grains.

We start by writing a <u>de-coupling condition</u>[25]

$$E_c > n\, E_J \tag{1}$$

where $E_c = e^2/2C$ is the charging energy between two superconductors
with capacitance C, $E_J = I_c \phi_o/2\pi$ is the Josephson coupling energy
with maximum supercurrent I_c, ϕ_o is the flux quantum and n is the
number of nearest neighbors. By including the number of nearest
neighbors this condition is less stringent than the condition originally considered by Abeles. Recent calculations by McLean and
Stephen[26] for a three dimensional granular system also confirm that
the Abeles condition is too restrictive.

It is useful to write the de-coupling condition of Eq. 1 at $T = 0$
in the form

$$R_\square^N > R_\square^J = n\pi\Delta(0)C\, R_o/2e^2 \tag{2}$$

where $R_\square^J$ can be regarded as a <u>maximum Josephson coupling resistivity</u>
for Josephson square arrays, $\Delta(0)$ is the zero temperature energy gap
and $R_o = \hbar/e^2 = 4114\ \Omega$. Strong coupling corrections[27] have been
ignored. This resistivity $R_\square^J$ is a materials-dependent quantity;
proportional to the strength of the superconducting coupling, as
determined by $\Delta(0)$, and related to the spatial distribution of the
superconducting component in the insulating matrix, as determined by
C. Because our ion-beam deposited films are made with lead with
large $\Delta(0) = 1.4$ mV and because the tunneling is between clusters
with large C, one might expect that $R_\square^J > 30,000\ \Omega$. Accordingly, zero
resistance transitions should occur for films with $R_\square^N > 30,000\ \Omega$.

We can relate $R_\square^J$ to cluster size by writing the expression
$C = \epsilon\, \epsilon_o\, d_F\, \ell_c/d_{ox}$ for the capacitance between two square clusters

with sides ℓ_c in length, embedded in a film of thickness d_F and separated by an oxide of thickness d_{ox}. Incorporating this expression into the definition of $R_\square^J$ in Eq. 2 and using $n = 4$, $d_{ox}/\varepsilon_0 = 1 \, \text{Å}$ and $d_F = 250 \, \text{Å}$ we can calculate $R_\square^J \stackrel{\sim}{\sim} 50 \, \ell_c$ ohms for ℓ_c measured in Å. Thus, from the inequality of Eq. 2, we see that Josephson coupling would be quenched in an array of square clusters which have sides of lengths $\ell_c < R_\square^N/50$. For example, at $R_\square^N = 30,000 \, \Omega$ this occurs for clusters with sides $\ell_c < 600 \, \text{Å}$.

It is useful to write the de-coupling condition of Eq. 1 in yet another form;

$$R_\square^N > (n\beta/2)^{1/2} R_0 \tag{3}$$

where $\beta = 2\pi I_c R^2 C/\phi_0$ is the Stewart-McCumber damping parameter.[28] To first order the product $R_\square^N C$ and hence β is independent of cluster size. We can therefore estimate a typical value of β appropriate to our films from the I-V characteristics of the series-connected clusters of Fig. 2a. Direct calculation using the capacitance of a 20 μm long cluster boundary gives $\beta \stackrel{\sim}{\sim} 300$ whereas an estimate using the set-back current[28] of Fig. 2a gives $\beta \stackrel{\sim}{\sim} 100$. From this latter more conservative estimate of $\beta \stackrel{\sim}{\sim} 100$ we calculate from (3) and the results of the preceeding paragraph that Josephson coupling will not be quenched until $R_\square^N = 58 \, \text{k}\Omega$, provided the clusters are no smaller than $\ell_c \stackrel{\sim}{\sim} 1160 \, \text{Å}$.

The purpose of the numerical approximations of the preceeding two paragraphs is to give a plausibility argument for the existence of Josephson coupling in the presence of deleterious electrostatic charging energies for films with $R_\square^N$ well above $30,000 \, \Omega$. Our granular lead films are unique in this respect because of the hysteretic low damping (high β) Josephson tunneling which occurs between macroscopic-size clusters. Accordingly we ascribe the disappearance of zero resistance transitions observed in all of our films with $R_\square^N > 30,000 \, \Omega$ to the presence of localized electronic states. Adkins[29] has analysed a square array in which electrons are allowed to tunnel from site to site (cluster to cluster in our case) and has shown, using a straightforward physical argument based on the uncertainty principle, that at $T = 0$ a crossover from extended to localized states occurs when $R_0 \stackrel{\sim}{\sim} 4\hbar/e^2 \stackrel{\sim}{\sim} 16 \, \text{k}\Omega$. As both the pair and single particle tunneling probabilities for a given tunnel barrier are equivalent,[22] it is not surprising that the Josephson coupling would be affected in this same region of resistivity.

THE ONSET OF TEMPERATURE BROADENING

One of the more striking aspects of the resistive transitions in our granular lead films is the rapid onset of temperature broadening as $R_\square^N$ increases towards $30,000 \, \Omega$. We illustrate this feature in Fig. 5 which is a plot of the temperature ratio T_{2D}/T_{cg} vs. $R_\square^N$. For reasons which will soon become apparent, we define T_{2D} as the temperature at which zero resistance appears in two-dimensional films.

Because T_{2D} of the high $R_\square^N$ films is well below the 1°K limit of our pumped helium cryostat we found it necessary to estimate T_{2D}

137

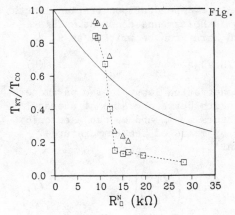

Fig. 5 Plot of the temperature ratio $T_{KT}/T_{\Delta R}$ vs. $R_\square^N$ for a sequence of resistive transitions on the same 2 mm long by 200 μm wide by 250 Å thick film. Estimates of T_{KT} were made using a 1% of $R_\square^N$ criterion (triangles) and extrapolations with power law fits (squares). The solid line is the Kosterlitz-Thouless prediction. We assume that $T_{\Delta R}$ is approximately equal to the BCS transition temperature of the film.

using a 1% of $R_\square^N$ criterion[3] (triangles of Fig. 5) and, for comparative reasons, by using power law fits of the form

$$R = R_o(T/T_{2D} - 1)^S \qquad (4)$$

to the resistive tails below $T_{\Delta R}$ (squares of Fig. 5). The data plotted in Fig. 5 represent these estimates obtained from nine resistive transitions exhibited by the same film after each successive anneal-measurement cycle. Two of these transitions are shown in Fig. 1. The use of power law fits is motivated by the predictions of percolation calculations which have been used by previous investigators to interpret resistive transitions of inhomogeneous superconductors.[5,30] The best fit parameters for the data of Fig. 1 were respectively; $T_{2D} = 0.86K$ and $S = 2.04 \pm .01$ for the $R_\square^N = 16.3$ kΩ data (squares) over the temperature range $1.19K < T < 5.0K$, and $T_{2D} = 0.48K$ and $S = 1.15 \pm .01$ for the $R_\square^N = 28.3$ kΩ data (triangles) over the temperature range $1.0K < T < 2.4K$. This latter value of S is in good agreement with the predictions of Straley[31] for percolation in two dimensions; a prescription which might be expected to apply to films in which the clusters are small compared to film dimensions. Similar exponents $S \gtrsim 1$ were found for three additional samples with equally broad transitions and high $R_\square^N$.

It would be misleading at this time to place much emphasis on such power law fits because the data for which percolation theory would be most relevant, that is small clusters and high $R_\square^N$, does not extend to low enough temperature. The important feature of the data as presented in Fig. 5 however is that the rapid onset in temperature broadening at $R_\square^N \simeq 15$ kΩ is insensitive to the method we use to estimate T_{2D}.

We now turn our attention to how this sudden onset relates to recent predictions[3,11] of a Kosterlitz-Thouless[10] vortex-antivortex dissociation transition in thin 2D superconductors. We proceed by defining the Kosterlitz-Thouless transition temperature $T_{KT} = T_{2D}$ by the relation[3,11]

$$K_B T_{2D} = (\phi_o/4\pi)^2 d_F /2\lambda^2_{eff}(T_{2D}) \qquad (5)$$

where λ_{eff} is the effective temperature-dependent penetration length of the superconducting film and K_B is Boltzmanns constant. This length λ_{eff} for a Josephson coupled array can be written as[32]

$$\lambda_{eff}^2 = \hbar c^2/8\pi e J_o a \tag{6}$$

providing $\lambda_{eff} \gg \lambda_L$, the London penetration length. The parameter J_o is the critical supercurrent density between grains of average size a. For a square array of clusters $a = \ell_c$ and we can ascertain the temperature dependence of λ_{eff} by means of the temperature-dependent Josephson critical current[22]

$$J_o \ell_c d_F = \frac{\pi\Delta(0)}{2\ e\ R_\square^N} \left[\frac{\Delta(T)}{\Delta(0)} \tanh\left(\frac{\Delta(T)}{2k_B T} \right) \right] \tag{7}$$

Combining equations (5) – (7) and using the BCS relation $\Delta(0) = 1.76\ k_B T_c$ to define the film transition temperature T_c we arrive at the final result:

$$\frac{T_{2D}}{T_c} = 2.18 \frac{R_o}{R_\square^N} \left[\frac{\Delta(T_{2D})}{\Delta(0)} \tanh\left(\frac{\Delta(T_{2D})}{2k_B T_{2D}} \right) \right] \tag{8}$$

It is interesting that this same relation can be derived using the extreme dirty limit formulas for λ_{eff}.[3] Accordingly, it is not surprising that the general result embodied in Eq. 8 for Kosterlitz-Thouless transitions in 2D superconductors should be model independent.

In comparing the theory with the data we assume for simplicity $T_c (BCS) \simeq T_{cg} \simeq T_{\Delta R}$ and superimpose the theoretical curve of Eq. 8 as a solid line on the data of Fig. 5. It is strikingly apparent that the theory does not account for the observed rapid onset in temperature broadening. This discrepancy is most probably due to the presence of localized electronic states which have not been taken into account.

CONCLUSIONS AND ACKNOWLEDGEMENTS

In conclusion, the results of Fig. 5 prompt us to speculate about the nature of the "zero resistance" state for $R_\square^N \gtrsim 15$ kΩ. If the appearance of localized states is in fact responsible for the pronounced broadening of the resistive transition, then we would predict that in this resistivity region the zero resistance transitions implied in the data of Fig. 1 do not occur and that the resistance at lower temperatures (T $\ll$ 1K) would flatten out and perhaps even start to increase.[33] This behavior would be consistent with our expectation that there should be a finite range to the superconducting coupling in the presence of these localized states and that this range determines the cluster size. It is clear however from out data that these localization effects are strong enough at $R_\square^N \simeq 30{,}000\ \Omega$, the maximum metallic resistivity, to quench the superconducting coupling over all length scales longer than the characteristic size of an isolated grain.

The author appreciates and acknowledges the fruitful collaboration with J. M. Vandenberg during the initial stages of this research. The very capable technical assistance of R. H. Eick and R. A. Hamm with regard to the technique of ion-beam deposition is also very much appreciated.

REFERENCES

1. A. F. Ioffe and A. R. Regel, Prog. Semicond. $\underline{4}$, 237 (1960).
2. For a recent review see Electrical Transport and Optical Properties of Inhomogeneous Media, AIP Conference Proceedings No. 40 ed. J. C. Garland and D. B. Tanner (American Institute of Physics, New York, 1978).
3. M. R. Beasley, J. E. Mooij and T. P. Orlando, Phys. Rev. Lett. $\underline{42}$, 1165 (1979).
4. D. C. Licciardello and D. J. Thouless, Phys. Rev. Lett. $\underline{35}$, 1475 (1975); and J. Phys. C. $\underline{8}$, 4157 (1975).
5. G. Deutscher and M. Rappaport, J. de Phys. $\underline{C6}$, 581 (1978).
6. For a review see W. J. Skocpol and M. Tinkham, Rep. Prog. Phys. $\underline{38}$, 1049 (1975).
7. G. Deutscher, Y. Imry and L. Gunther, Phys. Rev. $\underline{B10}$, 4598 (1974).
8. J. Rosenblatt, Rev. Phys. Appl. $\underline{9}$, 217 (1974).
9. S. A. Wolf, D. U. Gubser and Y. Imry, Phys. Rev. Lett. $\underline{42}$, 324 (1979).
10. J. M. Kosterlitz and D. J. Thouless, J. Phys. $\underline{C6}$, 1181 (1973).
11. L. A. Turkevich, J. Phys. C., Solid State Phys. $\underline{12}$, 385 (1979).
12. R. C. Dynes, J. P. Garno and J. M. Rowell, Phys. Rev. Lett. $\underline{40}$, 479 (1978).
13. R. N. Castellano, Thin Solid Films $\underline{46}$, 213 (1977).
14. A. F. Hebard and J. M. Vandenberg, to be published.
15. W. L. McClean, T. Worthington and M. Gershenson, Bull. Am. Phys. Soc. $\underline{22}$, 404 (1977).
16. E. Simanek, Phys. Rev. Lett. $\underline{38}$, 1161 (1977).
17. B. Abeles, Phys. Rev. $\underline{B15}$, 2828 (1977).
18. S. Nakahara, to be published.
19. M. Strongin, R. S. Thompson, O. F. Kammerer and J. E. Crow, Phys. Rev. $\underline{B1}$, 1078 (1970).
20. P. K. Hansma and J. R. Kirtley, J. Appl. Phys. $\underline{45}$, 4016 (1974).
21. A. F. Hebard and R. H. Eick, J. Appl. Phys. $\underline{49(1)}$, 338 (1978).
22. V. Ambegaokar and A. Baratoff, Phys. Rev. Lett. $\underline{10}$, 486 (1963); Erratum, Phys. Rev. Lett. $\underline{11}$, 104 (1963).
23. M. W. Young, J. M. D. Thomas, C. J. Adkins and J. W. Tate, J. de Phys. $\underline{C6}$, 448 (1978).
24. P. W. Anderson, Lectures on the Many Body Problem, Vol. 2, ed. E. R. Caianello (New York, Academic Press, 1964) p. 127.
25. This relation has been attributed to de Gennes; e.g., T. Worthington, P. Lindenfeld and G. Deutscher, Phys. Rev. Lett. $\underline{41}$, 316 (1978).
26. W. L. McLean and M. J. Stephen, Phys. Rev. $\underline{B19}$, 5925 (1979).

27. T. A. Fulton and D. E. McCumber, Phys. Rev. 175, 585 (1968).

28. W. C. Stewart, Appl. Phys. Lett. 12, 277 (1968); D. E. McCumber, J. Appl. Phys. 39, 3113 (1968).

29. C. J. Adkins, Phil. Mag. 36, 1285 (1977).

30. C. J. Lobb, M. Tinkham and W. J. Skocpol, Sol. State Comm. 27, 1273 (1978).

31. J. P. Straley, Phys. Rev. 15B, 5733 (1977).

32. B. Giovannini and L. Weiss, Sol. State Comm. 27, 1005 (1978).

33. E. Simanek, Sol. State Comm. 31, 419 (1979).

THE PHASE TRANSITION IN JOSEPHSON JUNCTION ARRAYS

Yoseph Imry*
Department of Physics and Astronomy,
Tel Aviv University
Ramat Aviv, Israel

ABSTRACT

The phase locking in both parallel connected Josephson junctions (or a large planar junction) and weakly coupled superconducting particles is discussed. Both systems are equivalent to the x-y model of phase transitions. Studies of the critical behaviour near the transition to the phase-coherent state, as well as the I-V characteristics, can probe the dynamics of the x-y model. This is of a special interest in the two-dimensional case where the Berezinskii-Kosterlitz-Thouless phase can be studied, along with the dynamics of vortices.

INTRODUCTION

For a weakly coupled array of small particles made of superconducting material, the superconducting transition can occur in two stages[1,2]. Around a nominal transition temperature, T_0 of the grain, each separate grain will exhibit a smeared (by finite size)[3,4] transition to a state where the modulus of the order parameter, $|\psi|$, builds up a non-zero value. At a lower transition temperature, T_c, the phases, θ_i, of the superconducting order parameters in the grains, $|\psi_i|e^{i\theta_i}$, will lock[1,2] due to the Josephson intergrain coupling, under suitable conditions, and the system will become a superconductor. This phase-locking transition is isomorphous to the x-y (n=2) model phase transition , and its sensitivity to external magnetic fields and currents makes it amenable to various interesting experiments. One useful feature of this transition is that the Ginzburg critical region[5] which is usually extremely small in continuous superconductors, can be made as large[2] as in ordinary nearest neighbour magnets. Thus, critical phenomena around this transition can be studied. On the other hand, for too small grains, further complications exist, due to the Coulomb interactions[6,7] and the discreteness of the single grain levels[8]. For grains larger than 50-100 A, these effects can be avoided, but disorder effects, due to possible inhomogeneities in the grain couplings and sizes, complicate the problem. These complications will be discussed towards the end of this paper and shown to be avoidable in the 2D (two-dimensional) case on which we shall mainly focus in this paper.

*Research supported in part by the U.S.-Israel Binational Science Foundation (B.S.F.), Jerusalem, Israel.

The question of the phase transition in 2D $n=2$ systems has recently undergone extremely interesting developments. While strict long range order is impossible in 2D systems with continuous symmetries[9], a low temperature phase with correlations which exhibit power law decays is possible[10]. The low temperature phase does not have thermally excited vortex excitations, and an appealing mechanism for the phase transition is the unbinding of bound vortex-antivortex pairs[11,12]. The latter exist in the low temperature phase. As the temperature is increased, the smaller pairs screen the interactions within the larger ones and at T_c the largest pairs unbind. In the superfluid case, the separate vortices above T_c lead to dissipation and eliminate superfluid flow. The theory of this transition has been quantitatively worked out[13,14]. The order parameter correlation function has a decay length, ξ, above T_c, which diverges like $\exp(\text{const}/\tau^{\frac{1}{2}})$ above T_c, where $\tau = (T-T_c)/T_c$. Below T_c the correlation function decays with distance like $r^{-\eta(T)}$ where $\eta \to 0$ as $T \to 0$ and $\eta \to \frac{1}{4}$ as $T \to T_c$. The latter is related to a predicted[15] universal jump in the superfluid density at T_c, which has been beautifully confirmed by experiments[16].

For the 2D superconductor[17,18] Coulomb effects change the vortex interactions[19] at large separations and should enable free vortices to exist at any temperature for a large enough system. However, for system sizes on the order of a centimeter these effects may not be felt for thin enough films so that they may practically exhibit the 2D transition[17]. Such a transition should exhibit an exponential divergence of the paraconductivity above T_c[18] and interesting dependences on the measuring current and frequency.

The advantage of the granular systems is that the correspondence to the x-y model and the meaning of the higher smeared transition T_o are obvious, the critical region is large and the Coulomb effects can be made to be small. Indeed, phase transitions were observed in such 2D systems, satisfying a typical scaling dependence on temperature and current[20].

A further system which is equivalent to an x-y model is an array of Josephson junctions coupled in parallel, or a large planar junction. This satisfies the sine-Gordon equation, and is thus also equivalent[14,21] to an x-y model. In fact, we show here how the study of such systems can give one interesting insights on such models.

We start this paper by reviewing the single "point" Josephson junction. The various couplings leading to the granular superconductor or to the sine Gordon system are discussed. The case of the latter in 1D is then treated, which clarifies some of the questions related to vortices. We then go on to discuss the 2D case. The various complications in real systems: Disorder and finite size, Coulomb energies and level discreteness are finally discussed and the results summarized.

THE SINGLE JUNCTION

A small Josephson junction[22], has a single degree of freedom. This is the ("gauge invariant") difference

$$\phi \equiv \theta_2 - \theta_1 \tag{1}$$

between the phases, θ_i, of the order parameters of the two superconductors. The latter will be taken to be large enough and/or at low enough temperatures (with respect to their bulk transition temperature T_c^o, so that the amplitudes, $|\psi_i|$, of their order parameters can be taken as constant in time. On the other hand, we shall first assume that the superconducting pieces or "grains" are small enough so that ψ (both amplitude and phase) is constant across each grain. The "potential" energy of the junction is

$$U(\phi) = E_J(1 - \cos\phi) \quad , \quad E_J = \hbar I_J / 2e \tag{2}$$

where I_J is the Josephson current amplitude. A useful model[23] for the junction's dynamics introduces the capacitive "kinetic energy"

$$Q^2/2C = (\hbar^2 C/8e^2) \dot{\phi}^2 \tag{3}$$

where C is the junction's capacitance and Q the charge transferred across it. The Josephson relation for the voltage V

$$V = (\hbar/2e)\dot{\phi} \tag{4}$$

has been used here. V yields a normal quasiparticle current which is modeled by

$$I_n = V/R_n \tag{5}$$

where R_n is possibly voltage (and frequency) dependent. Eqs.(2,3) yields the well-known Josephson current

$$I_s = I_J \sin\phi \tag{6}$$

The equation of motion for ϕ is that of a driven pendulum moving in a viscous medium

$$\ddot{\phi} + G\dot{\phi} + \sin\phi = I/I_J \tag{7}$$

with time measured in units of the inverse Josephson frequency ω_J, and $G \equiv (\omega_J RC)^{-1}$. Eq.7 can also be regarded as a lumped circuit model for the junction[23]. The I-V characteristics following from (7) have thoroughly been discussed in the literature[23].

Fluctuations were neglected at this stage. This is appropriate to the zero temperature case. Zero point quantum fluctuations[5] can be neglected as long as the junction's capacitance is large enough so that

$$\hbar\omega_T = (2e/\hbar)(E_J/C)^{1/2} \ll E_J \tag{8}$$

which is what we shall assume. At finite temperatures ϕ can fluctuate, and over a long enough time period average $\langle I \rangle$ to zero if V=0 or, alternatively, cause a non zero $\langle V \rangle = (\hbar/2e) \langle \dot{\phi} \rangle$ if $\langle I \rangle \neq 0$ is maintained. However, once $E_J \gg kT$, such fluctuations depend on an extremely small Boltzmann factor and are thus very rare. The noise voltage, <V>, can easily be too small to be measurable once $E_J/kT \gtrsim 20$, say. However, <V> is always non zero in principle for finite I, and the phases θ_1 and θ_2 are not locked. Expressions for <V>(<I>) were given in the literature[24,25] and studied numerically[26] The agreement with experiment[27] is very good. Note, however, that for $I_J \sim .1$ µA, E_J/k_B becomes $\sim 2°K$ and the noise resistance is so high that the Josephson effect is washed out. Our problem is how can phase coherence be restored due to interjunction interactions.

COUPLED ARRAYS OF JUNCTIONS

Here, one can visualize two different situations. (a) An array of coupled superconducting particles[1,2]. Here the Josephson interaction (2) couples the phases of the superconducting units. From the assumptions below, we thus have a system of phases θ_i coupled by nearest neighbour interactions $-E_J \cos(\theta_i - \theta_j)$. This is isomorphous[2] to the "x-y" (or n=2) model of phase transitions - an array of planar rotators whose angles, θ_i, are coupled via $-J \cos(\theta_i - \theta_j)$ terms. Thus, the results for the latter model can be used for our "granular superconductor". In particular, no phase transition exists in one dimension (1D), and a conventional phase transition exists in 3D, with "n=2" critical behaviour. The latter is the same as that of a bulk continuous superconductor, except that the size of the "critical region", where fluctuation effects are important, and which is negligible in the continuous case, can be made reasonably large[2] in the granular case. On the other hand, since the charging effects[6,7] can be made to be very small for large enough grains, one may be able to eliminate the electromagnetic coupling[28] which, in principle, should make the transition in the continuous superconductor first order. The 2D case, which is at a "marginal dimensionality" is of a special interest here. While no strict long range order can occur, an interesting phase transition to a quasi ordered phase[10-15] takes place. The granular superconducting film thus offers a realization of the 2D x-y model, where one can study the unusual properties of this transition. Again, charge effects can be eliminated with large enough superconducting particles. One particular manifestation of the charging effects which is possible will be mentioned later on. (b) When the junctions are coupled in parallel by normal inductions (the same coupling exists in large continuous junctions), the various phase differences ϕ_i of the junctions are coupled by interactions of the form[29,30]

$$\frac{1}{2} K \left(\phi_i - \phi_j\right)^2 \tag{9}$$

where $K = \psi_0 (2\pi L I_J)^{-1}$, with ψ_0 the flux quantum and L the normal inductance between the two junctions. With the $-E_J \cos \phi$ terms for the single junction, one has a so-called sine-Gordon model. This has been shown[14,21] to be similar in its critical behaviour again to the x-y model! So, we have another realization of the latter. Note however, that in this case only the 1D and 2D cases can be made. An interesting degree of freedom which exists here is a magnetic field parallel to the insulating barrier. Every flux unit threading thus the inductance,L, between two junctions tends to make the two phase differences differ by 2π, i.e., (10) is replaced by

$$\tfrac{1}{2} K (\phi_1 - \phi_2 - h)^2 \tag{10'}$$

where h is 2π times the number of flux units associated with the external field, H_{ext} through L. A continuous 1D or 2D large junction can be viewed as a large number of units coupled by (10). In the static continuum limit, this becomes the well-known continuous sine Gordon Hamiltonian, given for $H_{ext}=0$ by

$$\mathcal{H} = \int d^2x\, E_J \left[\tfrac{\Lambda_J^2}{2}(\nabla\phi)^2 - \cos\phi \right] \tag{11}$$

Λ_J being the Josephson penetration length of the junction[22]. Much of the physics of this model, including the effects of vortex excitations, which are crucial in the 2D case, can be appreciated by considering the 1D Sine–Gordon model. This is discussed in the next section.

"PARALLEL CONNECTED" CHAIN OF JUNCTIONS

Here, the equation of motion of the ith junction is[29,30]

$$\ddot{\phi_i} + G\dot{\phi_i} + \sin\phi_i + K(\phi_{i+1} - \phi_i + \phi_{i-1} - \phi_i) = I_i/I_J \tag{12}$$

Where I_i is the external driving current on the ith junction and the equations for i=1,N depend on the boundary conditions. For I_i=0 and no dissipation this is equivalent to a discrete version of the Sine-Gordon equation. No long range order will occur at finite temperatures. In this case the occurrence of the finite noise voltage can be given a rather vivid explanation. An important excitation of the Sine-Gordon chain is the soliton - a phase change of 2π connected with a quantum of flux, which can run across the chain. An external current drives this soliton in a given direction (Lorentz or Magnus force) and this yields an increase of the phase. It is interesting that steady soliton motion for finite I and G can be found[31]. In fact, the various soliton states yield branches in the I-V characteristics. For small I the soliton mobility μ_s is known to be proportional to the inverse of the product of G and the soliton restmass. The solitons move with a steady state velocity $\mu_s I$. The density, n_s, of thermally activated solitons is[34]

$$n_s = (8 E_0 / \pi k_B T)^{1/2} \exp(-E_0/k_B T) \tag{13}$$

with E_0 the soliton rest energy. Since each soliton advances the total phase of the chain by 2π, one gets[35] using (13) and (4)

$$\langle V \rangle = 2\pi n_s \mu_s I \tag{14}$$

i.e., a finite noise resistance. A more general expression,[35] for finite I, has been derived in ref.36. In the linear (small I) range their result has the same exponential, but a different prefactor from (13). The physics of the increase of $\partial\langle V\rangle/\partial\langle I\rangle$ with I was discussed by Landauer[33], in terms of nucleation theory[35].

Whenever one has such vortices - they will lead to a non zero voltage, under the influence of a current. Thus, a necessary condition for a resistanceless state is that no vortices be present at equilibrium. The lowest space dimension where this happens is two. This case is discussed in the next section.

TWO DIMENSIONAL ARRAYS OF JUNCTIONS

A two dimensional array of Josephson junctions should have a vortex-free phase[11],[12] below a certain critical temperature T_c^{2D}. Only bound pairs of vortices exist in this phase and they do not lead to a noise resistance in the limit $I \to 0$. We shall discuss two cases: a) The planar junction (or parallel connected array) and b) The planar system of weakly coupled grains.

a) The Planar Junction. Here the equations of motion in the discrete case are the 2D generalization of (12). In the continuous (large planar junction) limit, this becomes

$$\ddot{\phi} - \bar{c}^2 \Delta_2 \phi + G\dot{\phi} + \sin\phi = I(\vec{x})/I_J \qquad (15)$$

Here $\phi(\vec{x}, t)$ is the phase difference as a function of the 2D position vector $\vec{x}$ across the junction, $\bar{c}$ is the velocity of electromagnetic waves in the junction, G is a dissipation factor, $I(\vec{x})$ is the external driving current and Δ_2 the 2D Laplacian operator. The Hamiltonian in the case G=0, I=0 is just the Sine-Gordon 2D one, whose statistical mechanics is equivalent to that of the 2D x-y model[21]. Thus a vortex-free state exists below the T_c^{2D} of the latter model. The phase transition will also exist for small finite G. The $I \to 0$ noise resistance should vanish as $T \to T_c^{2D}$ from above in a 2D n=2-like manner (i.e. like $\exp(-\text{const}/\tau^{1/2})$, and remain zero below T_c^{2D}. The question of the nonlinear effects in the resistivity - its dependence on the measuring current density j is quite non-trivial and will be taken up in the discussion of the granular superconductor below.

b) An Array of Coupled Superconducting Particles. As explained before, this is equivalent when the grains are not too small to the classical x-y model. The latter should undergo at high enough dimensionality a regular n=2 phase transition to a superconducting phase coherent state. One should emphasize, however, that the basic unit, or x-y "spin" in this description is each superconducting particle. Thus for example the amplitude of the specific heat corresponds to a total entropy change on the order of a Boltzmann constant k_B, per superconducting grain. This can be rather small for large grains. The D.C. conductivity of the system should diverge as $T \to T_c$ from above, with a characteristic exponent, and stay zero below T_c as long as the current density, j, is below critical $j < j_c(T)$. This suggests[20] a usual scaling type dependence of the conductivity, or voltage on the temperature and measuring current:

$$V(I,T) \propto I^x \chi(\text{const} \cdot \tau/I^a) \qquad (16)$$

where χ is a scaling function, $\chi(0)=1$, $\chi(z) \sim z^\mu$ for large z, $R_{I \to 0} \sim \tau^\mu$, and

$$x - 1 = \lambda \mu \qquad (17)$$

Such a scaling relation should also hold in the special case of 2D, where the transition is to the unusual Berezinskii-Kosterlitz-Thouless phase. In fact, experiments[20] have confirmed (16,17) extremely well for 2D granular NbN films yielding the following values[20] for the exponents[37]:

$$\mu = 3.7 \pm 0.3 \; ; \; x = 3.0 \pm 0.2 \; ; \; \lambda = 0.57 \pm 0.1 \qquad (18)$$

While the conductivity does not seem to diverge exponentially as it might according to refs. 12 and 18, the large value $\mu \cong 4$ may in fact be not inconsistent with an exponential ($\mu \to \infty$) divergence. More decades in the $\tau \to 0$ limit are needed to sharpen this distinction (see, however, the remarks on finite-size effects below).

The value of the exponent λ, is consistent with the most naive picture of the critical current vanishing below T_c as

$$j_c(T) \propto |\tau|^{1/\lambda} \qquad (19)$$

which seems to hold experimentally for the NbN films that satisfy (17,18)[38]. We emphasize, however, that a non zero critical current below T_c may, strictly speaking, not exist in the special 2D case. In fact, intuitively appealing arguments[39] for the vortex-free phase of the 2D superfluid yield a vanishing j_c at all temperatures, with a non linear $\sigma(j) \alpha j^\zeta$, vanishing with j like a power ζ larger than two. The physics behind these calculations is that a finite, even arbitrarily small current, is able in principle, to unbind a bound vortex-antivortex pair. Such pairs exist in the quasi ordered 2D x-y phase[11][12]. The constant magnus force drives the vortex and antivortex in opposite directions and results in an effective repulsive potential which decreases linearly with the separation, r, of the pair for large r. This, of course, can overcome, in principle, any finite binding at small r. Once the pair unbinds, a finite flux-flow resistance, due to the steady change of phase difference with time, (eq.4) follows, as in type II superconductors. Assuming that the vortex distribution is essentially the same for small j as for j=0, yielded[39] a power law decay of the superfluid current and a $\sigma \alpha j^\zeta$ below T_c.

We should like to suggest, that while j_c may strictly vanish, as in the results of refs.39, it may be possible to have in practice an extremely small resistance for a finite range of currents $j \lesssim j_{c,eff}$. One way in which this may happen is that a given current j will easily unbind all vortex pairs with large enough separations and thus decrease T_c. At the same time more tightly bound vortex pairs, while unstable in principle, may survive for reasonable times, due to the energy barrier opposing their dissociation. This question certainly needs further theoretical study. It is interesting to remark that bound vortex-antivortex pairs ("breathers") are known to exist in the 1D long narrow junction or Sine-Gordon chain[40]. Their study in that simple case, where some exact results exist, may help to clarify these questions. Another factor which may be relevant in this connection is vortex pinning, say, by irregularities in the structure. The influence of the latter on static properties will be discussed in the next section.

A simple way to obtain information on vortex dynamics is through the I-V characteristics. Each "quantum" state of the system with a given number of vortices will yield a corresponding branch in the I-V characteristics. This structure is particularly simple in the 1D case[31]. The vortices can be due to an external magnetic field or thermally excited. In principle, vortices may also be trapped in metastable states of the system.

DISORDER,FINITE SIZE CHARGING AND DISCRETE LEVEL EFFECTS,CONCLUSIONS

Before summarizing the ideas presented in this paper, one should discuss four complications that may exist in real experimental systems.
a) Disorder Effects. A significant amount of disorder may certainly occur in a granular superconductor, and even in pressed systems of uniform superconducting particles. The Josephson coupling depends so sensitively on the properties of the weak intergrain contact, that any small nonuniformity of the latter throughout the system may yield substantial such variations, for example, of E_J. In addition, the grain sizes may not be uniform. In the case of a large planar junction,similar small variations in the oxide thickness are difficult to avoid. We are thus faced with the possibility that the disorder may affect the phase locking transition.

Obviously, nonuniformities over macroscopic scales can easily smear the transition. Assuming that those can be avoided, the question of nonuniformities with only short range correlation is still a very serious one. There appear to be cases in 3D systems where this can lead to percolation effects[41], when parts of the systems become ordered, and span the whole system prior to other parts. A general criterion for finding whether a small disorder is relevant near the phase transition was given by A. B. Harris[42]. This criterion is physically very appealing and is in agreement with the results of all the more sophisticated calculations performed thus far on phase transitions in disordered systems. It therefore appears very reasonable to use this Harris argument. The idea is that if the correlation length, ξ, diverges as $\tau^{-\nu}$, the relative fluctuation in T_c of a coherence volume is $\tau^{\nu d/2}$. To get a sharp transition one thus needs

$$\nu > 2/d \qquad (20)$$

i.e., when (20) is satisfied, the correlations grow _fast enough_ to average the effects of the microscopic disorder. Fortunately, (20) is satisfied with a very wide margin in the 2D x-y transition. The exponential divergence of ξ obtained by Kosterlitz and Thouless corresponds to $\nu = \infty$. This would mean that the system should be able to easily average, close to T_c, the effects of a finite, small, microscopic disorder.
b) Finite Size Effects. The exponential divergence of ξ makes it comparable with the linear system's size, L, not very far from T_c.

This yields a relatively large T_c smearing[4], $\Delta\tau_s$, due to finite size.

$$\Delta\tau_s \propto (\ln L)^{-2}$$

(21)

which is a serious limitation on getting "asymptotically close to T_c"!

c) Charging Effects. If the superconducting particles are small enough so that eq.(8) is almost satisfied, important changes occur in the Josephson effect. In fact, Anderson[6] has demonstrated that once $E_c > E_J$ the Josephson effect in a single junction is washed out by quantum fluctuations. Abeles[7] has raised the possibility that the same effect can be responsible for the destruction of superconductivity in granular systems with small enough grains. The problem has been treated by McLean and Stephen[43] and Simanek[44] who found that in the granular case, even large values of $E_c/E_J \sim 10$ can be tolerated. In the former calculation the charging energy appears like quantum corrections to a lattice Debye Waller factor[45]. This raises the interesting possibility that in 2D, where the correlation function[10] of $\cos\phi$ decreases at low temperatures like $r^{-\eta}$, η will increase due to the quantum effects. This can also lower T_c, for the same intergrain coupling for smaller grains, if $\eta(T_c)$ is assumed to retain its universal value.

d) Level Quantization Effects. For metallic grains that are not much larger than about 30 A, the level separation due to the finite size at the Fermi energy becomes comparable to $k_B T_c$. This will lower the nominal T_o of the grains. This effect has been calculated in ref.[46]. Intergrain tunneling will broaden these levels. Once this broadening is less than $k_B T_c$, the above T_c depression will occur for the phase locking of the whole system[47]. This should happen for R $\sim 10\Omega$. Interestingly, this condition is related to the one for Anderson localization[48] to start to be felt[49].

Conclusions: Phase locking in the large planar junction is a realization of the Sine-Gordon model. The granular superconductor is isomorphous to the x-y model. Both models are equivalent and should display the interesting quasi long range order in two dimensions. Measurements of the critical behaviour of the resistivity (and specific heat) and its dependence on external magnetic fields and currents, as well as the I-V characteristics, can illuminate and examine the questions of phase locking and vortex dynamics in these systems.

REFERENCES

1. G. Pellam, G. Dousselin, H. Cortes and J. Rosenblatt, Solid State Comm. 11, 427 (1972).
2. G. Deutscher, Y. Imry and L. Gunther, Phys. Rev. B10, 4598 (1974).
3. B. Mühlschlegel, D. J. Scalapino and R. Denton, Phys. Rev. B6, 1767 (1972).
4. Y. Imry and D. J. Bergman, Phys. Rev. A3, 1416 (1971).
5. V. L. Ginzburg, Sov. Phys. Solid State 2, 1824 (1960).

150

6. P. W. Anderson, in Lectures on the Many Body Problem, E. R. Cal-
   aniello (Academic, New York, 1964) Vol.2, p.127.
7. B. Abeles, Phys. Rev. $B15$, 2828 (1977).
8. P. W. Anderson, J. Phys. Chem. Solids, 11, 26 (1959).
9. P. C. Hohenberg, Phys. Rev. 158, 383 (1967).
10. See e.g., Y. Imry, CRC Reviews on Solid State Science, p.157
    (1979) and references contained therein.
11. V. L. Berezinskii, Sov. Phys. JETP, 32, 493 (1971); 34, 610
    (1972).
12. J. M. Kosterlitz and D. J. Thouless, J. Phys. $C6$, 1181 (1973).
13. J. M. Kosterlitz, J. Phys. $C7$, 1046 (1974).
14. J. V. José, L. P. Kadanoff, S. Kirkpatrick and D. R. Nelson,
    Phys. Rev. $B16$, 1217 (1977).
15. D. R. Nelson and J. M. Kosterlitz, Phys. Rev. Lett. 39, 1201
    (1977).
16. D. Bishop and J. D. Reppy, Phys. Rev. Lett. 40, 1727 (1978);
    I. Rudnick, Phys. Rev. Lett. 40, 1454 (1978); see, however,
    J. G. Dash, Phys. Rev. Lett. 41, 1178 (1978).
17. L. A. Turkevich, J. Phys. $C12$, L385 (1979); M. R. Beasley,
    J. E. Mooij and T. P. Orlando, Phys. Rev. Lett. 42, 1165 (1978).
18. S. Doniach and B. A. Huberman, Phys. Rev. Lett. 42, 1169 (1979);
    B. I. Halperin and D. R. Nelson, J.Low Temp. Phy. 36, 599 (1979).
19. J. Pearl, J. Low Temp. Phys. 9, 566 (1964).
20. D. U. Gubser, S. A. Wolf and Y. Imry, Phys. Rev. Lett. 42,
    324 (1979).
21. S. T. Chui and J. D. Weeks, Phys. Rev. $B14$, 4978 (1976).
22. B. D. Josephson, Adv. Phys. 14, 419 (1965).
23. W. C. Stewart, Appl. Phys. Lett. 12, 277 (1968); D. E. McCum-
    ber, J. Appl. Phys. 39, 3113 (1968).
24. V. Ambegaokar and B. I. Halperin, Phys. Rev. Lett. 22, 1364
    (1969); R. Stratonovich, Topics in the Theory of Random Noise,
    Gordon and Breach, N.Y., (1963).
25. D. M. Falco, W. H. Parker, S. E. Trullinger and P. K. Hansma,
    Phys. Rev. $B10$, 1865 (1974).
26. J. Kurkijärvi and V. Ambegaokar, Phys. Lett. $31A$, 314 (1970).
27. J. T. Anderson and A. M. Goldman, Phys. Rev. Lett. 23, 128
    (1969).
28. B. I. Halperin, T. C. Lubensky and S.-k. Ma, Phys. Rev. Lett.
    32, 296 (1974).
29. J. A. Blackburn, J. P. Leslie and H. J. Smith, J. Appl. Phys.
    42, 1047 (1971).
30. Y. Imry and P. M. Marcus, IEEE Trans. Magn. MAG-13, 868 (1977).
31. P. M. Marcus and Y. Imry, submitted to Solid State Comm.;
    D.W.McLaughlin and A. C. Scott, Phys. Rev. $A18$, 1659 (1978).
32. M. B. Fogel, S. E. Trullinger, A. R. Bishop and J. Krumhansl,
    Phys. Rev. $B15$, 1578 (1977).
33. R. Landauer, private communication.
34. K. Kawasaki, Progr. Theor. Phys. 55, 2029 (1976).
35. M. Buttiker and R. Landauer, IBM preprint (1979).
36. S. E. Trullinger, M. D. Miller, R. A. Guyer, A. R. Bishop,
    F. Palmer and J. A. Krumhansl, Phys. Rev. Lett. 40, 206, 1603
    (1978).

37. However, J. L. Berchier and D. H. Sanchez, Rev. Phys. Applique, in press, obtained different values of the exponents for rather small arrays of proximity effect bridges.

38. D. U. Gubser, et al., these proceedings.

39. B. A. Huberman, R. J. Myerson and S. Doniach, Phys. Rev. Lett. $\underline{40}$, 780 (1978); V. Ambegaokar, B. I. Halperin, D. R. Nelson and E. D. Siggia, Phys. Rev. Lett. 40, 783 (1978).

40. A. R. Bishop, J. Phys. $\underline{C11}$, L329 (1978).

41. M. L. Rappaport and G. Deutscher, these proceedings; see also G. Deutscher and M. L. Rappaport, J. de Physique C6-581 (1978), $\underline{40}$, L219 (1978).

42. A. Brooks Harris, J. Phys. $\underline{C7}$, 1671 (1974).

43. W. L. McLean and M. J. Stephen, Phys. Rev. $\underline{B19}$, 5925 (1979).

44. E. Simanek, Solid State Comm. $\underline{31}$, 419 (1979).

45. G. Deutscher and Y. Imry, Phys. Lett. $\underline{42A}$, 413 (1973).

46. M. Strongin, R. S. Thompson, O. K. Kammerer and J. E. Crow, Phys. Rev. $\underline{B1}$, 1078 (1970).

47. Y. Imry and M. Strongin, to be published.

48. D. J. Thouless, Phys. Reports $\underline{13}$, 93 (1974).

49. R. C. Dynes, J. P. Garno and J. M. Rowell, Phys. Rev. Lett. $\underline{40}$, 479 (1978).

152

B. Giovannini, D.H. Sanchez and J.L. Berchier
DPMC - Geneva University - GENEVA - Switzerland

ABSTRACT

We discuss results on n x n 2D arrays of proximity effect junctions from the point of view of Josephson arrays.

INTRODUCTION

The possible occurrence of cooperative effects in systems consisting of a large number of Josephson junctions has already attrac-
ted a lot of attention. Most of the experimental work published so
far has been done on disordered systems (pressed spheres [1] and granular films [2]), so we started a study on arrays of proximity effect junctions in order to test ideas about collective phenomena on a regular
lattice of Josephson junctions. Here we review briefly experimental [3,4,5] and theoretical [6,7] work at Geneva University on proximity
effect arrays from the point of view of Josephson arrays.

THE SAMPLES AND GENERAL FEATURES

The arrays consist of n_0 x n_0 (n_0 = 10, 20, 30 and 40) In squares
separated by regions of Au/In (Fig. 1). The length of the In square
sides d_S (In) varied from about 4.5 μm to 16 μm with film thicknesses
w from 370 Å to 710 Å. The regions of Au/In separating two In squares
are of widths d_N(Au/In) from 1.5 μm to 11 μm and the Au film thicknesses from 230 Å to 250 Å. Details on sample preparation are given
in references 4, 5 and 8 and on measuring equipment in references 5,9.

From the V-I characteristics of these
devices we obtained the DC resistance at
the origin R(T) vs.T. A typical curve is
shown in Fig. 2, together with the normalized resistance of a control sample consisting of a square of Au of sides (20 d_S
+ 19 d_N) in contact with the In film. This
control sample (aC 16P) was done simultaneously with the array (aR 16P 20 x 20).

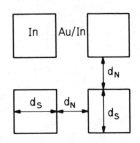

FIGURE 1 - Schematic pic-
ture of the structure of
an array.

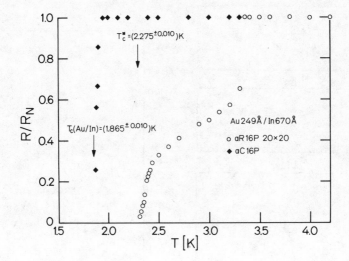

FIGURE 2 - Typical normalized resistance of an array and its control sample, as a function of temperature.

The array R vs. T curve indicates two transition temperatures, one at about $T_c(In)$, and another at T_c^* to a resistanceless state. The second transition at T_c^* occurs at higher T's than $T_c(Au/In)$ (as measured by the control sample) when ℓ film (In) $\gtrsim 0.5$ μm.

Between $T_c(Au/In)$ and T_c^*, and for T not too close to T_c^*, the arrays behave as SNS junctions with a Bardeen-Johnson law for the critical current, i.e.

$$Ic \ (array, \ T) = Ic \ (array) \ exp(-\beta \ (array) \ T)$$

EXPERIMENTAL EVIDENCE FOR A PHASE TRANSITION AT T_c^*

At present it is difficult to prove beyond doubt from the experiments that a phase transition occurs at T_c^* (3). But there is evidence that this is the case:

1) The critical current versus T deviates systematically from an exponential behaviour near T_c^*; these deviations have been analysed assuming that $J_c \sim (T_c^* - T)^{1/\lambda}$.

2) Near T_c^*, the arrays follow the scaling equation proposed by Wolf et al.[10], who also predict the behaviour of the critical current for $T < T_c^*$ when $T \rightarrow T_c^*$.

Figure 3 shows an example on how this formalism is followed by these devices, and Table I gives typical "critical exponents" found for two pairs of simultaneously made samples.

154

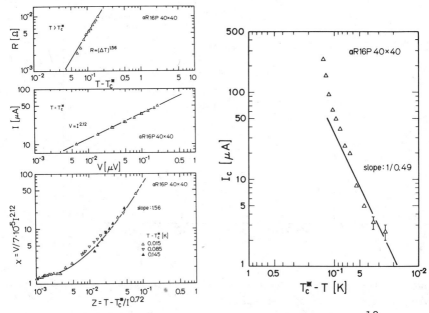

FIGURE 3 - Example on how the arrays follow Wolf et al.'s[10] formalism at T_c^*.

From Table I we observe that: i) x > 1, and in consequence the
condition to apply this formalism is satisfied; ii) λ and θ are about
the same, as proposed by Wolf et al.[10]; iii)μ varies between 0.7 and
1.6

2D In squares in finite arrays of SNS junctions					
Samples	$d_S(In\ (\mu m)$ $d_N(Au/In)(\mu m)$	μ	x	λ	θ
eR40G 20×20 230Å Au 500Å In	6 4	0.77	1.31	0.40	0.54
eR16G 20×20 230Å Au 500Å In	15 11	0.87	1.86	0.98	0.92
aR16P 40×40 249Å Au 670Å In	12.5 5.2	1.56	1.80	0.51	0.42
aR16P 20×20 249Å Au 670Å In	11 5.8		2.12	0.72	0.49

TABLE I - Typical "critical exponents" found when the formalism
of Ref. 10 is applied to simultaneously made samples.

THEORETICAL FRAMEWORK AND COMPARISON WITH EXPERIMENTS

First we shall consider a 3D system. According to the ideas of Rosenblatt [1] an array of Josephson junctions in three dimensions should undergo two phase transitions: the superconducting phase transition of the individual grains and a paracoherent-ferrocoherent (pf) transition analogous to a superconducting phase transition for the whole system.

The similarity between superconducting and pf transitions can be understood for example by considering the array in the strong coupling model of superconductivity. In this model, the Hamiltonian is written as [11]:

$$\mathcal{H} = -2\varepsilon_f \sum_\nu S_z^\nu + \gamma \sum_\nu (S_z^\nu)^2 - v \sum_\nu \{S_+^\nu S_-^\nu + S_-^\nu S_+^\nu\}$$
$$- v \sum_{\nu,\nu'} (S_+^\nu S_-^{\nu'} + S_+^{\nu'} S_-^\nu) \quad , \tag{1}$$

where
$$\vec{S}^\nu = \sum_k \vec{\sigma}^{k,\nu} \quad . \tag{2}$$

Here S_z^ν is essentially the charge on grain ν, and γ the inverse capacitance. ε_f is the Fermi energy; V the BCS interaction; $\sigma^{-k,\nu}$ (a Pauli Matrix) which creates a pair k in grain ν and v is a tunnelling matrix element. The third term of this Hamiltonian induces a phase transition in each grain at a temperature $T_{CBCS} \sim Vn$ (n : number of superconducting electrons in each grain) with the formation of a magnetic moment in the x-y plane (gap) of the order n, the total magnetic moment for the whole system being of order $\sqrt{N} \cdot n$ (N : number of grains); at a temperature $T_{CJ} \simeq Zvn^2$ (Z : number of nearest neighbours), the last term of $\mathcal{H}$ will induce a phase transition with the formation of a total moment in the x-y plane of order nN. So if $Zvn \leqslant V$, there will be a paracoherent region in the phase diagram. If $\gamma \gg v$ (small capacitance) the Hamiltonian (1) is related to the plane rotator model, whereas for $\gamma \ll v$, it is related to the x-y model.

A pf transition should be characterized by the appearance of a London equation; if one defines Q (qω) by

$$J_\alpha(q\omega) = -Q_{\alpha\beta}(q\omega) A_\beta(q\omega)$$
$$Q_{\alpha\beta}(q\omega) = \frac{q_\alpha q_\beta}{q^2} Q^\ell(q\omega) + (\delta_{\alpha\beta} - \frac{q_\alpha q_\beta}{q^2}) Q^t(q\omega) \quad , \tag{3}$$

one should have below T_{CJ}

$$\lim_{q\to o} \lim_{\omega\to o} Q^t(q\omega) = \frac{c}{4\pi} \frac{1}{\lambda_J^2} \quad . \tag{4}$$

We tried to prove, without success, and present therefore as a conjecture, that

$$\lambda_J^{-2} = \frac{8\pi\,edJ(T)}{\hbar c^2 d_s w} \tag{5}$$

where d is the distance $(d_N + d_s)$ and $J(T)$ is the critical current between any two grains as function of temperature with all many body effects included (except vortex motion), and $\lim J(T) = 0$ as $T \to T_{cJ}$.

If the resulting total magnetic field is less than both the critical field for the whole system and the field necessary to induce diffraction and interference phenomena between the different junctions, and if λ_J is larger than the size of the system, $J(T)$ is also the observed critical current of the (3D) system. The relation of $J(T)$ to the order parameter is shown by noting that for the corresponding magnetic system, the term in front of $(\nabla\phi)^2$ in the free energy is essentially the stiffness constant C which can be written [12]

$$C = \frac{M^2}{q^2 \chi^{\perp}(q,o)} \tag{6}$$

and [13]

$$\chi^{\perp}(q,o) \sim q^{-2} \tag{7}$$

So one has

$$\lambda_J^{-2} \sim C \sim M^2$$

where M is the magnetization of the whole system and so the critical current between two adjacent grains is proportional to the square of the order parameter of the array.

If we denote by $\rho_s{}^a$ the quantity corresponding to $\rho_s = |\Psi|^2$ in a superconductor, one has (provided (5) is correct)

$$\rho_s{}^a = J(T) \frac{dm}{e\hbar d_s w} \tag{8}$$

In two dimensions the situation is more complicated, and we shall discuss our results in the framework of the Kosterlitz-Thouless theory, ignoring all the many complications that one can think of and will have to be investigated (quasiparticle currents, effect of the macroscopic order on the state of each grain and so on).

According to equation (8) and reference 14 we should observe that $J(T)$ tends to a constant

$$\lim_{T \to T^-_{kT}} J(T) \to \frac{kT_{kT}}{\hbar} \frac{2e}{\pi} \frac{d_s}{d} = 1.3\ 10^{-8}\ A \times T_{kT}\ (^ok) \times \frac{d_s}{d} \tag{9}$$

The relation of $J(T)$ to the observed critical current is not clear in that case, given the influence of "ionization" of vortex pairs [16].

Assuming that $J_c(T) = n_o J(T)$, equation (9) would, for a 20 x 20 array, give a critical current $J_c \sim \frac{1}{4}10^{-6}$ A, which is smaller than we could measure.

The resistivity in a KT transition was calculated by Doniach and Huberman [15] and by Halperin and Nelson [16]. The first authors find

$$\ln \frac{R}{R_N} \sim - \frac{\tilde{\mu}o}{kT} (t + xt^{\frac{1}{2}})^{-1} \quad ,$$

where

$$t = \frac{T}{T_{kT}} - 1 \quad .$$

and predict also a large magnetoresistance.

Halperin and Nelson find

$$\ln \frac{R}{R_N} \sim t^{-1} \quad .$$

We have carried out recently preliminary measurements in $H_\perp$ (see reference 17 for more complete results), of which figure 4 shows the experimental $\ln(R/R_N)$ vs.t.

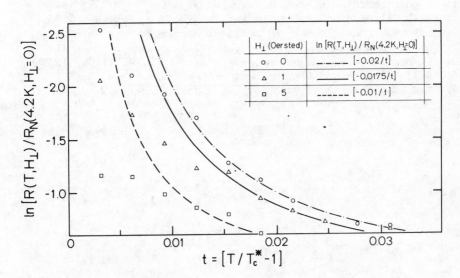

FIGURE 4 - Experimental $\ln(R/R_N)$ vs.t, measured in the fR 40P (20 x 20) sample (Ref. 16).

We see that the experimental points fall into an hyperbola, in qualitative agreement with theoretical calculations. It is difficult at present to say if they follow a $(1/t)$, or a $(1/t + xt^{\frac{1}{2}})$ dependence. The apparent change in the curve is also subject to caution (it correspond to the smallest resistance points and in consequence the larger error bars).

CONCLUSION

There are good indications that the second transition temperature T_c^* which we observe in $n_0 \times n_0$ proximity arrays might be interpreted as a Kosterlitz-Thouless transition. Several points however are still unclear and further work is necessary to confirm our results.

REFERENCES

1. J. Rosenblatt, Rev. Phys. Appl. 9, 217 (1974); J. Rosenblatt, A. Raboutou, P. Pellan, Low Temp. Phys - LT14, Ed. by Matti Krusius and Matti Vuorio (North-Holland Pub. Co.) Amsterdam (1975) 361.
2. D.U. Gubser & S.A. Wolf, J. Phys. Coll. 39, C6-579 (1978).
3. D.H. Sanchez & J.L. Berchier, to be published.
4. J.L. Berchier & D.H. Sanchez, Rev. Phys. Appl. 14, 757 (1979).
5. J.L. Berchier, Ph. D. Thesis (Geneva, Sept. 1979).
6. B. Giovannini & L. Weiss, Sol. State Commun. 28, 1005 (1978).
7. S.E. Barnes, Phys. Lett. 66A, 422 (1978).
8. J.L. Berchier & D.H. Sanchez, Rev. Sci. Instrum. 49, 1452 (1978).
9. J.L. Berchier & D.H. Sanchez, to be published.
10. S.A. Wolf, D.U. Gubser and Y. Imry, Phys. Rev. Lett. 42, 324 (1979).
11. B. Giovannini & L. Weiss, Helv. Phys. Acta 51, 716 (1978).
12. B.I. Halperin and P.C. Hohenberg, Phys. Rev. 188, 898 (1969).
13. S.K. Ma, Modern theory of critical phenomena (Benjamin 1976).
14. D.R. Nelson and J.M. Kosterlitz, Phys. Rev. Lett 39, 1201 (1977).
15. S. Doniach & B.A. Huberman, Phys. Rev. Lett. 42, 1169 (1979).
16. B.I. Halperin and D.R. Nelson, J. Low Temp. Phys. 36, 599 (1979).
17. D.H. Sanchez & J.L. Berchier, this conference.

Superconductivity in 2D Granular NbN

D.U. Gubser, S.A. Wolf, T.L. Francavilla, and J.L. Feldman
Naval Research Laboratory, Washington, DC 20375

ABSTRACT

The systematics of superconductivity in 2D granular NbN are reported as a function of variable intergranular coupling strength $J_{gg'}$. The characteristics of the resistive transition, the critical currents and the dynamical I-V response are markedly altered by variations in $J_{gg'}$. The results of this study are consistent with previous investigations of 2D granular NbN where three critical temperatures T_{cg} (superconducting transition of individual grains), T_{cj} (2D phase ordering transition) and T* (sudden increase in I_c) were identified. As the coupling $J_{gg'}$ decreases, the critical fluctuation region above T_{cj} increases in magnitude and in temperature span. Similarly, the temperature T* moves to lower temperatures relative to T_{cj} as $J_{gg'}$ decreases. Examination of the I-V response curves revealed a hitherto unidentified characteristic temperature T_s which marks a change in the dynamic response of these 2D NbN films.

INTRODUCTION

The superconducting properties of granular NbN differ from other granular superconductors in several respects. First, since the coherence length ξ_o is approximately 50 A in NbN, the isolated NbN grains of nominal diameter $d \sim 2 \xi_o$ become superconducting at a characteristic temperature T_{cg}.[8] In most other granular systems (i.e. Al,[1] Pb,[2] or Hg[3]), the grain size is substantially less than the coherence length, i.e. $d_g \ll \xi_o$; hence, the grains themselves do not become fully superconducting. The development of a superconducting state in these other granular materials requires a moderately strong intergranular interaction which creates regions or clusters where the grains act collectively to nucleate the superconducting state. A second important difference from other granular systems is that NbN is a high T_c (15.5K) superconductor. The higher T_c brings interesting features of the granular superconducting transition into experimentally accessible temperature regions and permits clear separation of various temperature regimes where different interactions dominate the character of the transition. A third difference between the 2D NbN granular system reported here and other granular systems is the relatively uniform coupling between grains due to the fabrication procedure (anodization of polycrystalline NbN films).

160

Granular films prepared either by evaporation in an oxygen or inert gas atmosphere or by co-evaporation with an insulating material have more random coupling between grains. The dynamics of the superconducting transition are different for these two types of coupling. Uniform coupling in granular NbN leads to a phase-ordering transition at T_{cj} while nonuniform coupling leads to a transition dominated by percolation effects.

Previous publications have examined the temperature intervals 1) $T > T_{cg}$ where zero dimensional (OD) characteristics of the individual NbN grains were observed[4,5], 2) $T \simeq T_{cj}$ where the dynamics of the 2D superconducting transition were investigated,[5-7] and 3) $T < T_{cj}$ where the critical current dependence $I_c(T)$ in the superconducting state was reported.[8] The latter investigation revealed an unusual increase in I_c at a characteristic temperature designated T^*. In this article, we present measurements on 4 granular NbN films possessing significantly different intergranular coupling strengths J_{gg}, in order to study the systematics of the variations of T^* and T_{cj} with J_{gg}. The data revealed the presence of yet another characteristic temperature below T_{cj} which is designated T_s and which indicates a change in the dynamical response of the sample.

EXPERIMENTAL DETAILS

Polycrystalline NbN films were prepared by reactively sputtering onto heated quartz cylindrical substrates which were continuously rotated during the sputtering process to provide uniform thickness films, typically 100A to 200A thick. Grain size in these films was varied by changing either the substrate temperature or film thickness and was estimated from line widths of x-ray crystallographic reflections.

The granular region was produced by partially anodizing the polycrystalline film in an electrolytic cell containing a concentrated solution of boric acid.[9] The nominal film thickness t of the remaining layer of unanodized NbN was estimated by monitoring the anodization voltage across the cell. When t was reduced below approximately 70 A, the grains began to separate since anodization proceeds fastest along the grain boundaries. Samples under investigation were anodized to

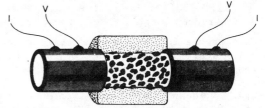

Fig. 1 - A schematic illustration of a cylindrical sample. The NbN film is deposited on a 1 mm diameter quartz rod. The central portion is anodized which leaves the NbN grains embedded in an oxide matrix. Current and voltage leads are attached as indicated.

nominal film thickness's of 30A at which point the grains were separated by an insulating oxide barrier of approximately 10A to 20A. Figure 1 is a schematic diagram of the sample showing the anodized 2D granular region and the unanodized NbN ends which serve as current-voltage contacts.

The samples were mounted in a dilution refrigerator which could span temperatures from 30 mk to room temperature. The resistance $R(T)$, current-voltage $(I-V)$, and critical current $I_c(T)$ characteristics of the various films were determined by a dc 4 terminal technique in which all leads to the sample were rf shielded and filtered. Similarly the dilution refrigerator in which the samples were located was surrounded by both magnetic and superconducting shields which provided a stable, low magnetic field, $H<10^{-6}$ tesla, environment. Such shielding precautions were necessary for measurements of samples with small intergranular coupling interactions since rf noise significantly lowered T_{cj}, changed the curvature of $R(T)$ near T_{cj}, and reduced $I_c(T)$ in the region below T_{cj}.

Current densities in the granular sample used for measuring resistance in the $I \longrightarrow 0$ limit were of the order of 10^3 amp/m^2 (0.1 amp/cm^2). Critical currents $I_c(T)$ in the superconducting state were taken to be the current value corresponding to the first detectable onset of resistance which was essentially a 0.1 μV voltage criteria set by the sensitivity limit of the voltmeter.

EXPERIMENTAL RESULTS

Figure 2 shows the sheet resistance vs temperature $R_\square(T)$ for 4 different granular NbN films. Two of these samples (B and D) have a grain size of approximately 150 A nominal diameter $(d_g > 2\xi_o)$ while the other two samples (A and C) have a grain size of approximately 75A diameter $(d_g < 2\xi_o)$. All samples possessed activated resistance at temperature $T \gg T_{cg}$, i.e. all increased in resistance as the temperature was lowered. The peak resistance for sample D was 400 $\Omega/\square$ which was only a few percent larger than the room temperature value (note in Fig. 2, 10R$_\square$ is plotted to aid resolution) while the peak resistance for sample A was 50,000 $\Omega/\square$, a 10 fold increase over its room temperature value. This activated behavior is consistent with a model whereby the grains are assumed isolated from one another by a non-metallic oxide barrier and electron transport is controlled by a thermally activated tunneling of electrons. This single particle tunneling and, hence, $R_\square$ is proportional to the spacing s between grains.

As the temperature of the sample nears T_{cg}, effects due to the superconducting properties of the individual grains became apparent. In the large grained samples (D and B) this effect is easily observable as a drop in resistance occurring at the transition temperature of the grains ($T_{cg} \approx 13.5$K). The effects

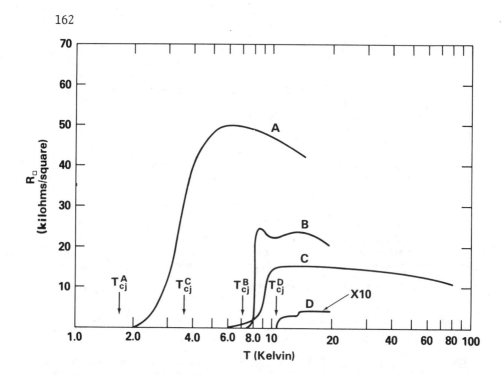

Fig. 2. - Resistance transitions of 4 different 2D granular NbN films. T_{cj} of the individual films are marked for reference.

due to superconductivity in the isolated grains is more subtle in the small grained specimens since superconductivity in these grains is weakened when $d_g < 2\xi_o$. Nevertheless, the effects on $R_\square(T)$ of superconductivity associated with individual grains are present in samples A and C as evidenced by the observation of zero dimensional (OD) superconducting fluctuations in the temperature interval $T_{cg} < T < 2 T_{cg}$,[4,5]. The OD character of these fluctuations is further evidence that the properties of the overall system are determined by the electronic properties of small individual grains weakly coupled to one another across insulating barriers.

At temperatures $T < T_{cg}$ the grains begin to strongly interact with one another, due to the Josephson or pair particle tunneling interaction, and the overall resistance of the film drops rapidly. The strength of this Josephson coupling interaction J_{gg}, controls the character of the curve and is dependent on both the intergranular spacing s, which predominantly influences $R_\square$, and the grain size d_g which effects the magnitude of the pair wave function in the grains. For the strongest coupled sample D (i.e. small $R_\square$ and large grains d_g), one observes a relatively sharp transition to the R=0 state at T_{cj}. This type of overall transition is characteristic of most other granular systems. As one reduces the coupling interaction by increasing the separation between grains, (i.e. increasing $R_\square$), the transition temperature T_{cj} is lowered and a small resistance "tail" begins to appear prior to the completed transition at T_{cj}. The small grained sample C has a weaker Josephson coupling than the large grained sample B i.e. $J_{gg}^C, < J_{gg}^B$, even though $R_\square^C < R_\square^B$. The reduction of Josephson coupling due to a decrease in grain size more than compensates for the tendency of the interaction to increase as s becomes smaller. Sample C has a smaller T_{cj} and a larger resistive tail than either samples D or B. The weakest coupling sample A is produced by increasing the separation s between grains in the small grained film. In this sample, T_{cj} has been reduced to 1.6K and the resistive tail is very pronounced.

The resistance tails about T_{cj} increase in magnitude and in temperature range as the coupling $J_{gg},$ decreases and they have a universal temperature dependence which is accurately represented by a power law function,

$$R(T) \; \alpha \; (T-T_{cj})^\mu \qquad , \qquad (1)$$

where μ is 3.7 ± 0.3. Such power law resistance dependences are expected within critical fluctuation regions near phase transitions. The temperature width for the critical region above a 2D granular phase ordering transition increases as $J_{gg}^{-1},$, which is also consistent with the observed increase in the resistance tail portion of the transition curve. Lack of a significant resistance tail in sample D is interpreted as evidence that the critical region for the phase ordering transition in this film with large intergranular coupling is smaller than experimental resolution.

Previous publications[4-6] have demonstrated that the current-voltage characteristics within the resistance tail region obey the stringent mathematical rules predicted from critical phenomena theory. Namely, current-voltage measurements within this region are accurately described by the scaling equation

$$V = bI^\nu \chi(z) \qquad bI^\nu \chi\left(\frac{d(T-T_{cj})}{I^\lambda}\right) \qquad , \qquad (2)$$

where b and d are sample dependent constants, ν and λ are sample independent exponents and χ is a universal function of $z = d(T-T_{cj})/I^\lambda$ The exponents and constants in this expression are obtained from the two limits

164

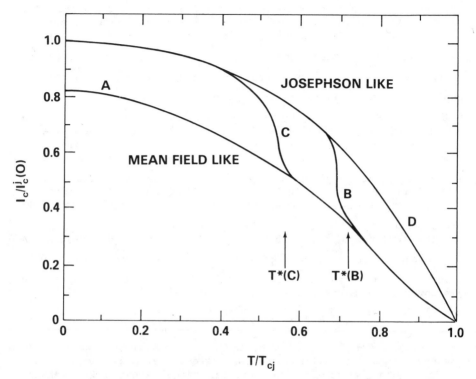

Fig. 3. - Reduced critical current vs temperature plots of the 4 NbN films shown in figure 2. Curves are normalized to $I_c^J(0)$ and T_{cj}. T* for samples C and B are marked. T* for sample D is essentially 1 while T* for sample A is zero.

$$(V/I)_{I \longrightarrow 0} = R = a \Delta T^{\mu} = a(T-T_{cj})^{\mu}$$

and   (3)

$$V_{\Delta T \longrightarrow 0} = bI^{\nu}$$

along with the relations $\nu - \lambda\mu = 1$ and $d^{\mu} = a/b$. The critical exponents characteristic of granular NbN are $\mu = 3.7 \pm 0.3$, $\nu = 3.0 \pm 0.2$ and $\lambda = 0.57 \pm .1$. Similarly, using the same formalism, the critical current $I_c(T)$ below T_{cj} can be uniquely determined

$$I_c = d(T_{cj}-T)^{1/\lambda} \qquad , \qquad (4)$$

where d and λ are the same constants that appear in Eq. 2. This temperature dependent form for I_c is valid for sample currents which obey Eq. 2 i.e. for currents small enough that critical fluctuations above $T_c(I)$ still exist. Equation 4 has previously been experimentally verified.[7] The temperature exponent $1/\lambda$ for the critical current is 1.7 $\pm$ 0.2 which is near the Ginzburg-Landau mean field result of 1.5. The consistency of the V-I-T measurements with critical phenomena scaling theories is further support of our interpretation that the characteristics of the transition near T_{cj} are dominated by critical fluctuations around a 2D phase order- ing superconducting transition.

A complete mapping of $I_c(T)$ below T_{cj} reveals qualitative differences in the shapes of the curves for samples A through D. Figure 3 shows the reduced critical current vs reduced temperature curves for these samples. The strongest coupled sample D had a Josephson temperature dependence[10] $I_c^J(T)$ over almost all the temper- ature range below T_{cj}. Only very near T_{cj} at small I_c did the data slightly deviate from the Josephson temperature dependence. Sample B, for which the coupling was weaker, had a Josephson like tempera- ture dependence at low temperatures, but at temperatures approaching T^*, I_c rapidly fell and the dependence above T^* was approximately mean field like, $I_c^{MF}(T)$, approaching T_{cj} with a $\Delta T^{1.7}$ power depen- dence. Sample C was sequentially weaker in coupling than D or B and was Josephson like $I_c^J(T)$ at low temperature but the cross-over temperature T^* to the mean field like temperature dependence I_c^{MF} occurred at a lower reduced temperature. The weakest coupling sample A remained mean field like $I_c^{MF}(T)$ to temperatures less than 0.05K; however, indications (see below) of a cross over to the Josephson like dependence were apparent at the lowest temperatures making it possible to normalize the data to $I_c^J(0)$ as with the other curves.

The I-V characteristics as well as $I_c(T)$ change markedly as the temperature is reduced (see Fig. 4). At temperatures T < T_{cj} the I-V curves are smooth and non-linear possessing a finite critical current I_c. As the temperature is reduced, the I-V curves change in character at a temperature T_s where a small voltage discontinuity or step begins to appear (not discernable with resolu- tion shown in figure 4) and the I-V curves have a linear differ- ential resistance at high voltages. At temperatures T<T^*, the voltage step increases in size, the finite resistance at currents below the step rapidly diminishes (creating the earlier noted I_c fall), and the voltage above the step falls on the same straight line possessing a finite current intercept.

The insert in Fig. 4 shows the $I_c(T)$ dependence of sample C indicating the various characteristic temperatures. The temperature dependence of the current where the step occurs is given by $I_c^J(T)$ even at temperatures above T^* (dashed line). For sample A, the lowest measured temperature of 0.05 K was below T_s; hence, $I_c^J(0)$ could be experimentally determined.

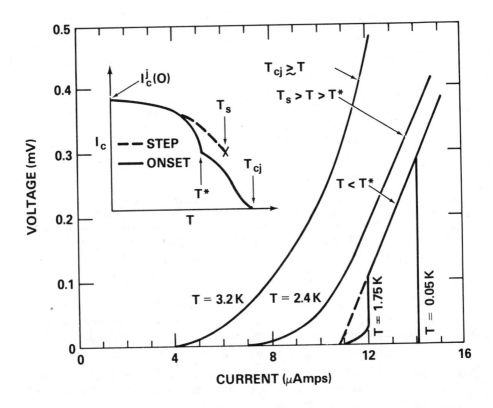

Fig. 4. - Current-Voltage characteristics for sample C taken at 4 different temperatures. Insert in the figure is a schematic drawing of the $I_c(T)$ curve to indicate the relative position of the various critical temperatures.

DISCUSSION

Interpretation of the various critical temperatures, T_{cg}, T_{cj}, T^*, and T_s, in terms of a microscopic theory has proven difficult. T_{cg} is fairly well understood as the mean field superconducting transition temperature of the individual grains. The scaling laws observed near T_{cj} indicate that a phase transition is occuring at T_{cj} but the details of the interaction leading to this transition are not clear. Some arguments[11] have been presented suggesting that T_{cj} is a 2D topological phase transition of the type described by Kosterlitz and Thouless.[12] The two transitions at T^* and T_s are less clear from a microscopic viewpoint although a previous publication[8] has associated T*, rather than T_{cj}, with the 2D topological phase transition.

Superconductivity in 2 dimensions is predicted to result from a binding of thermally excited vortex-antivortex pairs at T_c^{2D}. At temperatures above T_c^{2D}, a flux flow resistance due to unbound vortices will be present in the film until at a higher temperature, called T_c^{BCS}, the film begins to return to the normal state.[11,13,14] Theories of the 2D vortex-antivortex transition in superconductivity treat the region above T_c^{2D} as a critical region for vortex fluctuations and calculate the number of unbound vortices, and consequently the flux flow resistance, within the framework of fluctuation theory. Halperin and Nelson[14] obtain near T_c^{2D} a resistance of the form

$$R = K_1 \, e^{-K_2/(T-T_c^{2D})^{1/2}} . \tag{5}$$

Attempts to fit our data on 2D granular NbN to a resistance of this functional form were unsuccessful using either T* or T_{cj} as T_c^{2D}. However, if T_s is identified with T_c^{2D} then the resistance, which becomes measureable only above T_{cj}, can be fit accurately to Eq. 5 although the constants K_1 and K_2 are larger than theoretical estimates. If T_s is T_c^{2D}, then T_{cj} would be associated with T_c^{BCS} (as previously suggested in reference 8). T* may be a dimensionality cross-over similar to the type described by Klemm, Luther and Beasley.[15] The change in critical current dependence at T* is thought to be due to the formation of well-defined Josephson vortices with cores confined to the region between the grains. Further experimental input and theoretical analysis are needed to clarify these concepts.

REFERENCES

1. W.L. McLean, T. Chui, B. Bandyopadhyay, and P. Lindenfeld, see article in this proceedings.
2. A.F. Hebard, see article in this proceedings.
3. E. Epstein, A.M. Goldman, E.D. Dahlbert, and R. Mikkelson, see article in this proceedings.
4. S. Wolf and W.H. Lowrey, Phy. Rev. Lett. 39, 1038 (1977).
5. D.U. Gubser and S.A. Wolf, J. Phys. (Paris), Colloq. 39, C6-579 (1978).

6. S.A. Wolf, D.U. Gubser, and Y. Imry, Phy. Rev. Lett. $\underline{42}$, 324 (1979).

7. S.A. Wolf, D.U. Gubser, J.L. Feldman, and Y. Imry, Proc. of the "d&f Band Superconductivity Conference" (1979).

8. D.U. Gubser and S.A. Wolf, Solid State Comm. $\underline{32}$, 449 (1979).

9. S. Wolf, J. Kennedy, and M. Nisenoff, J. Vac. Sci. Technol. $\underline{13}$, 145 (1976).

10. V. Ambegaokar and A. Baratoff, Phys. Rev. Lett. $\underline{10}$, 486 (1963).

11. B.A. Huberman and S. Doniach, see article in this proceedings.

12. J.M. Kosterlitz and D.M. Thouless, J. Phys. $\underline{C6}$, 1181 (1973).

13. M.R. Beasley, J.E. Mooij, and T.P. Orlando, Phys. Rev. Lett. $\underline{42}$, 1165 (1979).

14. B.I. Halperin and D.R. Nelson, J. Low Temp. Phys. $\underline{36}$, 599 (1979).

15. R.A. Klemm, A. Luther, and M.R. Beasley, Phys. Rev. B$\underline{12}$, 877 (1975).

GRANULAR WEAK LINK JOSEPHSON DEVICES

by

J. H. Claassen, E. J. Cukauskas, and M. Nisenoff
Naval Research Laboratory, Washington, DC 20375

ABSTRACT

Weak links incorporating granular Aℓ, Nb, and NbN
have exhibited a variety of Josephson phenomena and show
high promise as SQUID elements, mm-wave detectors, and
possibly switching devices. Current theoretical ideas
indicate that a vortex-flow model should be used to explain
these results. Several pieces of experimental evidence are
in conflict with this model, and suggest that a true
Josephson effect is involved.

Josephson devices have been intensively studied ever since the
discovery of the effect. To produce such a device it is necessary to
"weakly couple" two superconducting electrodes. In the classical
realization of the effect, the coupling is via electron tunneling
across a thin insulating layer. However, the material separating the
electrodes is by no means limited to an insulator - semiconductors,
semimetals, normal metals, and a second superconductor have all been
used successfully as the intervening layer. In this paper we will
consider the prospects of using a granular superconductor as the
separating region, in the "weak link" geometry. We will see that the
existing theoretical approach predicts that an "ideal" Josephson effect
should be difficult to realize in this case, although many Josephson-
like phenomena should be present. Experimental evidence, however,
increasingly supports the idea that a true Josephson effect can be
obtained with relative ease.

Figure 1a illustrates the weak-link geometry that is to be discussed. The bridge region serves to partially decouple the superconducting wave functions of the electrodes. If its thickness is comparable to that of the electrode films, the requirement of weak
coupling implies that its transition temperature T_c should be less
than that of the banks. (For simplicity we are ignoring the weakening
effects that occur as a result of current concentration in the plane of
the electrode films, as occurs in a Dayem bridge.) Alternatively the
thickness of the bridge can be made much less than the electrodes. The
latter option turns out to be much more desirable from a device stand-
point,[1] and has been widely studied in the last few years. Inevitably
as the thickness of the weak link film is reduced it will become
granular in nature, to the extent that local variations in thickness
become the main determinant of local properties of the film.

Although granular materials are quite effective in decoupling the
electrodes, they have been one of the least studied weak link materials
to date. One reason for this has to do with another requirement for

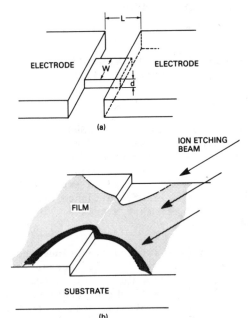

Figure 1. (a) Schematic drawing of a weak link. (b) Representation of a technique to produce weak links whose length L is as small as a few hundreds of angstroms. The ion beam selectively thins the film along the step riser, thereby defining the weak link region. The width W is established by conventional photolithography, and is $\gtrsim 1$ μm.

realization of the Josephson effect, that the superconducting electrons that "leak" from one electrode to the other must retain their memory of the initial wave function (that is, certain correlations must remain). Existing theory[1] for metallic weak link structures shows that this requires that the electrodes not be separated by much more than the coherence length of the weak link material, given by $\xi = .36$ $(\hbar v_F \ell / k \Delta T)^{\frac{1}{2}}$ in dirty materials. Here ℓ is the electron mean free path in the weak link material, and ΔT is the difference between the operating temperature and the critical temperature T_c of the weak link. In granular materials the apparent mean free path is very small. Critical field measurements seem to show that the above expression for ξ remains valid in this limit - i.e., the Ginzberg-Landau theory remains valid in granular materials with very short effective mean free paths.[2] In granular Aℓ, for example, coherence lengths of ~100Å at T = 0 have been inferred,[3] compared to ~10^4 Å for the metal. The requirement that the weak link length L be $\lesssim \xi$ thus becomes extremely difficult to meet in practice.

In the above discussion we have used the most stringent definition of the Josephson effect, that the supercurrent that flows across the weak link depends sinusoidally on the difference in phase of the order parameter in the electrodes. This is frequently referred to as the dc Josephson effect. In weak links that are longer than a few times ξ the current-phase relationship (CPR) becomes reentrant (multiple valued)[1] rather than sinusoidal. Another mechanism then takes over that can mimic many of the phenomena associated with an ideal Josephson junction. It becomes possible for a vortex (unit of

quantized flux) to exist in the weak link.[1] At a critical value of
the current density, vortices are nucleated at the film edge and
move across the film transverse to the current flow.[4] By the well-
known ideas of flux-flow in Type II superconductors,[4] a voltage must
then appear across the electrodes in the form of a series of pulses
(each corresponding to nucleation of another vortex). If there is a
single line of vortices in the weak link, the frequency of the pulses
is 2eV/h where V is the average voltage. Superposition of an ac current at a frequency commensurate with the natural rate of formation
of vortices should tend to correlate them. This results in steps in
the I-V characteristic at voltages mhf/ne, where f is the impressed
frequency and m and n are integers.

All of the effects mentioned above are associated with the "ideal"
Josephson effect as well. For them to be seen in a vortex flow
geometry two requirements must be met:[4] (1) the electromagnetic size
of the vortex, $\lambda_\perp$, should be greater than the separation between
electrodes, and (2) pinning forces on the vortices should be negligible. Granular materials satisfy both requirements easily. In a Nb
film which has been thinned by anodization to the onset of granular
behavior, $d \approx 50$ Å, we have $\lambda_\perp = 2\lambda^2/d \cong 1.5\,\mu m\ (T_c/\Delta T)$, where λ is the
penetration depth. It is a well-known feature of granular films,
moreover, that the pinning forces are much smaller than in bulk
films.[2]

Virtually all calculations of the performance of practical
devices utilizing the Josephson effect[5,6] have assumed that "ideal"
junctions are used. It is widely acknowledged that the ultimate performance of these devices is obtained only for ideal junctions. On
the other hand, it is clear that a vortex-flow device should work
with some degree of success in many applications - rf and dc SQUIDs,
microwave mixers, and low power switching devices, for example. In
the absence of detailed calculations we have very little idea how
much the performance is degraded when a flux-flow junction is used in
place of an ideal junction. It may very well be that granular weak
links provide advantages that outweigh a slight loss in performance.
A case in point is the rf SQUID application. Here the biggest
practical difficulty in using a weak link is to obtain a low enough
critical current. The low critical current density of granular
materials greatly eases this problem.[7] Experience indicates[8] that
adequate SQUID performance can be obtained from weak links having a
reentrant CPR. To take advantage of the ultimate capability of an
ideal junction, on the other hand, would require operation at quite
high frequencies (>10 GHz) and the availability of an extremely low
noise preamplifier.[8]

The vortex-flow picture of granular weak links discussed above
can be described as the "official" view, based as it is on the
Ginzberg-Landau theory of weak links.[1] This theory has been quite
successful in accounting for much of the behavior of metallic weak
links.[9] There is, however, a growing body of evidence that the

vortex flow picture is not correct for granular weak links, and that they may be closer to ideal Josephson junctions than has been suspected. Most dramatic is the direct measurement by the Cornell group[10] of a nearly sinusoidal current-phase relationship in a granular Nb weak link shown in Fig. 2. If vortices could exist in the weak link we would expect a highly reentrant CPR (large critical phase angle). A rough estimate of the GL coherence length for the device in Fig. 2 gives $\xi \sim 60\text{Å}$ $(T_c/\Delta T)^{\frac{1}{2}}$. The GL theory predicts that the weak link CPR is single-valued (critical phase angle $<\pi$) only if $L < 3.5 \, \xi$. This would only occur for $(\Delta T/T_c) < 10^{-4}$, whereas in fact a sinusoidal CPR is observed down to $\Delta T/T_c \simeq 0.2$.

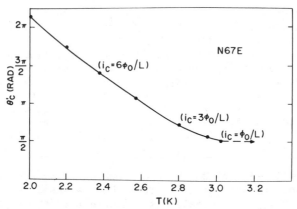

Figure 2. A direct measurement of the current-phase relationship of a granular Nb weak link. A critical phase angle of $\pi/2$ implies a nearly sinusoidal CPR, while the value π signals the onset of a multiple-valued CPR. In addition a direct measurement of the intrinsic noise of a SQUID incorporating this device was made[10] and found to agree with the Kurkijarvi-Webb calculation[6] for temperatures which gave a sinusoidal CPR. T_c of the weak link was ~3.6K.

Further indirect evidence of a sinusoidal CPR comes from measurements of granular weak links in the rf SQUID configuration. A particular parameter, the step slope ratio α, has been shown to figure importantly in the noise performance of rf SQUIDs Both experimental and theoretical evidence[8] imply that excess values can be attributed to non-sinusoidal CPRs. Figure 3 shows the measured values of α for a number of granular weak link SQUIDs along with the predicted dependence assuming a sinusoidal CPR.[11] All of these devices, according to the GL theory, should be in the vortex-flow regime.

Recently, we have been studying the current-voltage characteristics of granular NbN weak links. Step structure induced by microwave frequencies as high as 25 GHz has indeed been seen in some devices that were fabricated by the same technique that yielded good

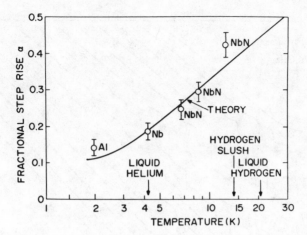

Figure 3.   The step slope ratio α is plotted as a function
of operating temperature for a number of rf SQUIDs using a
granular weak link.   The critical current and inductance
were approximately the same in each case.   The solid line is
a theoretical prediction assuming a sinusoidal CPR.[8]

SQUID response.[12]   However a vortex-flow mechanism, as outlined above,
cannot completely be ruled out in explaining this data.   A complicating factor in interpretation of I-V results arises from the
increased power dissipation that is involved, in comparison to SQUID
measurements.   It can be presumed that granular material is a rather
poor conductor of heat, so that large local temperature increases
could occur at a modest power level.

A novel technique has recently been used in our laboratory to
make weak links that are much shorter than can be achieved by conventional photolithographic techniques.[13]   Its essential features are
illustrated in Fig. 1b.   Using NbN, weak link lengths as small as
~750Å have been produced.   Although the thinning procedure was different than was used in the SQUID devices (ion beam erosion rather
than anodization) there is strong evidence that the weak link is
granular.[13]   Reducing the length of the bridge in this manner should
improve the cooling, allowing a higher bias voltage to be investigated.
Note, however, that the weak link is still many times longer than the
coherence length, ~40Å in this case.

In Fig. 4 we show some initial results for one of these short
granular weak links.   Very well defined steps in the I-V curve are
seen with application of 70 GHz microwaves.   Several features of
these curves cannot be reconciled with existing predictions based on
the vortex flow model.[4]   The model indicates that the microwave-induced
step heights should increase monotonically with the microwave current.
Our data, on the other hand, clearly show steps which oscillate in

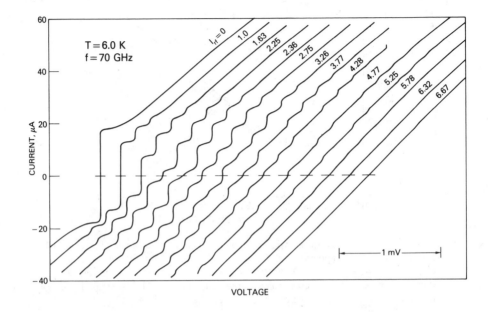

Figure 4. A family of current-voltage characteristics of a short granular NbN weak link, with increasing levels of 70 GHz radiation. The units of rf current are arbitrary. This device was fabricated by the technique illustrated in Fig. 1b, and has nominal weak link dimensions 1.5 μm x 750 Å.

size as the rf level is increased. Moreover, we see steps only at integral multiples of hf/2e while the model predicts additional "sub-harmonic" step structure. It has been found[13] that many features of the I-V curves in Fig. 4 can be fit rather well using the Resistively Shunted Junction model. In this model a sinusoidal CPR is assumed even at very high frequencies, and it follows from the GL theory of metallic weak links only if L << ξ.[1]

Finally, we note the work of Hu et al.[14] wherein the barrier in sandwich structure was formed by co-evaporation of Sn and Ge. The full range of Josephson phenomena, including steps in the I-V curve induced by 100 GHz radiation, were observed in devices with 600 Å thick barriers. It would not be surprising if these barrier films constitute a granular Sn system, especially in view of results that have been obtained by Deutscher et al.[15] for similarly prepared Ge-Pb, Ge-In, and Ge-Aℓ.

In conclusion, we feel that the mechanism for Josephson coupling between superconducting electrodes via granular material is an important unsolved problem. Treatment of thin granular films using the GL theory for dirty type II superconductors does not seem to be an adequate approach. More experimental information is clearly required, especially regarding the upper frequency limits in the short weak links and their current-phase relationships.

Whatever the physics of the short granular weak link shown in Fig. 4 may be, there is little doubt of its potential technological importance. Its resistance is 30-100 times greater than is usually reported for metallic weak links, and is at a convenient level for matching to a microwave network. The critical current is low enough for use in rf and dc SQUIDs. We are not aware of any other thin film weak link device that has shown nearly ideal step response at this high a frequency (70 GHz). Operation is not restricted to temperatures close to T_c. Finally the RI_c product, which is an important overall figure of merit,[5] is quite respectable at ~0.5 mV. These advantages make granular weak links prime contenders for use in low-noise mm-wave receivers, SQUIDs, and even micropower switching devices.

The authors would like to acknowledge many useful conversations with S.A. Wolf, who also performed some of the early SQUID measurements. One of us (JHC) thanks D. Prober for helpful advice about step edge fabrication techniques.

REFERENCES

1. K. K. Likharev, Rev. Mod. Phys. 51, 101 (1979).
2. B. Abeles, Applied Solid State Sci., Vol. 6, ed. Raymond Wolfe (Academic Press, NY, 1976).
3. B. Abeles, Roger W. Cohen, and W. R. Stowell, Phys. Rev. Lett. 18, 902 (1967).
4. K. K. Likharev, Sov. Phys. JETP 34, 906 (1972).
5. A.N. Vystavkin, V. N. Gubankov, L. S. Kuzmin, K. K. Likharev, V. V.Migulin, and V. K. Semenov, Res. Phys. Appl. 9, 79 (1974).
6. J. Kurkijarui and W. W. Webb, in Proc. Appl. Superconductivity Conf., Annapolis, MD, IEEE Pub. No. 73 VHO682-5-TABSC (IEEE, NY, 1972), p. 581.
7. G. Deutscher, in Future Trends in Superconductive Electronics, AIP Conf. Proc. No. 44, (American Institute of Physics, NY, 1978), p. 397.
8. L. D. Jackel and R. A. Buhrman, J. Low Temp. Phys. 19, 201 (1975).
9. V. N. Gubankov, V. P. Koshelets, and G.A. Ovsyamikov, Sov. Phys. JETP 44, 181 (1976).
10. R.A. Buhrman, private communication.
11. S.A. Wolf, E.J. Cukauskas, F.J. Rachford, and M. Nisenoff, IEEE Trans. Mag. MAG-15, 595 (79).
12. E. J. Cukauskas, J.H. Claassen, M. Nisenoff, C.H. Galfo, R.L. Steiner, and B.S. Deaver, this conference.
13. J. H. Claassen and M. Nisenoff, to be published.
14. E.L. Hu, L.D. Jackel, A.R. Strmad, R.W. Epworth, R.F. Lucey, C.A. Zogg, and E. Gormik, Appl. Phys. Lett. 32, 584 (1978).
15. G. Deutscher, M. Rappaport and Z. Ovadyahu, Sol. State Comm. 28, 593 (1978).

PINNING EFFECTS IN PERIODIC SUPERCONDUCTING
STRUCTURES

P. Martinoli
Institut de Physique, Université de Neuchâtel
CH-2000 Neuchâtel, Switzerland

J. R. Clem
Ames Laboratory-USDOE and Department of Physics,
Iowa State University, Ames, Iowa 50011, USA

ABSTRACT

Pinning effects in superconducting films with periodically
varying thickness in one dimension are reviewed. Peak structures in
the critical current vs magnetic field curves and Josephson-like
quantum phenomena in the flux-flow régime are described with models
based on the interaction of the vortex lattice with the periodic
potential created by the thickness modulation.

INTRODUCTION

The study of pinning phenomena in a variety of physical systems
where a lattice of coupled "particles" interacts with a periodic
force field has become a topic of considerable interest at the present time. In this paper we discuss pinning effects in type-II superconducting films whose thickness is periodically modulated in one
dimension. Some years ago we pointed out [1] that such a film structure
creates a periodic pinning potential for the vortex lattice induced
by a transverse magnetic field $H \approx B$. The resulting interaction gives
rise to pronounced peak structures in the critical current curves [1],
$j_c(B)$, and to Josephson-like quantum phenomena [2,3] in the flux-flow
régime. The physical picture emerging from these effects is excee-
dingly simple for a particular set of configurations the vortex
lattice assumes in the periodic film structure, but is surprisingly
complex in general. In this connection, we shall see that models
based on the formation of a superlattice of flux line dislocations
prove to be very useful in explaining some of the features characterizing periodic pinning structures.

STATIC INTERACTION - CRITICAL CURRENTS

Thickness modulated layers with a periodicity, λ_g, of the
order of ~ 1 µm were fabricated from oxygen-doped Al-films using
combined photolithographic and holographic techniques [1,4]. Typical
critical current data obtained for current flow parallel to the
grooves of the grating-like film profile are shown in Fig. 1 for a
layer having $\lambda_g = 1.1$ µm. The peaks appearing in the j_c vs. B curve
reflect the occurence of particular configurations assumed by the
vortex lattice in the periodic film structure. In the discussion

which follows we shall distinguish between two classes of configurations, namely matching and non-matching configurations.

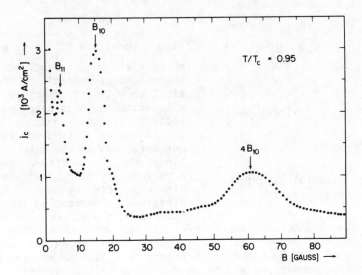

Fig. 1   Critical current density vs transverse magnetic
field for a modulated film (λ_g = 1.1 μm).

In a matching configuration the vortex lattice is in registry with the periodic pinning structure. This occurs whenever $\vec{q} = \vec{g}$, $\vec{q}$ being the wave vector of the thickness modulation (q = $2\pi/\lambda_g$) and $\vec{g}$ a reciprocal vector of the triangular vortex lattice. In terms of B this condition becomes [5]

$$B_{n_1 n_2} = (\sqrt{3}/2)\,(\varphi_0/\lambda_g^2)\,(n_1^2 + n_2^2 + n_1 n_2)^{-1} \qquad (1)$$

where φ_0 is the flux quantum and n_1, n_2 are integers. Obviously, for j = 0 the vortices are located at the bottom of the potential wells represented by the thickness minima[1]. When j gradually increases from zero, all vortices, under the influence of the Lorentz driving force $\vec{F}_L = \vec{j} \times \vec{\varphi}_0$, are uniformly shifted from the bottom of the corresponding wells by a distance u determined by the equilibrium condition $\vec{F}_L + \vec{F}_P = 0$, where $\vec{F}_P = \vec{F}_{P0} \sin qu$ is the periodic pinning force. This can be written in the form

$$j = j_{cM} \sin \varphi \qquad (2)$$

a relation which shows how the vortex lattice adjusts its phase φ = qu with respect to the periodic pinning structure as j varies from zero (φ = 0) to the critical value $j_{cM} = F_{P0}/\varphi_0$ ($\varphi = \pi/2$). On account of the highly coherent nature of the pinning interaction resulting from the absence of lattice restoring forces in matching configurations [5], j_{cM} is the largest supercurrent the vortex lattice

178

can sustain in modulated films. Using Eq. (1), the j_c-maxima at B_{10} and B_{11} in Fig. 1 can indeed be assigned to the fundamental matching configurations shown in Fig. 2.

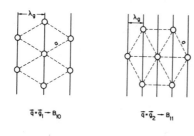

$\vec{q}\cdot\vec{q}_1 - B_{10}$ $\vec{q}\cdot\vec{q}_2 - B_{11}$

Fig. 2   Fundamental matching
configurations.

The case of non-matching configurations ($B \neq B_{n_1 n_2}$) is more complex and only recently has been the object of preliminary theoretical work [5,6]. To simplify the discussion, in this paper we shall neglect the two-dimensional nature of the vortex lattice and restrict our attention to the case of a linear chain of vortices placed in a periodic pinning structure [4]. Although suffering from obvious limitations in describing the true situation of our experiments, the one-dimensional model considered here has the merit of clearly showing the essential aspects of the pinning problem. Recently, a similar model has been used by Sacco and Sokoloff [7] to discuss pinning phenomena in charge density wave systems and superionic conductors.

As shown in Ref. 4, relaxation of an originally unperturbed vortex chain, of natural lattice parameter a, into the periodic potential results in the formation of a vortex-defect superlattice if the vortex array is commensurate with the pinning structure, i.e. if $a/\lambda_g = M/N$ where M and N are integers. The period of the superstructure is given by $\lambda_s = M\lambda_g = Na$, provided M and N have no common factor. The chain defects, whose average spacing is $\lambda_D = \lambda_s/|M-N| = a\lambda_g/|a-\lambda_g|$, turn out to be vacancies if M > N, or interstitials if M < N, and may be thought of as one-dimensional dislocations.

To describe the superlattice further, we need an expression for the pinning induced restoring force, F_{Rm}, exerted by the chain on the vortex m. For convenience, we first consider the case of a Hooke's law interaction force of the form :

$$F_{Rm} = \mu \, (u_{m+1} - 2u_m + u_{m-1}) \qquad (3)$$

where μ is the force constant. The true long-range interaction among vortices in thin superconducting films will be considered later on. Using Eq. (3), the equilibrium conditions $\vec{F}_L + \vec{F}_{Pm} + \vec{F}_{Rm} = 0$ for the N vortices forming the basis of an elementary cell of the superlattice are expressed by a set of N coupled non-linear equations of the form :

$$j/j_{cM} + \sin \varphi_m - \beta(\varphi_{m+1} - 2\varphi_m + \varphi_{m-1}) = 0 \qquad (4)$$

supplemented with periodic boundary conditions. In Eq. (4) $\beta = \mu/qF_{Po}$ is a parameter measuring the relative strength of the pinning force with respect to that of the interaction force. Thus, a pinning structure is said to be weak or strong according to whether $\beta \gg 1$ or $\beta \ll 1$.

We first discuss the case j = 0. If β is large enough ($\beta \gtrsim 1$), the phase displacement φ varies slowly over distances of the order of λ_g. Accordingly, one can use a continuum approximation, where the set (4) reduces to a "sine-Gordon" equation. Its solution φ(x) is a stair-shaped function [4] representing a regular sequence of dislocations with period λ_D, each dislocation extending over a range of the order of $\lambda_g\sqrt{\beta}$. Therefore, if $\lambda_g\sqrt{\beta} \ll \lambda_D$, the dislocations are well resolved and φ changes rather abruptly by 2π at the defect sites. In the opposite limit ($\lambda_g\sqrt{\beta} \gg \lambda_D$) the dislocations interact strongly with each other. As a result, they are washed out leaving a nearly harmonically distorted chain.

The situation is more delicate if one considers the critical currents of the vortex chain. In this connection, we first notice that j_c vanishes in the continuum approximation discussed above. As a matter of fact, in this limit the energy of the vortex array turns out to be independent of its position relative to the periodic pinning structure. This clearly indicates that, to decide whether the vortex chain is pinned or not, it is essential to take into account the discrete nature of the lattice. To compute j_c, one must therefore determine the critical positions of the vortices from the set (4) using numerical techniques. Critical currents for various commensurate configurations of the vortex chain are shown in Fig. 3. The following features emerging from this graph are worthwhile mentioning.

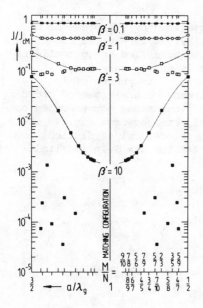

Fig. 3 Critical currents of a vortex chain in a harmonic pinning potential for a Hooke's law interaction force.

(i) For a given (rational) value of a/λ_g (and, consequently, of λ_D/λ_g) j_c decreases as β becomes larger and larger. Recalling our previous discussion, one is thus led to the conclusion that the presence of well resolved flux line dislocations is essential to produce a significant pinning effect.

(ii) For strong pinning structures ($\beta \ll 1$) j_c is largely independent of a/λ_g. This can be easily understood if one realizes that in this case j_c is essentially determined by the stability of a single dislocation, vortex chain defects being well isolated from each other over the whole range of a/λ_g. It can be shown that in this regime j_c is given by $j_c/j_{cM} = 1 - \beta'$, where $\beta' = 2\pi\beta$. Our numerical data are in good agreement with this expression.

180

(iii) For weak pinning structures ($\beta \gg 1$) we distinguish two diffe-
rent régimes. If a/λ_g is such that $\lambda_D < \lambda_g\sqrt{\beta}$, j_c shows profound oscillations as one proceeds through the set of configurations defined by
the ratio M/N. This is a manifestation of the basically different
response of commensurate (N finite) and incommensurate (N → ∞) vortex
chains to the Lorentz driving force $\vec{F}_L$. While a commensurate state
appears to be pinned ($j_c \neq 0$), an incommensurate chain can slide
freely ($j_c = 0$) if the pinning structure is sufficiently weak [4,7].

For $\lambda_D > \lambda_g\sqrt{\beta}$, a condition always satisfied if one is close
enough to a matching configuration (λ_D → ∞), the oscillations disap-
pear and j_c, as expected on the basis of the single dislocation picture outlined under (ii), saturates towards a constant value. This
suggests that there is a critical value, β_c, of β, given approximately by $\lambda_D \approx \lambda_g\sqrt{\beta_c}$, below which a distinction between commensurate and
incommensurate phases becomes irrelevant. Physically, β_c corresponds
to the onset of an appreciable interaction among dislocations.

In our experiments (Fig. 1) j_c-oscillations associated with com-
mensurate-incommensurate transitions were not observed. In this connection, it should be noticed that in real films the discrete nature
of the j_c-curves resulting from a strictly periodic pinning structure
is blurred by unavoidable inhomogeneities randomly distributed in the
metallic layer. For this reason we speculate that a more realistic
behaviour of j_c is that represented by the smooth dotted curves of
Fig. 1.

(iv) Weak pinning structures are characterized by the presence of
j_c-peaks at $a/\lambda_g = M/2$ (or, more generally, at $2\vec{q} = \vec{g}$), a condition
defining a particular set of configurations, called Bragg configura-
tions [5]. The origin of these structures is easily understood if one
considers the expansion of the chain energy [5] in powers of $1/\beta$. In
this expression Bragg configurations already occur in second order
(N = 2) and are therefore more strongly pinned than commensurate configurations of higher order. This clearly emerges from Fig. 4, where
numerical results are compared with the theoretical predictions
$j_c/j_{cM} = 1/8\beta$ for N = 2 and $j_c/j_{cM} = 1/24\beta^2$ for N = 3 in the limit
$\beta \gg 1$.

There are several indications
for the pinning mechanism operating in our modulated films to be
of moderate strength ($\beta \gtrsim 1$). Accordingly, the satellite structure
appearing at $B \approx 60$ G = 4 B_{10} in
Fig. 1 can be assigned to the
Bragg configuration $2\vec{q} = \vec{g}_1$. The
presence of higher harmonics in
the Fourier spectrum of the film

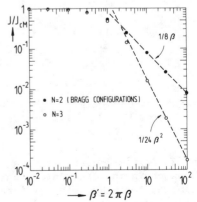

Fig. 4 Critical currents of the
2nd and 3rd order commensurate
configurations of the vortex chain.

profile [1,4], however, requires a certain precaution in attributing the total intensity of the Bragg peak at $4B_{10}$ to the effect predicted by Fig. 3.

(v) In Fig. 3 the onset of a matching configuration is characterized by a discontinuity in j_c, whereas the experimentally observed matching transitions are smooth (Fig. 1). One is tempted to interpret the finite width of the j_c-peaks at B_{10} and B_{11} in terms of a "statistical" matching effect reflecting the influence of random background pinning. However, a certain ambiguity arises if one realizes that an additional degree of freedom enters the problem of a two-dimensional vortex lattice interacting with a one-dimensional periodic potential. In this case the theoretical possibility of an intrinsically smooth registry transition cannot, a priori, be excluded. If this proves to be the case, then part of the width should be correlated with the elastic properties of the vortex lattice.

The critical current curves of Fig. 3 are symmetric about $a = \lambda_g$, a feature contrasting with the shape of our matching peaks (Fig. 1) and of those observed by Fiory et al. [8] in Al-films perforated by a triangular lattice of microholes. It can be shown that the symmetry characterizing Fig. 3 is a direct consequence of the particular form chosen for F_{Rm}. If, instead of Eq. (3), we introduce for a flux line located at x_m the Coulomb-like restoring force

$$F_{Rm} = (\varphi_0/2\pi)^2 \sum_n (x_m - x_n)^{-2} \tag{5}$$

appropriate for vortices in thin superconducting films (in the limit $|x_m - x_n| \gg \Lambda$, where Λ is an effective penetration depth), then our numerical analysis of the set (4) leads to the results shown in Fig. 5, where β' is now given by $\beta' = (\varphi_0/2\pi)^2 (\lambda_g/a^3 F_{P0})$. Most of the features previously discussed in connection with Fig. 3 are still present in Fig. 5. The j_c-curves, however, are no longer symmetric about a matching configuration. As a consequence of the Coulomb-like repulsion described by Eq. (5), dislocations created by interstitial vortices ($a < \lambda_g$) turn out to be less stable than those associated with vacancies ($a > \lambda_g$). Accordingly, when the vortex lattice slightly deviates from a matching configuration, j_c decreases more rapidly for $a < \lambda_g$ than for $a > \lambda_g$. As shown by Fig. 1

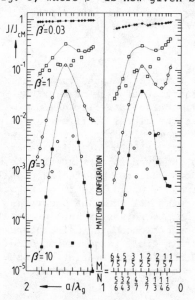

Fig. 5 Critical currents of a vortex chain in a harmonic pinning potential for a Coulomb-like interaction force.

this is the behaviour actually observed in our experiments.

DYNAMIC INTERACTION - QUANTUM EFFECTS

When j exceeds j_c a particular flux-flow régime occurs for matching configurations. As a matter of fact, dynamic coupling of the vortex lattice with the periodic pinning potential results in this case in a highly coherent velocity oscillation of the vortices [2,3]. This collective oscillation of the flux lines modulates the uniform motion of the lattice which would exist in the absence of pinning.

In terms of the uniform phase φ of the vortices defined in the previous section, their equation of motion can be written as

$$\gamma \, d\varphi/dt = j/j_{cM} + \sin \varphi \qquad (6)$$

where $\gamma = \eta/qF_{po}$ and η is the viscosity coefficient related to the flux-flow resistivity ρ_f by $\eta = B\varphi_0/\rho_f$. It is readily seen that Eq. (6) is identical to that governing the time-dependent phase in a resistively shunted Josephson junction. As shown by one of us [5], there is in fact a close analogy between flux-flow phenomena in periodic pinning structures and ac Josephson effects in arrays of superconducting weak links. Under ideal conditions (no random pinning), thickness modulated films in the dynamic matching state are equivalent to series arrays of highly synchronized resistive junction oscillators acting in phase and frequency coherence (superradiant state).

The pinning induced quantum oscillation of the vortex lattice in the dynamic matching state gives rise to an oscillating electric field $E(t) = B\dot{\varphi}(t)/q$, whose presence can be revealed by a sensitive detection system [3]. Since $E(t)$ has spectral components at frequencies, f_m, given by $f_m = mE_{dc}/B\lambda_g$, with a detector tuned at f_D radiofrequency (RF) signals associated with the voltage oscillation are expected whenever the condition $f_m = f_D$, i.e.

$$E_{dc} = \lambda_g f_D B/m \qquad (7)$$

is satisfied. Recorder traces of the RF detector output, tuned at $f_D = 45$ MHz, are shown in Fig. 6 as a function of E_{dc} for B-values about the matching field $B_{10} = 5$ G of a modulated Al-film having $\lambda_g = 1.9$ μm. It is readily verified that the signal positions agree with those predicted by Eq. (7) by setting m = 1. This shows that we have detected the fundamental component of $E(t)$. So far, higher harmonics of the oscillation have not been observed in our experiments.

As predicted by Eq. (7), Fig. 6 shows that the emitted RF signals shift linearly with B. In this connection, we would like to point out that for a strictly sinusoidal pinning potential RF signals corresponding to the quantum oscillation of the moving vortex lattice should appear only for $B = B_{n_1 n_2}$. However, although reduced in their intensity, RF signals were detected over a certain field range surrounding B_{10}. This is considered as further evidence for the statistical matching effect discussed in the previous section in connection with random pinning.

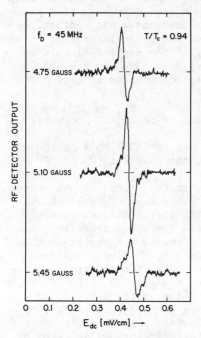

Fig. 6 RF signals emitted at 45 MHz by a thickness modulated Al-film (λ_g = 1.9 μm) about the matching field B_{10} = 5 G.

The largest RF power detected in our experiments amounts to about 10^{-14} W. This is several orders of magnitude smaller than that calculated from the superradiant model and the transmission characteristics of the detection system (about 10^{-10} W). This drastic RF power reduction is clearly due to partly uncorrelated vortex motion caused by random pinning.

A simple method providing indirect evidence for the collective oscillation of the vortices consists in exposing thickness modulated films to RF radiation. Pinning induced coupling at RF frequencies [2,4,5,9] gives rise to interference phenomena between the natural oscillation of the vortex lattice and the applied radiation field similar to those arising from ac quantum interference in superconducting weak links. As a result of a phase-locking mechanism, interference steps are expected in the RF-excited current (I)-voltage (V) characteristics of thickness modulated films. Fig. 7 shows I-V curves of two Al-films

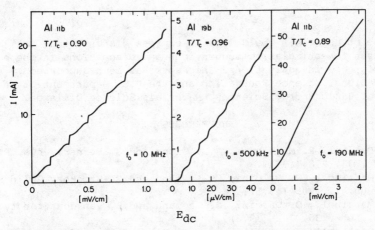

Fig. 7 I-V characteristics of thickness modulated Al-films exposed to RF radiation. λ_g is 1.1 μm and 1.9 μm for Al11b and Al19b respectively. The transverse magnetic field is B_{10}.

184

exposed to RF radiation of different frequencies. For all curves the
matching configuration is that defined by $\vec{q} = \vec{g}_1$ (Fig. 2). Step transitions occur whenever the frequencies mf associated with vortex motion in the various harmonic components of the periodic pinning structure become multiples of the frequency f_o of the applied electromagnetic field. Since the fundamental frequency f is given by $f = v/\lambda_g =$
$E_{dc}/B\lambda_g$ (where v is the flux-flow velocity), the steps of Fig. 7 are
located at

$$E_{dc} = (n/m)\lambda_g f_o B . \qquad (8)$$

The magnitude of the steps is found to be an oscillating function of
the RF power [2], in qualitative agreement with calculations of
Russer [10] based on Eq. (6).

The interference effect is sensitive to deviations of the vortex
lattice from a matching configuration. For $B \neq B_{n_1 n_2}$ dynamic excitation of strongly damped deformations of the vortex lattice causes
broadening of the interference transitions. For large flux-flow velo-
cities and frequencies it has been shown [5] that under certain conditions the important deformations affecting the interference effect
are harmonic and correspond to transverse modes of the vortex lattice.
In this case the width of the interference transitions turns out to
be proportional to the shear modulus [11] of the vortex lattice. As
shown in the previous section, however, the pinning induced lattice
distortions usually deviate quite strongly from a sinusoidal shape.
In this case, vortex motion is probably better described in terms of
moving flux line dislocations. However, on account of the high com-
plexity of the dynamic equations [4] for superimposed dc and RF driving
currents, a quantitative description of their influence on the interference effect appears to be a rather difficult problem.

ACKNOWLEDGMENTS

One of us (P.M.) would like to express his gratitude to
J.L. Olsen for stimulating suggestions and discussions in the early
stage of these investigations. This work has been supported by the
Swiss National Science Foundation and the U.S. Department of Energy,
Office of Basic Energy Sciences, Materials Science Division.

REFERENCES

1. O. Daldini, P. Martinoli, J.L. Olsen and G. Berner, Phys. Rev.
   Lett. 32, 218 (1974).
2. P. Martinoli, O. Daldini, C. Leemann and E. Stocker, Solid State
   Commun. 17, 205 (1975).
3. P. Martinoli, O. Daldini, C. Leemann and B. van den Brandt, Phys.
   Rev. Lett. 36, 382 (1976).
4. P. Martinoli, J.L. Olsen and J.R. Clem, J. Less-Common Metals 62,
   315 (1978).
5. P. Martinoli, Phys. Rev. B17, 1175 (1978).

6. V.L. Pokrovsky and A.L. Talapov, Phys. Rev. Lett. $\underline{42}$, 65 (1979).
7. J.E. Sacco and J.B. Sokoloff, Phys. Rev. $\underline{B18}$, 6549 (1978).
8. A.T. Fiory, A.F. Hebard and S. Somekh, Appl. Phys. Lett. $\underline{32}$, 73 (1978).
9. A.T. Fiory, Phys. Rev. Lett. $\underline{27}$, 501 (1971).
10. R. Russer, J. Appl. Phys. $\underline{43}$, 2008 (1972).
11. A.T. Fiory, Phys. Rev. $\underline{B8}$, 5039 (1973).

LAYERED SUPERCONDUCTORS

M. R. Beasley
Department of Applied Physics
Stanford University
Stanford, California 94305

ABSTRACT

The theory and experiment of layered superconductors are reviewed with emphasis on those aspects which relate to the quasi-two-dimensional, Josephson-coupled nature of these materials.

INTRODUCTION

One of the unifying themes of this conference is the concept of coupled superconductors, that is, superconducting elements of reduced dimensionality coupled together to form systems of higher dimensionality. In this paper we are concerned with the specific case of layered superconductors. In general such systems can be thought of as consisting of a stacked array of two-dimensional superconducting layers (see Fig. 1) coupled together via some

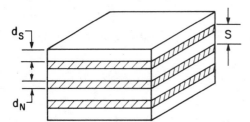

Fig. 1. Schematic of a layered superconductor.

Josephson coupling mechanism, for example, tunneling, the proximity effect, or even microshorts. Although they are similar in spirit to many of the other systems discussed elsewhere in these proceedings, there are certain features of two-dimensional systems that make them particularly interesting.

First, from the materials point of view there appears to be a wide variety of layered superconducting systems. These include the naturally occuring layer compounds and their intercalates,[1,2] lamellar eutectic alloys,[3] and vapor deposited multilayer thin-film structures.[4-7] Second, from the theoretical point of view such systems have the attraction that in many situations of interest the "hard part of the theory" (i.e. the discrete coupling between the layers) reduces to a one-dimensional problem. This has made detailed theoretical calculations tractable for many physical situations of interest. Finally, in light of the recent recognition of the possible presence of several Kosterlitz-Thouless-type transitions in the phase diagram of two-dimensional superconductors,[8] the question naturally arises — what related effects might there be in the quasi-two-dimensional layered systems?

In this paper we review the status of layered superconductors from both the theoretical and experimental points of view with emphasis on those aspects with the greatest bearing on the field of inhomogeneous superconductors as a whole. Finally at the end we mention some of the other equally interesting aspects of these systems and speculate about future directions.

THEORY OF JOSEPHSON-COUPLED LAYERED SUPERCONDUCTORS

The Josephson-coupled model of layered superconductors was first introduced by Lawrence and Doniach[9] in the context of a theory of the superconducting layered compounds. In their model the authors assumed that the individual layers were well-defined super-conductors obeying a 2-D Ginzburg-Landau (GL) theory and coupled together via Josephson coupling. More specifically they assumed a free energy functional of the form

$$F = \sum_{i,j} \left[\int d_x d_y \left\{ \alpha |\psi_i|^2 + \frac{\beta}{2} |\psi_i|^4 + \frac{\hbar^2}{2m^*} |\nabla_{2D}\psi_i|^2 \right\} + \eta |\psi_i - \psi_j|^2 \right] \quad .(1)$$

In their original work and in all subsequent work by others based on this model any possible 2-D critical phenomena were neglected. As intimated in the introduction this assumption probably should be reexamined in light of the recent work of Kosterlitz and Thouless, and we shall return to this point later.

As noted by Lawrence and Doniach, near T_c where the inter-plane coherence length $\xi_z(T)$ [see below] is large compared to the layer repeat distance s, the difference term in Eqn. (1) can be replaced by a gradient term and the free energy reduces to the simpler 3-D anisotropic (or effective mass) GL theory. In this case the effective mass in the z-direction becomes

$$M = \frac{\hbar^2}{2s^2\eta} \tag{2}$$

and, by the usual GL analysis, the coherence length perpendicular to the layers is given by

$$\xi_z^2(T) = \frac{\hbar^2}{2M\alpha} \propto \eta \quad . \tag{3}$$

Clearly then, neglecting critical phenomenon and strong anisotropy per se, the most novel physical properties in layered superconductors presumably arise away from T_c where for sufficiently weak coupling $\xi_z(T)$ becomes less than the layer separation. Here the long-wavelength, effective-mass approximation used by Lawrence and Doniach breaks down, and it is necessary to

188

consider the full Josephson coupled theory, Eqn. (1). With this
point in mind a number of the properties of layered superconductors
have been calculated using the LD theory. These include the
fluctuation conductivity[9] and diamagnetism[10] above T_c , and the
upper[11-13] and lower[13] critical fields below T_c . In most cases
these properties have also been calculated with appropriate
generalized theories based on the microscopic Gorkov theory of
superconductivity.[14-17] The general picture that emerges from
these studies is illustrated in Fig. 2.

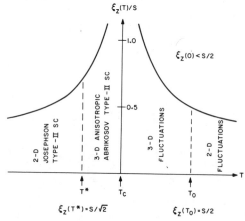

Fig. 2. Expected regimes and
crossover behavior in layered
superconductors.

From this figure we see that there are several regimes of
behavior expected, depending on the relative magnitudes of $\xi_z(T)$
and s , as temperature is reduced through the superconducting
transition. Well above T_c , where $\xi_z(T) < s$, 2-D fluctuation
behavior is expected crossing over to 3-D behavior at a crossover
temperature T_0 defined by the relation $\xi_z(T_0) = s/2$. Such
fluctuation crossover behavior is a common feature of systems of
quasi-reduced dimensionality. The more interesting behavior arises
below T_c where there can be novel dimensional effects when
$\xi_z(T)$ again becomes shorter than s , even though 3-D long range
order in the conventional sense is expected to hold even for
arbitrarily weak coupling. This was first recognized independently
by Klemm, Beasley, and Luther[11] and by Bulaevskii[12] who, motivated
by the very large critical fields observed in the superconducting
layered compounds, calculated the upper critical field H_{c2} using
the Josephson-coupled model.
     The essential results of these calculations are illustrated in
Fig. 3. In terms of the interlayer coupling parameter
$r = (4/\pi)(2\xi_z(0)/s)^2$, it is seen that for very weak ($r \to 0$) or very
strong ($r \gg 1$) coupling, the parallel critical field behavior is
either 2-D, thin-film-like [$H_{c2}(T) \propto (T_c - T)^{1/2}$] or 3-D, bulk-like
[$H_{c2}(T) \propto (T_c - T)$], respectively. However for intermediate coupling
($r \sim 1$) there is a dimensional crossover at the temperature T^*
defined by the relation $\xi_z(T^*) = s/\sqrt{2}$ at which $H_{c2\parallel}$ goes from
being 3-D to 2-D-like as temperature is reduced.

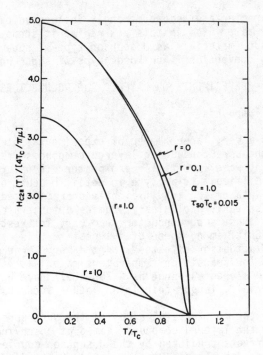

Fig. 3. Predicted critical field behavior $H_{c2||}$ based on the Josephson-coupled model [from Ref. 11].

This novel result can be understood as follows. For $T^* < T < T_c$, the interlayer coherence length extends over many layers and the bulk anisotropic GL results pertain. Correspondingly H_{c2} is given by the effective mass model.[18] For $T < T^*$ where $\xi_z(T) < s$ the normal cores of the vortices, which normally fill the superconductor at H_{c2}, can effectively fit between the layers where they have no pairbreaking effect. More precisely one should say the vortices have gone from being Abrikosov-like to Josephson-like. In any event, below T^* the orbital pairbreaking associated with the applied field becomes ineffective and H_{c2} is then determined by residual intralayer pairbreaking mechanisms. For the curves shown Pauli paramagnetic (i.e. spin) pairbreaking has been assumed with the specific parameters indicated.[16] Deutscher et al.[19] have considered the case of finite layer thickness. In the absence of any intralayer pairbreaking H_{c2} formally becomes infinite at T^*.

In summary then, based on the Josephson-coupled model, layered superconductors should not only exhibit highly anisotropic superconductivity but also an entirely new class of type-II superconductivity at temperatures below T^* where the vortices take on a

Josephson character and become strongly influenced by the periodic nature of the material. In this new regime it seems appropriate to refer to such materials as Josephson type-II superconductors as opposed to conventional Abrikosov type-II superconductors.

EXPERIMENTS ON LAYERED SUPERCONDUCTORS

A. Layered Compounds

Although a very large number of experimental studies have been reported on the superconducting layered compounds (see Ref. 1 and 2 for a review), many were essentially exploratory in nature and are consequently difficult to analyze in detail because of the limited experimental data or the insufficiently characterized nature of the samples. These early preliminary studies demonstrated clearly, however, that these superconductors had very interesting physical properties. Chief among these of interest to this conference were perhaps the fluctuation effects[20] and the very large critical fields found in such low transition temperature materials.[21] For example critical field slopes as large as $\sim$ 280 kOe/K have been observed[22] in these materials, larger than in any other known bulk superconductor.

Probably the most careful study of the superconducting properties of the layered compounds aimed at observing the two-dimensional effects predicted by the Josephson-coupled model is that of Prober, Schwall and Beasley (PSB) who studied the fluctuation diamagnetism above T_c[23] and the upper critical field H_{c2} below T_c[24] in several intercalated layer compounds. In their fluctuation study these authors found that only for the case of $TaS_2(pyridine)_{1/2}$ were the data of sufficient quality to warrant comparison with theory and that in this particular case the fluctuations were three-dimensional (albeit highly anisotropic) in nature. Moreover, these results were found to be in satisfactory agreement with the theory[14,15] using the measured material parameters. Although a crossover to two-dimensional fluctuations was expected sufficiently far above T_c, the predicted crossover temperature T_0 was unfortunately above the maximum temperature at which the fluctuations could be accurately measured. Thus a "text book" demonstration of dimensional crossover behavior in the superconducting layered compounds does not exist, although there appears little doubt that such a phenomenon occurs at high enough temperatures. More favorable materials with larger layer separations exist, but not yet in the high-quality large samples required for such fluctuation experiments.

Following their fluctuation study, PSB undertook a careful study of the upper critical fields of the superconducting layered compounds.[24] The compounds studied included TaS_2 and $TaS_{1.6}Se_{0.4}$ intercalated with collidine, pyridine, or aniline, and the unintercalated compounds $TaS_{1.6}Se_{0.4}$ and $NbSe_2$. Although the samples employed in these experiments were probably among the best ever prepared, the experimental results were not free of a variety of complicating features. Many peculiar effects were

observed, and while by no means could even all the qualitative
features of the data be properly explained, the following general
picture emerged. Based on estimates of the GL coherence lengths
in these materials derived from the H_{c2} data near T_c , it was
found that the interlayer zero-temperature GL coherence lengths
$\xi_z(0)$ are sufficiently small ($\sim 3 - 7$ Å) in some of the inter-
callated compounds that the anisotropic GL theory (or more generally
the anisotropic Gorkov theory) definitely must breakdown at low
temperatures. Moreover, assuming the Josephson-coupled model is
correct, the coherence lengths were such that the crossover behavior
predicted by this model should arise in these particular compounds.

Direct evidence for this crossover was found in the case of
$TaS_2(aniline)_{3/4}$ by virtue of the distinct upturn observed in $H_{c2||}$
at the lowest temperatures. (See Fig. 4). However, for the

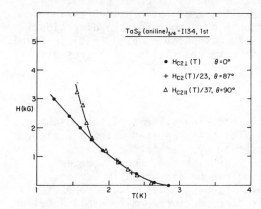

Fig. 4. Measured critical
fields H_{c2} in $TaS_2(aniline)_{3/4}$.
Note upturn in $H_{c2||}$ at low
temperatures.

other materials the data are less clear and the interpretation more
delicate because distinct upturns were not observed, and PSB had
to resort to theoretical curve fitting in order to establish the
crossover. In the end, precise, quantitative agreement with the
theory was not possible. However, as emphasized by PSB the
theory does account nicely for the systematic trends observed in
$H_{c2||}(T)$ for the intercalated compounds taken as a whole, i.e. the
systematic changes in the shapes of the curves are in accord with
theory. The most persistent anomaly in the data is a definite upward or positive curvature in $H_{c2}(T)$ near T_c which can be seen
in Fig. 4. This curvature is observed in both the perpendicular
and parallel critical fields and therefore is not related to the
crossover phenomenon predicted by the theory. Similar anomalies
have been noted previously by others[25] and they remain unexplained.
Unfortunately it is not even certain whether they are an intrinsic
effect or a consequence of imperfect samples.

The results of PSB also show that the parallel critical fields
observed in the layered compounds (both the intercalated ones and
also the unintercalated compound $NbSe_2$) are too large to be
consistent with the conventional theory of Pauli paramagnetic pairbreaking, even including the moderating effects of random spin-orbit

scattering. Specifically the spin-orbit scattering rates $1/\tau_{so}$ found necessary to explain the high-field data exceed estimates of the total electron scattering rate $1/\tau$ - a physically impossible situation. They conclude that new or additional mechanisms for reducing Pauli paramagnetic pairbreaking are required. Several very interesting possibilities have been suggested in the literature, including the existence of an inhomogeneous partially-depaired state for nonspherical Fermi surfaces (i.e. an anisotropic generalization of the original Fulde-Ferrell partially-depaired state),[26] triplet pairing between electrons on adjacent layers[27] or due to the effect of an incipient lattice instability,[28] and a coherence spin-orbit interaction with the crystal potential in the absence of the inversion symmetry center.[29] Another, perhaps more prosaic, but important possibility is the effect of strong electron-phonon coupling, which has recently been shown by Orlando, et al.,[30] to have a very large effect on Pauli paramagnetic pair-breaking. Thus, in the final analysis reasonable support for the dimensional crossover behavior predicted by the Josephson coupled model is found, but the ultimate magnitude of the observed fields still presents theoretical problems.

B.   Artificial Layered Systems

In addition to the naturally occuring systems discussed above, artificial layered systems have also been prepared using a variety of approaches. The advantage of such systems is that their perfection and regularity can be very high and, more importantly, the layer thicknesses and coupling can be more readily varied. Examples include multilayered S/S´ (superconductor/superconductor) vapor deposited systems,[4] S/N (superconductor/normal metal) lamellar eutectic alloy systems,[3] and vapor deposited S/Semi (superconductor/semiconductor)[6,7] and S/I (superconductor/insulator)[5] systems. Some even newer approaches are described in the paper by Schuller and Falco at this conference.[31] Unfortunately, however, in most of these studies either the superconducting layers or the nonsuperconducting barrier layers were too thick, so that the layers themselves were not two dimensional (yielding 3-D fluctuations and low H_{c2}'s) or the superconducting layers exhibited no Josephson coupling. Thus, although these systems all showed interesting properties, particularly with regard to flux pinning, for the most part they were not suitable for investigating the Josephson type-II superconducting effects predicted by the Josephson-coupled model.

The one exception is the work of Ruggiero, Barbee, and Beasley[7] who have recently reported multilayer Nb/Ge composites where the Nb and Ge layers were varied in thickness from ~ 10 Å up to ~ 100 Å. The samples were deposited using a novel sputtering system developed previously by Barbee. Their most recent results[32] in fact clearly demonstrate a crossover from 3-D to 2-D in the parallel critical fields both as a function of the coupling strength ($r \gg 1 \rightarrow r \ll 1$) and as a function of temperature for intermediate ($r \simeq 1$) coupling strengths. The results are illustrated in Fig. 5. The solid lines show the fit to the theory of Ref. 16. Similar composites using Aℓ and Ge layers have been made using sputtering by Haywood and Ast,[6] but in their samples the Ge thickness was never thin enough to allow Josephson coupling.

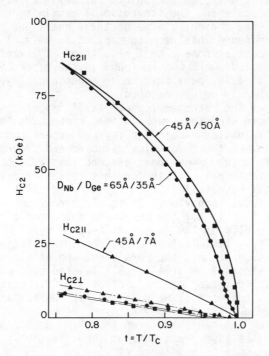

Fig. 5. Critical fields of Nb/Ge multilayer composites as a function of Ge layer thickness. Note dimensional crossover effects.

In summary then it appears that the novel superconductivity expected in Josephson-coupled layered superconductors exists both in the layered compounds and multilayer artificial composites, although admittedly stronger evidence in the former case would be desirable. It will be interesting to see now how the other physical properties of these systems differ from conventional type-II superconductors.

OTHER PROBLEMS AND FUTURE PROSPECTS

In the discussion above we have emphasized the Josephson-coupled features of layered superconductors. These are hardly the only interesting aspects of such materials, however. For example, in the Josephson-coupled model all the effects of layering on the transition temperature T_c , the energy gap Δ , and the density of states $N(E)$ of the superconductor are absorbed into phenomenological parameters. But these properties are of fundamental interest for their own sake. One would particularly like to understand the effects on T_c of the periodic layering, not to mention the influence of the superconductor/nonsuperconductor interfaces, particularly when the nonsuperconductor is a semiconductor or an organic molecule and the conventional proximity effect theory does not apply. The present status of these questions in the case of the layered compounds has been summarized in Refs. 1 and 2. For multilayered composites some recent results on T_c variations and references to previous work can be found in the paper by Granqvist and Claeson.[33] It is evident that these aspects of layered superconductors have hardly been scratched.

Also, even at the phenomenological level important questions remain. As we have stressed several times above, the implications of the Kosterlitz-Thouless ideas for layered superconductors must be addressed. In all the theoretical studies and interpretation of experiments to date it has been assumed that 2-D superconductors are entirely conventional. It is for this reason, for example, that in the theoretical results for H_{c2}, the perpendicular critical fields, show no unusual behavior. It is clear now, however, that almost certainly this is not the case, and one expects that at some level the results of the Josephson-coupled model will need modification. It is tantalizing to say the least, but entirely speculative, to suggest that the persistent and similar anomalies[25] seen in the experimental H_{c2}'s of all layered systems studied to date may be a manifestation of these effects.[6] Of particular note in this regard is the work of Haywood and Ast where large anomalies were seen which depended both on the number of layers and the separation between them, even though no Josephson coupling between the layers was present. Qualitatively similar results have been seen by Ruggiero, et al.[32]

In conclusion, then, we see that all the way from the microscopic to the phenomenological levels, the field of layered superconductors remains full of interesting questions for further research.

This work was carried out under the support of the National Science Foundation.

REFERENCES

1. F. R. Gamble and T. H. Geballe, Treatise on Solid State Chemistry, ed. by N. Bruce Hannay (Plenum, N.Y., 1976) Vol. 3.

2. L. N. Bulaevskii, Sov. Phys. Usp. 18, 514 (1976).

3. A. J. Bevolo, E. D. Gibson, J. D. Verhoeven, and D. K. Finnemore, Phys. Rev. B14, 114 (1976); J. M. Dupart, R. A. Brand, J. Baixeras, and O. Bethoux, J. Phys. (Paris) 38, 393 (1977).

4. H. Raffy, J. C. Renard, and E. Guyon, Solid State Commun., 11, 1679 (1972).

5. R. E. Howard, M. R. Beasley, T. H. Geballe, C. N. King, R. H. Hammond, R. H. Norton, J. R. Salem, and R. B. Zubeck, IEEE Trans. MAG-13, 138 (1977).

6. T. W. Haywood and D. G. Ast, Phys. Rev. B 18, 2225 (1978).

7. S. Ruggiero, T. W. Barbee, and M. R. Beasley, Bull. Am. Phys. Soc. 24, 357 (1979).

8. See paper by B. Huberman in these proceedings.

9. W. E. Lawrence and S. Doniach, in Proceedings of the 12th International Conference on Low-Temperature Physics, ed. by E. Kando (Academic Press of Japan, Kyoto, 1971), pg. 361.

10. T. Tsuzuki, Phys. Lett. 37A, 159 (1971); K. Yamaji, ibid 38A, 43 (1972).

11. R. A. Klemm, M. R. Beasley, and A. Luther, J. Low Temp. Phys. 16, 607 (1974).

12. L. N. Bulaevskii, Sov. Phys. JETP 37, 1133 (1973).

13. N. Boccara, J. P. Carton, and G. Sarma, Phys. Letters 49A, 165 (1974).

14. R. A. Klemm, M. R. Beasley, and A. Luther, Phys. Rev. B8, 5072 (1973).

15. R. R. Gerhardts, Phys. Rev. B9, 2945 (1974).

16. R. A. Klemm, A. Luther, and M. R. Beasley, Phys. Rev. B 12, 877 (1975).

17. L. N. Bulaevskii, Sov. Phys. JETP 38, 634 (1974); L. N. Bulaevskii and A. A. Guseinov, Sov. Phys. JETP Lett. 19, 382 (1974); also see Ref. 2.

18. D. R. Tilley, Proc. Phys. Soc. 86, 289 (1965); D. R. Tilley, ibid 86, 678 (1965).

19. G. Deutscher and O. Entin-Wohlman, Phys. Rev. B 17, 1249 (1978).

20. T. H. Geballe, A. Menth, F. J. DiSalvo and F. R. Gamble, Phys. Rev. Letters 27, 314 (1971).

21. S. Foner, E. J. McNiff, Jr., A. H. Thompson, F. R. Gamble, T. H. Geballe, and F. J. DiSalvo, Bull. Am. Phys. Soc. 17, 289 (1972); R. C. Morris and R. V. Coleman, Phys. Rev. B7, 991 (1973).

22. D. E. Prober, M. R. Beasley, and R. E. Schwall, Bull. Am. Phys. Soc. 20, 342 (1975).

23. D. E. Prober, M. R. Beasley, and R. E. Schwall, Phys. Rev. B15, 5245 (1977).

196

24. D. E. Prober, R. E. Schwall, and M. R. Beasley, submitted for publication.

25. J. A. Woolam, R. B. Somoano, and P. O'Connor, Phys. Rev. Lett. 32, 712 (1974).

26. K. Aoi, W. Dieterich, and P. Fulde, J. Phys. 267, 223 (1974).

27. K. B. Efetov and A. I. Larkin, JETP 41, 76 (1975).

28. K. B. Efetov, JETP 46, 1020 (1977).

29. L. N. Bulaevskii and A. I. Rusinova, JETP Lett. 21, 66 (1975).

30. T. P. Orlando, S. Foner, E. J. McNiff, Jr., and M. R. Beasley, Phys. Rev. B 19, 4545 (1979).

31. I. K. Schuller and C. M. Falco in these proceedings.

32. S. T. Ruggiero, T. W. Barbee, and M. R. Beasley, to be published.

33. C. G. Granqvist and T. Claeson, Solid State Communication, 31, 33 (1979).

LAYERED ULTRATHIN COHERENT STRUCTURES*

Ivan K. Schuller and Charles M. Falco
Solid State Science Division
Argonne National Laboratory, Argonne, Illinois 60439

ABSTRACT

We describe a new class of superconducting materials, Layered Ultrathin Coherent Structures (LUCS). These materials are produced by sequentially depositing ultrathin layers of materials using high rate magnetron sputtering or thermal evaporation. We present strong evidence that layers as thin as 10 Å can be prepared in this fashion. Resistivity data indicates that the mean free path is layer thickness limited. A strong disagreement is found between the experimentally measured transition temperatures T_c and the T_c's calculated using the Cooper limit approximation. This is interpreted as a change in the band structure or the phonon structure of the material due to layering or to surfaces.

INTRODUCTION

One of the most fascinating areas of solid state physics is the artificial production and stabilization of new materials that do not occur naturally. The possibility of fine tunning band structures, phonon spectra etc. by artificially layering materials seems very attractive and promising. In particular, layered superconductors have been studied for some time.[1] The study of layered superconductors can shed light on the role of the interfaces on surface superconductivity and on the Cooper limit problem.

We have prepared ultrathin layers of niobium (Nb) and copper (Cu) with layer thicknesses ranging from 10 Å - 2500 Å. It is found that in fact this system grows in layered form and that diffusion does not destroy the LUCS structure. We find extremely good reproducibility in the sample preparation, mean free paths limited by layer thicknesses and T_c's smaller than predictions based on a simple Cooper[2] limit calculation.

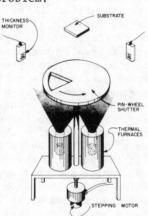

Figure 1. Experimental setup using two thermal furnaces.

SAMPLE PREPARATION AND CHARACTERIZATION

Samples can be prepared in two completely different ways. Figure 1 shows the experimental setup for

*Work supported by the U. S. Department of Energy.

thermal evaporation[3] of LUCS. Two thermal evaporation sources are located close to each other. The substrate on which the sample is prepared is located between the two sources roughly 15 inches above them. A rotary shutter exposes the substrate alternately to the two evaporated metal beams. The evaporation rate in each thermal source is controlled and monitored using a quartz crystal based feedback system. This system is used for the preparation of samples that are used in our tunneling studies.

The sputtering system is based on two high rate magnetron sputtering guns. The two guns are located roughly 15 inches from each other. The substrate is held against a rotating table which alternately moves it from one beam to the other. The sputtering is performed with 6 mtorr of argon pressure and the sputtering rates are controlled by keeping sputtering pressure and power constant. Since the energy of sputtered atoms is distributed in a much narrower range (due to thermalization by the Ar sputtering gas) the sputtered sample growth is closer to a single crystal than the thermally prepared samples. On the other hand, the preparation of tunnel junctions is difficult in sputtering systems where high energy ions can destroy the tunneling barrier. To illustrate the methodology we will describe the properties of sputtered Nb/Cu LUCS.

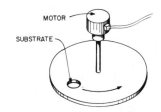
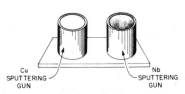

Figure 2. Experimental setup using two sputtering guns.

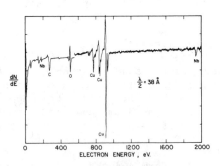

Figure 3. Auger spectrum for a 38 Å Nb/Cu LUCS

To characterize the sample Ion Mill Auger Spectroscopy was performed. Auger spectroscopy allows the study of the composition of the films 15 Å - 30 Å from the surface. This, in combination with ion milling, allows depth profiling of the chemical composition. It should be pointed out that since the escape depth of the Auger electrons is larger than one atomic layer it is expected that this measurement will be characteristic of an average composition over the escape depth. Figure 3 shows a derivative curve of the number of Auger electrons as a function of energy for a sample having a layer thickness $\lambda/2 = 38$ Å, and overall thickness of 1 μm.

Notice the presence of characteristic peaks of Carbon, Oxygen, Niobium, and Copper. Backstreaming from the diffusion pump is probably responsible for the residual Carbon. The large Cu peak indicates that the first layer is of Cu.

To depth profile the chemical composition of the samples, they are bombarded with 1 KeV Xe ions. This slowly mills the surface of the films, while simultaneously the Auger spectrum is analyzed. Figure 4 shows a graph of the peak to peak height of the Cu LMM Auger electron at ∿ 910 eV versus time. Since the ion milling is presumed to be performed at a constant rate this graph illustrates the change in Cu concentration versus depth. We should point out that attempts to depth profile films with $\lambda \leq 30$ Å were unsuccessful. This probably is due to the fact that the energetic Xe ions stir up the surface of the material. In addition the Auger electrons have an escape depth somewhere in the neighborhood of 30 Å so this kind of a measurement becomes insensitive for determining chemical compositions for films with smaller layer spacings. Figure 4 shows that the variation in Cu concentration is periodic with depth.

Detailed X-ray studies also indicate that the material is layered. A detailed account of the diffraction and Laue patterns will be published elsewhere.[4]

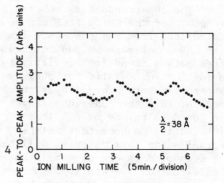

Figure 4. Depth profile of the Cu concentration for the Nb/Cu LUCS shown in Figure 3.

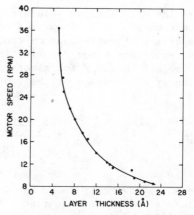

Figure 5. Superlattice wavelength versus speed of driving motor.

The reproducibility of sample preparation is indicated in Figure 5, where the superlattice wavelength derived from X-ray measurements is plotted against the speed of the driving motor.

Notice that the wavelength is proportional to the inverse of the motor speed indicating that sputtering pressure and power fluctuations do not significantly affect the results.

TRANSPORT PROPERTIES

The layered nature of the Nb/Cu LUCS manifests itself also in the various transport properties. Figure 6 shows the variation of

residual resistivity versus the inverse of the layer thickness.
As expected, the resistivity depends linearly on $1/\lambda$ indicating
that the mean free path is limited by the layer thickness.

The superconducting coherence
length ξ of the Nb/Cu LUCS can be
calculated from the coherence length
$\xi = 380$ Å[5] of pure Nb and the mean
free path ℓ found from resistivity
using $\xi = \sqrt{\xi_0 \ell}$[5] valid for a dirty
superconductor. For a layer thick-
ness of 10 Å the coherence length
is found to be $\xi = 62$ Å. It is
interesting to note that in the
normal state this material will behave
as decoupled layers of metals because
the electrons are confined to move
inside each layer. On the other
hand, below the transition temperature, this material should behave
as a homogeneous superconductor
since $\xi > \lambda$.

The existence of a supercon-
ductor where $\xi > \lambda$ allows a direct
comparison of experiment to Cooper limit calculation of the effective electron-phonon coupling (N_oV). It was shown many years ago
by Cooper[2] that N_oV for a material such as our Nb/Cu LUCS will be
given by the average of the two attractive interactions.

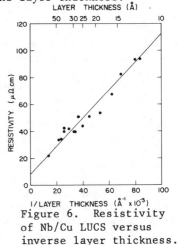

Figure 6. Resistivity
of Nb/Cu LUCS versus
inverse layer thickness.

$$(N_oV)_{Nb/Cu} = \frac{N_1V_1(N_1d_1) + N_2V_2(N_2d_2)}{N_1d_1 + N_2d_2} \qquad (1)$$

where 1 and 2 refer to Nb and Cu respectively and $d = \lambda/2$ is the
thickness of either Nb or Cu. Notice that if $d_1 = d_2$ (our case),
N_oV will be independent of thickness as long as $\xi > \lambda$. A lower
limit for the transition temperature of such a sandwich can be calculated from[7]

$$1.45 \ T_c = \theta_D \exp(- 1/N_oV) \qquad (2)$$

where the density of states in each material can be determined from
the experimentally measured specific heat coefficient γ using.

$$N_o = 3\gamma/2\pi^2 k_B^2 \quad . \qquad (3)$$

The various parameters used in the calculation of T_c are shown in Table 1.

TABLE I

Relevant parameters for Nb and Cu

Element	Z	γ [mJ/moleK^2]	N_0 [states/eVcm^3]	V [eVcm^3]	θ_D [°K]	T_c [°K]	$N_0 V$
Nb	5	7.66[8]	0.90x10^{23}	0.34x10^{-23}	241[9]	9.2	0.306
Cu	1	0.69[8]	0.125x10^{23}	0.512x10^{-23}	342[8]	<0.01	0.072[10]

We find using Eqs. (1), (2), and (3) and the value from Table I that the transition temperature of the Nb/Cu LUCS should be T_c = 5.4°K in the short wavelength limit ($\xi > \lambda$). Experimentally it is found that below $\lambda/2$ = 20 Å the transition temperature of the Nb/Cu LUCS is almost layer thickness independent and that $T_c \cong 2.5$°K. The strong disagreement, of over a factor of two, between experiment and theory implies that layering strongly affects the band structure and hence V or N_0 in these layered materials. Since Nb has a peak in the density of states at the Fermi surface we expect layering to affect N_0 more strongly than V, which would imply changes in the phonon structure.

In summary, we have been able to prepare Layered Ultrathin Coherent Structures (LUCS) where the layer thickness approaches interatomic spacings. All measurements to date, structural as well as transport, indicate that the material is layered at the atomic level. Resistivity measurements show that the mean free path is layer thickness limited. The disagreeement between the T_c's theoretically calculated and the ones experimentally determined imply the possibility of strong band structure effects.

A more detailed account of X-ray results, critical field versus temperature and angle, and T_c versus wavelength will be published elsewhere.

ACKNOWLEDGMENT

We would like to thank Dr. Dan Dahlberg for running the Auger spectra. Our thanks to R. T. Kampwirth for help in the initial stages of this work. Many thanks to S. K. Sinha and L. Guttman for stimulating discussions.

REFERENCES

1. Myron Strongin et. al., Phys. Rev. Letters $\underline{21}$, 1320 (1968).
2. L. N. Cooper, Phys. Rev. Letters $\underline{6}$, 689 (1961); IBM Journal $\underline{6}$, 75 (1962).
3. J. E. Hilliard in Modulated Structures - 1979, edited by J. M. Cowley, et. al., AIP Conference Proceedings No. 53, pg. 407.
4. Ivan Schuller to be published.
5. C. Kittel, Introduction to Solid State Physics, pg. 425, Fourth Edition, J. Wiley and Sons, Inc., N.Y. (1971).
6. P. G. deGennes, Superconductivity of Metals and Alloys, pg. 225, W. A. Benjamin, Inc., N.Y. (1966).
7. G. Gladstone, M. A. Jensen, and J. R. Sehrieffer in Superconductivity, Edited by R. D. Parks, Marcell Dekker, Inc., N.Y. (1969).
8. K. A. Gschneider, Sol. St. Phys. $\underline{16}$, 275 (1964).
9. Y. Heine, Phys. Rev. $\underline{153}$, 674 (1967).
10. E. Krätzig, Sol. St. Commun. $\underline{9}$, 1205 (1971).

MAGNETIC FIELD DEPENDENCE OF THE PAIR POTENTIAL IN INHOMOGENEOUS SUPERCONDUCTORS

D. K. Finnemore and T. Y. Hsiang
Ames Laboratory-USDOE and Department of Physics
Iowa State University, Ames, Iowa 50011

ABSTRACT

The depairing effects of an applied magnetic field have been studied for inhomogeneous superconductors by measuring the critical currents of SNS junctions. Critical currents are found to decrease exponentially with increasing H over 3 orders of magnitude change in I_c. If the depairing parameter is taken to be $\alpha = D_N eH/c$, one finds a diffusivity of 0.22 $m^2 s^{-1}$ which agrees with the value from resistivity to an accuracy of about 30%.

INTRODUCTION

With the recent advances in casting techniques there is now available a new family of inhomogeneous superconductors with performance characteristics which are well suited for large scale dc magnets in the 8 to 14 Tesla range. These composites are formed by arc casting dendritic Cu-Nb alloys,[1] drawing the alloy to wire, tin plating the wire and reacting to form very long, thin filaments of Nb_3Sn in a Cu matrix. Typically the Nb_3Sn filaments are long ribbon shaped structures approximately 10 nm thick, 200 nm wide, and several cm long. Because the filaments are discontinuous and separated by a Cu layer on the order of 100 nm thick the proximity effect may play a central role in the critical current. For applications where the magnet can be operated in steady field these supercurrents through the Cu matrix are very beneficial but for ac or pulsed field applications the proximity coupling can lead to large eddy currents within the wire and the concomitant losses.

The purpose of the experiments reported here is to study the magnetic field dependence of the induced pair potential in the normal metal region by measuring the superconducting critical currents for SNS triple layer junction. The Pb-Cd-Pb composite was chosen as a prototype system because the pair potential of Cd at the Pb-Cd interface is approximately the same as the pair potential in Cu at the Nb_3Sn-Cu interface, about 0.5 meV. In addition, the pair potential decay lengths are comparable and there are no interdiffusion problems providing that a small amount of Bi is added to the Pb to ensure a short coherence distance, ξ. The solubility of both Pb and Bi in Cd is less than 0.03 at .% at room temperature. In all of this work, emphasis is placed on the thick-clean limit for the Cd.

RESULTS AND DISCUSSION

The current-voltage (I-V) curves for these junctions show zero voltage ($<10^{-13}$ volts) out to some critical current, I_c, where the voltage abruptly rises and roughly obeys the $V = (I^2 - I_c^2)^{1/2}$ behavior of

0094-243X/80/580203-04$1.50 Copyright 1980 American Institute of Physics

the resistivity shunted junction model[2] over most of the temperature and magnetic field range studied. There were no hysteretic or broadening effects as might be expected if inhomogeneous flux pinning were a problem. In zero applied field the temperature dependence of the critical current obeys the relation from the deGennes-Werthamer theory[3] $I_c = I_0 (1-T/T_{cS})^2 e^{-K_N d_N}$ where I_0 is a constant, T_{cS} is the Pb transition temperature, d_N is the Cd thickness and $K_N^{-1} = \hbar v_F (2\sqrt{3}\pi k_B T)^{-1}$, is the order parameter decay length. Here v_F is the Fermi velocity taken to be 7.7×10^7 cm/sec. There is a rather good quantitative fit over the entire range from 1.5 to 7K.

With the application of a magnetic field, I_c decreases exponentially with increasing H as shown in Fig. 1. Although there is considerable scatter in the data, this exponential behavior is the domi-

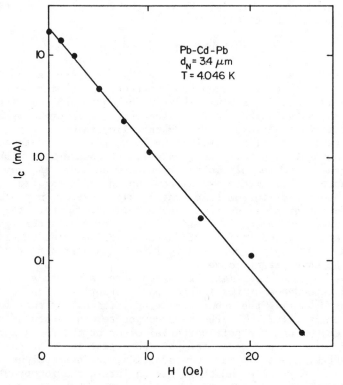

Pb-Cd-Pb
$d_N = 3.4 \ \mu m$
T = 4.046 K

Fig. 1. Magnetic field dependence of the critical current.

nant effect at low fields. A plot of the data on a linear or log-log scale clearly does not give a straight line. If the data are fit to an equation of the form $I_c = I_0 e^{-H/H_0}$, one finds that the slope of Fig. 1 is temperature dependent and roughly obeys $H_0 = AT^{-1}$ where A is a constant equal to $12.8 K^{-1}$. Fig. 2 shows a plot of H_0 for a 3.4 μm thick junction.

In view of the good fit of the zero field data to the deGennes-Werthamer theory[3] and the apparent exponential fall of J_c with H it

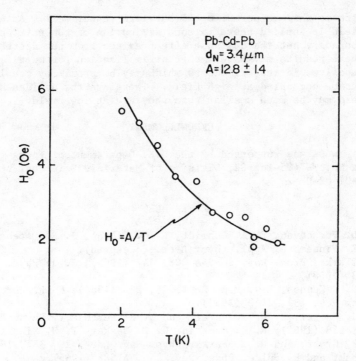

Fig. 2. Temperature dependence of the decay constant for applied fields.

seems reasonable to analyze the results in terms of a multiple pair breaking model.[4] Krähenbühl and Watts-Tobin[5] have shown that one can extend the dGW theory[3] to the case of a dirty superconductor and a clean normal metal barrier by replacing the diffusivity $D = 1/3 \ v_F \ell$ by an effective diffusivity $\tilde{D} = v_F^2(6)^{-1}(|\omega| + v_F/2\ell)^{-1}$ where $\omega = (2n+1)\pi k_B T/\hbar$ and ℓ is the electron mean free path. If one uses $K_N^2 \xi_N^2$ as the depairing parameter associated with the normal metal barrier and $\alpha = D_N e H/c$ as the depairing parameter for the applied field, the decay length is found to be.

$$K_N^{-1} = \xi_N [6(\frac{1}{2} + \frac{\alpha}{\pi k_B T})]^{-1/2} \ . \tag{1}$$

Substituting this into the J_c equation, the leading term for small magnetic fields is found to be.

$$I_c = I_0 \exp[-2\sqrt{3} \ d_N D_N e H (\hbar v_F c)^{-1}] \ . \tag{2}$$

Fitting this expression to the data for a 3.4 µm thick junction at 4.2K gives $D_N = 0.22 \ m^2 s^{-1}$ whereas the D_N derived from the electrical resistivity is $0.15 \ m^2 s^{-1}$. Considering the uncertainties in determining the mean free path from the resistivity this is good agreement.

CONCLUDING REMARKS

A multiple pair-breaking model describes the suppression of

supercurrents through normal metal barriers rather well. As a magnetic field is applied there is some diminution of the pair potential at the boundary but the dominant effect arises from the decrease of K_N^{-1}. These results may have important implication for multifilamentary composites in that filaments which may be proximity coupled in low H can be decoupled at high field. Therefore the ac losses at high field may be much smaller than they are at low field.

ACKNOWLEDGMENT

This work was supported by the U.S. Department of Energy, contract No. W-7405-Eng-82, Division of Materials Sciences, budget code AK-01-02-02-2.

REFERENCES

1. J. D. Verhoeven, F. A. Schmidt, E. D. Gibson, J. E. Ostenson, and D. K. Finnemore, Appl. Phys. Lett. (accepted).
2. J. Clarke, Proc. Roy. Soc. A 308, 447 (1969); J. de Phys. 29, C2-3 (1968).
3. P. G. deGennes, Rev. Mod. Phys. 36, 225 (1964); N. R. Werthamer, Phys. Rev. 132, 2440 (1963).
4. J. J. Hauser, H. C. Theuerer, and N. R. Werthamer, Phys. Rev. 142, 118 (1964); R. P. Guertin, W. E. Masker, T. W. Mihalisin, R. P. Groff, and R. D. Parks, Phys. Rev. Lett. 20, 387 (1968); M. Maki and P. Fulde, Phys. Rev. 140, A1586 (1965).
5. Y. Krähenbühl and R. J. Watts-Tobin, J. Low Temp. Phys. 35, 569 (1979).

SUPERCONDUCTING DIAMAGNETISM OF TaSe$_3$ AND NbSe$_3$

R. A. Buhrman, C. M. Bastuscheck, J. C. Scott, and J. D. Kulick
Cornell University, Ithaca, N.Y. 14853

ABSTRACT

The superconducting transitions of the highly anisotropic metals TaSe$_3$ and NbSe$_3$ were investigated using SQUID magnetometers. The observed diamagnetic susceptibility showed similar unusual field and temperature dependences for both materials. In particular, the susceptibility of the samples in low fields increased greatly at temperatures far below the transition temperature of the material (as indicated by the onset of temperature dependent diamagnetism and the upper limit of flux trapping). The measurements suggest the presence of a second transition at low temperatures where small superconducting regions of the sample become coupled throughout larger volumes.

INTRODUCTION

Compounds of tantalum and niobium with the chalcogens S, Se, and Te are of interest because the metal ions of these compounds are coupled much more strongly in one or two dimensions than in the remaining dimension(s). Tantalum triselenide and niobium triselenide are of particular interest because they show highly anisotropic metallic conduction to low temperatures. In addition, NbSe$_3$ shows two distinct charge density wave transitions[1] (at 144 and 59 K) while TaSe$_3$ shows none, even though the materials have similar structures.

There is confusion in the literature as to whether or not (or in what way) these compounds become superconducting. TaSe$_3$ has been reported to become superconducting around 2.2K on the basis of resistance and critical field measurements.[2,3] However, many, if not all, of the samples examined exhibited non-zero resistance to the lowest temperatures reached, and the report of superconductivity is in conflict with the reported absence of a diamagnetic transition in TaSe$_3$.[4]

In NbSe$_3$ two low temperature resistive anomalies have been reported.[5] The first is centered at approximately 2 K, the second at about .25 K. Again the possible superconductive nature of these transitions is obscured by the observation of non-zero resistance to the lowest temperatures obtained. Magnetic studies of NbSe$_3$ have been reported[4] which indicate that no diamagnetic transition occurs in this material until pressures in excess of .5 Kbar are applied.[6] Finally there has been a recent report[7] of a sharp resistive drop at about 1.5 K in NbSe$_3$ which has been alloyed with 5% TaSe$_3$. While a residual resistance apparently remained below this transition, on the basis of critical field studies this alloy material was labeled an anisotropic three-dimensional superconductor.

In this paper we describe the results of high resolution magne-

0094-243X/80/580207-09$1.50 Copyright 1980 American Institute of Physics

tization measurements of $TaSe_3$ and $NbSe_3$ in the temperature range of the low temperature resistive anomalies. In the case of $NbSe_3$ resistive measurements have also been made as a function of temperature, magnetic field and current density. Diamagnetism associated with these anomalies has been observed which clearly is due to the existence of superconducting long range order within these materials. However, the nature of these transitions is not in accord with that of bulk homogeneous superconductors.

In the first section of this paper the materials and samples are described, and the experiments are briefly explained. The second section presents observations of the diamagnetic transitions in the two materials. In the third section mechanisms are suggested which could account for the unusual diamagnetism.

SAMPLES AND EXPERIMENTAL TECHNIQUES

Tantalum and niobium triselenides are grown by heating stoichiometric amounts of the elements in an evacuated quartz tube for several weeks.[8] The materials form long, fine fibers (millimeters long and tens of micrometers cross-dimension) in which the long dimension coincides with the direction of high conductivity (crystallographic b-axis). Structural determinations show that the compounds can be thought of as chains of the metal ions (each at the center of a triangular prism defined by six half selenium atoms) linked most strongly along the fiber axis. The unit cell of $TaSe_3$ contains[9] four such chains while that of $NbSe_3$ contains six.[10] The compounds are expected to be highly anisotropic in the plane perpendicular to the b direction.

The $TaSe_3$ examined here was grown by W. Fisher. The composition was checked by x-ray diffraction for the presence of $TaSe_2$ and none was found. Under an optical microscope the material appeared as small clusters (0.5 to 3 mm diameter) of randomly oriented interpenetrating fine needles and striated ribbons. These crystals varied from 0.1 to 3 mm length, with cross-dimensions from 1 to 20 micrometers. The ends of the ribbons were generally split. About 100 mg of this material was loosely assembled in a volume approximately 1.5 x 3 x 8 mm. In analyzing the data the magnetization was referred to the sample volume, and no filling fraction correction was applied.

Three samples of $NbSe_3$ were prepared from material grown in this lab to investigate the effect of changing the sample morphology. The material as grown appeared similar to $TaSe_3$ under an optical microscope: clumps of randomly oriented long narrow ribbon-like crystals. Under an electron microscope these ribbons appeared to be composed of fibers on the order of several hundred angstroms wide: crystal ends were always frayed into these smaller fibers. From this material three samples were made:

Sample A: 94 mg of the material as-grown, loosely assembled into a volume 3 x 4 x 10 mm.

Sample B: 90 mg of the material compacted using an hydraulic press to form a cylinder 3 mm long x 2.5 mm diameter.

Sample C: 135 mg of similarly compacted material, but the fibrous
            $NbSe_3$ was etched in dilute H_2SO_4, rinsed, and dried
            before compaction.

The magnetic susceptibilities of these samples were measured
using SQUID magnetometers in two separate cryostats, one cooled with
a ^{3}He pot, the other by a dilution refrigerator. The static magnetization, M_{dc}, was measured by sweeping temperature in constant magnetic field H; the static susceptibility is defined as M_{dc}/H. The
temperature and field dependent ac susceptibility χ_{ac} was determined by measuring the magnetization response to a small ac field
($\leqslant 2$ mOe at 0.08 Hz) applied parallel to the static field with a
separate small solenoid.

Conventional four probe low frequency ac resistance measurements were made on single ribbons of $NbSe_3$ as a function of temperature, applied magnetic field, and current density. Although these
samples appear visually and in an SEM to be single crystals the
microscopic morphology has not been fully elucidated. The current
direction in all cases was along the crystallographic b axis (the
high conductivity direction) and magnetic fields up to 40 kOe were
applied parallel to the b axis and to the a* axis.

EXPERIMENTAL RESULTS

The low temperature diamagnetic susceptibilities of $TaSe_3$
and $NbSe_3$ are quite similar, and
appear to depend strongly on the
sample morphology. Important
features common to both materials
are 1) the susceptibility is very
small near the temperature where
the (upper) resistive transition
is observed (below 2.5 K), 2) the
susceptibility increases strongly
at temperatures far below this
transition temperature, 3) the ac
susceptibility is much greater
than the dc susceptibility (as
defined above) at low temperatures,
and 4) χ_{dc} decreases very quickly
with increasing field while χ_{ac}
is affected only slightly by small
fields, falling to half its zero
field value around 100 Oe.

As samples of $TaSe_3$ and $NbSe_3$
are cooled below the temperature
where the resistive transition is
observed to begin (~2.5K) a small
diamagnetic susceptibility is observed. Figures 1 and 2 show this
onset. The susceptibility shows
no thermal hysteresis, but flux

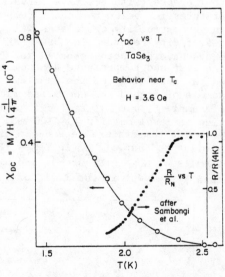

Figure 1. Onset of temperature dependent diamagnetism in $TaSe_3$ shown with
the first published resistive transition
drawn to the same temperature scale.
The resistance does not drop to zero
(baseline of graph). The solid line
guides the eye. $-1/4\pi$ represents total
flux exclusion from the sample.

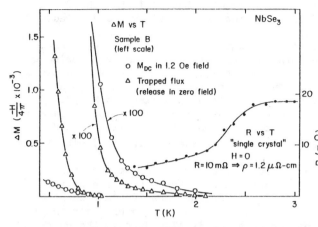

Figure 2. M_{dc} traces flux expulsion from the compacted sample of NbSe$_3$ during cooling. Below 0.5 K the field was removed. As the sample was warmed, trapped flux was released (same ΔM scale). Also shown is low temperature resistive anomaly measured on a crystal grown in this lab. The lines guide the eye.

trapping has been observed in all samples. Flux trapping is shown in Fig. 2 for one of the NbSe$_3$ samples, where it is seen to persist to above 2 K. Such flux trapping is proof of the existence of long range phase coherence and hence of the existence of superconductivity in NbSe$_3$.

As the temperature is decreased the susceptibility continues to increase (with positive curvature in the χ vs T plots) to temperatures far below the onset temperature. This continuous increase in susceptibility correlates well with the continuous decrease in resistivity reported in NbSe$_3$ (Fig. 3). Low temperature measurements have not been reported for TaSe$_3$. Figure 3 also shows that the size and temperature dependence of the susceptibility depends on the morphology of the sample. The corresponding curve for the sample of etched and compacted material is similar in shape to that of sample B, but χ_{dc} is larger and shows some indication of beginning to level out for T < 100 mK (Figure 4).

The temperature dependence of the ac susceptibility is very similar to that of χ_{dc} in TaSe$_3$ (Figs. 5 and 7), and in the several samples of NbSe$_3$ (Figures 4 and 6). However, χ_{ac} is much larger than χ_{dc} except in the limit of very small applied fields.

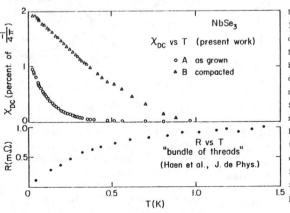

Figure 3. Upper portion shows low temperature increase of diamagnetic susceptibility of NbSe$_3$. Measurements were made below 1 K and the zero offsets determined by matching measurements made in the ^{3}He cryostat. Susceptibility of the as-grown material above 0.5 K is small but not zero. Lower portion of the figure reproduces the second low temperature drop in resistance for the lowest current density (1.3 mA/mm^2) reported by Haen et al.

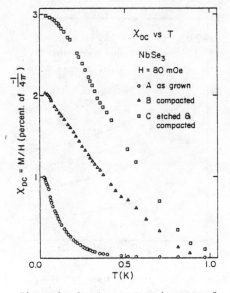

Figure 4. Low temperature increase of diamagnetic susceptibility for three samples of NbSe$_3$ (see text).

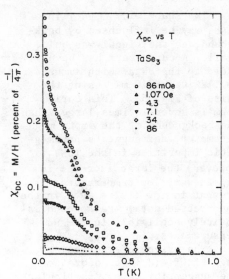

Figure 5. Low temperature increase of diamagnetic susceptibility for TaSe$_3$ (as grown material) in several dc fields.

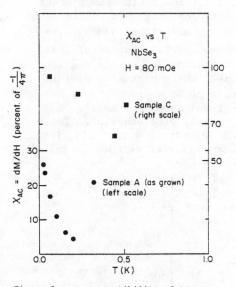

Figure 6. ac susceptibility of two samples of NbSe$_3$ at low temperature. χ_{ac} and χ_{dc} plots are similar in shape, but $\chi_{ac} \gg \chi_{dc}$. The baseline is zero for both vertical scales.

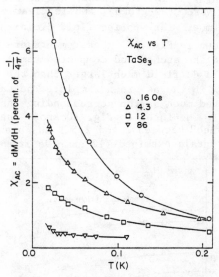

Figure 7. Low temperature ac susceptibility of TaSe$_3$ in several applied dc fields. χ_{ac} is larger than χ_{dc} and increases strongly at lower temperatures. Note different temperature scales for Figs. 5 and 7.

The shape of χ_{dc} vs T for TaSe$_3$ may be influenced by background, as the signal was quite small. A curie term has been added to the data which amounts to .12%/Oe at 10 mK (using the units of Fig. 5). This Curie term is several times larger than the background of the empty magnetometer, and suggests paramagnetic impurities in the TaSe$_3$. However, the large increase in χ_{dc} at very low temperatures is present in low fields even in the uncorrected data. Background is entirely negligible in the ac measurements.

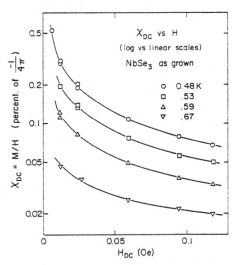

Figure 8. χ_{dc} vs H_{dc} curves for NbSe$_3$ constructed from χ_{dc} vs T measurements. χ_{dc} is not constant in low fields. Vertical scale is logarithmic.

The effect of increasing magnetic field is to decrease the susceptibilities, particularly the dc susceptibility. The measurements of χ_{dc} vs T in various fields can be replotted as χ_{dc} vs H for several temperatures. This has been done in Fig. 8 for low field measurements in NbSe$_3$ (as-grown), and is clearly not constant, even in fields of 20 mOe. The applied field diminished χ_{ac} much less than χ_{dc}, as shown in Fig. 9. Measurements are shown for two samples of NbSe$_3$, and the etched and compacted sample maintains χ_{ac} nearly constant to a dc field much larger than the field which begins to diminish χ_{ac} in the as-grown sample. The sample of TaSe$_3$ (not shown) behaved much as the corresponding (as-grown) sample of NbSe$_3$.

The inset to Fig. 10 shows the typical $\rho(T)$ behavior. The "knee" between 2 and 2.5 K has been observed, in zero field, in all crystals examined (12 samples from two different batches). Below

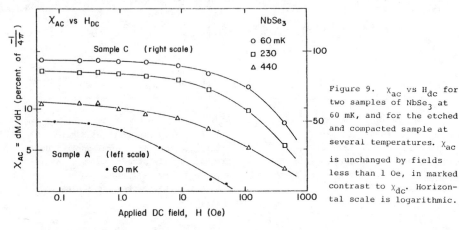

Figure 9. χ_{ac} vs H_{dc} for two samples of NbSe$_3$ at 60 mK, and for the etched and compacted sample at several temperatures. χ_{ac} is unchanged by fields less than 1 Oe, in marked contrast to χ_{dc}. Horizontal scale is logarithmic.

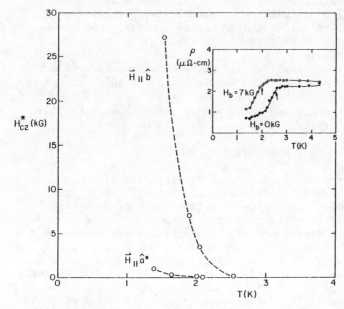

Figure 10. Effective parallel (H∥b) and perpendicular (H∥a*) critical fields $H^*_{C2}(T)$ for NbSe$_3$. The inset shows how the resistive anomaly is depressed in a field (H∥b) and indicates the temperature at which a 10% drop in resistance has occurred. This temperature is used to construct the main figure.

2 K the resistance levels off at a value which is highly sample dependent, varying from 30% to 90% of the 4.2 K resistance. So far no correlation has been found between the magnitude of the resistance drop and any other property of the samples, e.g. crystal dimensions, room temperature resistance, residual resistance ratio, history, etc.

The temperature at which the knee occurs is depressed by a magnetic field. The value of the field, H^*_{C2}, required to lower the temperature of the anomaly is depicted in Fig. 10. There is considerable anisotropy in this field dependence, characteristic of superconductors of reduced dimensionality. Fig. 11 shows the field

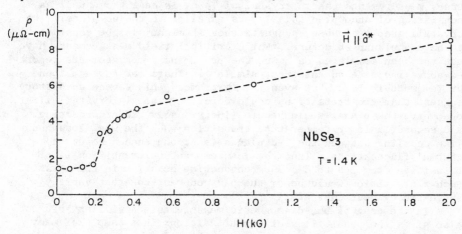

Figure 11. Field dependence (H∥a*) of the resistivity of NbSe$_3$ at 1.4 K. Current density was 5×10^{-3} A/cm^2.

dependence of the resistivity at a fixed temperature of 1.4 K. There is a well defined transition to normal state behavior at a field of 200 Oe applied perpendicular to the current. The corresponding transition is at a field of order 10 kOe for the parallel field, and is much broader.

It should be emphasized that all these measurements were made using currents less than 500 nA in samples of about 10^{-5} cm^2 cross-section (i.e. current densities less than 5 x 10^{-2}A/cm^2). Non-linear I-V characteristics are observed for current densities in excess of 10^{-1} A/cm^2 (i.e. 1 μA).

DISCUSSION

The onset of temperature dependent diamagnetism with the resistivity drop near 2.5 K indicates a superconducting transition in both TaSe$_3$ and NbSe$_3$ at this temperature. This is made certain by the observation of flux trapping in all samples. However, the temperature and field dependence of the susceptibility cannot be explained simply in terms of a superconducting transition near 2.5K. While the non-constancy of the dc susceptibility in weak fields and the difference between the ac and dc susceptibilities could be interpreted as extreme type II behavior, such an interpretation would explain neither the positive curvature of χ vs T nor the strong increase of χ at temperatures far below the superconducting transition temperature.

The observations are suggestive of a transition in which separate small regions of dimension much smaller than the superconduting penetration depth are individually superconducting below about 2.5 K and become coupled over much larger regions when the thermal energy k_BT becomes less than the coupling energy between regions. Two possibilities are coupling between portions of a single crystal and coupling between the small crystals which make up the sample.

Yamamoto[3] has suggested on the basis of critical field anisotropy measurements that a crystal of TaSe$_3$ is best thought of as consisting of uncoupled thin layers parallel to the bc plane. The crystallography of NbSe$_3$ suggests that it might also be considered to have a planar structure. While critical field measurements have not yet been completed on NbSe$_3$ the preliminary measurements reported above indicate an anistropy similar in character to that found by Yamamoto in TaSe$_3$ but even more extreme. This severe anisotropy suggests that two transitions could occur in a single crystal: first, one where the planes would become (individually) superconducting, and second, a lower temperature transition when the weak Josephson-like coupling between the 2-d planes is strong enough to overcome thermal fluctuations. Thus the low temperature transition is a transition from 2-d to 3-d superconducting behavior in the crystal. Such a transition would be of the paracoherent-coherent variety suggested by Deutscher et al.[11]

In the case of the diamagnetic measurements a similar argument also gives the possibility of two transitions in a sample of many weakly coupled crystals. In this model the first transition occurs when individual crystals become superconducting, the second when the inter-crystal superconducting coupling becomes established. While this second possibility cannot be ruled out, its likelihood is diminished by the requirement that the penetration depth of these materials must be very large, greater than 10 μm, in order to explain the small diamagnetism near the first resistive anomaly. This latter explanation also does not account for the non-zero residual resistance routinely observed in these materials.

While not conclusive, the experimental evidence tends to support the concept of weakly coupled 2-d superconducting planes within the $TaSe_3$ and $NbSe_3$ crystals. If so, the inter-phase coupling is much weaker than that normally found in the dichalcogenides with the 3-d ordering here occurring far below T_c. Thus these materials may well be the best examples available of 2-d superconductivity. Further work on these materials is in progress.

This research was supported by the National Science Foundation under grant number DMR77-09879 and by NSF through the Cornell University Materials Science Center, grant number DMR76-81083.

REFERENCES

1. R. M. Fleming, D. E. Moncton, D. B. McWhan, Phys. Rev. B 18, 5560 (1978).
2. T. Sambongi, M. Yamamoto, K. Tsutsumi, Y. Shiozaki, K. Yamaya, Y. Abe, J. Phys. Soc. Jap. 42, 1421 (1977).
3. M. Yamamoto, J. Phys. Soc. Jap. 45, 431 (1978).
4. P. Haen, F. Lapierre, P. Monceau, M. Nunez Regueiro and J. Richard, Sol. St. Comm. 26, 725 (1978).
5. P. Haen, J. M. Mignot, P. Monceau and M. Nunez Regueiro, J. de Phys. (Paris) 39, C6-703 (1978).
6. P. Monceau, J. Peyrard, J. Richard, P. Molinie, Phy. Rev. Lett. 39, 161 (1977).
7. W. W. Fuller, P. M. Chaikin, N. P. Ong, Solid St. Comm. 30, 689 (1979).
8. A. Meerschaut and J. Rouxel, J. Less Common Metals 39, 197 (1975).
9. E. Bjerkelund and A. Kjekshus, Acta. Chem. Scand. 19, 701 (1965)
10. J. L. Hodeau, M. Marezio, C. Roucau, R. Ayroles, A. Meerschaut, J. Rouxel and P. Monceau, J. Phys. C 11, 4117 (1978).
11. C. Deutscher, Y. Imry, L. Gunther, Phys. Rev. B 10, 4598 (1974).

A SEARCH FOR NEW MECHANISMS OF SUPERCONDUCTIVITY IN ULTRA
THIN FILMS: THE EFFECT OF INTERFACE AND FLUCTUATION PHENOMENA

Myron Strongin
Brookhaven National Laboratory, Upton, New York 11973

ABSTRACT

A discussion is given of superconductivity in ultra-thin films
with emphasis on various phenomena which affect the T_c of these
films. The effects of the substrate and interface are discussed
and are shown to have a great influence on the T_c in many cases.

INTRODUCTION

Thin film superconductors have always been somewhat mysterious
with the promise of high transition temperatures and phenomena
that would be characteristic of the two-dimensional nature of the
system, and also the unique interactions that could possibly occur at
interfaces and surfaces. Unfortunately, there has been little evidence of intrinsic interactions that are special to films. On the
other hand superconducting films have provided a rich medium for
studying fluctuation phenomena, the physics of two-dimensional
systems, and I think there might also be some evidence of unique
interface phenomena on semiconducting surfaces that deserve further
study. Preparing this talk has given me a chance to look back over
our work at Brookhaven and has allowed me some perspective in
viewing the evidence for new mechanisms in films, and in guessing
about what future directions may be profitable.

EPITAXIAL Al ON Si

To begin with the simplest system, although probably the most
difficult experiment,[1] I would like to discuss thin films of Al on
Si. We chose this system since for all practical purposes the
silicon is non-conducting at liquid helium temperatures and it was
known from previous work[2] how Al epitaxes on Si. In figure 1 we
show how first a 1/3 monolayer structure must be grown when Al is
deposited on the (111) face of Si, and then the structure of Al is
evident as the next layers are deposited. These films were covered
with Ge and when removed from the vacuum system and put in the
cryostat, the $T_c \sim 1.4$K. Other films had somewhat higher T_c's;
however the case shown in figure 2 is interesting. Both transitions
are of films made at the same time and both films have the same
transition defined by the $\frac{1}{2}R$ point which we call T_{C_1}. However the
transition is broader and the zero resistance point[2] is lowered in
the large $R_\square$ film, as one would expect from fluctuations. We
define this transition point for the purposes of the discussion, as
T_{C_0}. In both cases the grain size must be very large (as it must
be to get a LEED pattern) and the T_{C_1} is determined by the T_c in
the grain, which is near 1.4K. Of course it is also fascinating

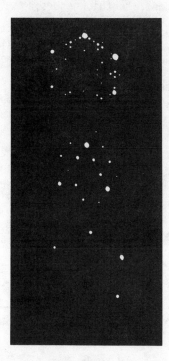

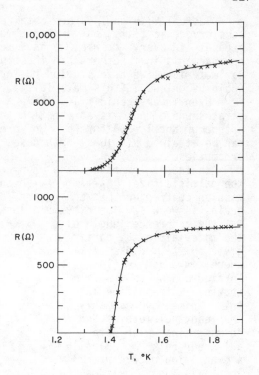

Fig. 1. Top, LEED "7" pattern characteristic of clean
Si(111) surface [Si(111)-7
pattern]. Electron
beam energies are in
the range of 40 to 50 eV.
Middle, LEED $\sqrt{3}$ Al pattern
characteristic of 1/3 monolayer Al structure on Si(111)
surface [Si(111)-$\sqrt{3}$ Al pat-
tern]. Bottom, Al structure.

Fig. 2. Top, transition of "nonepi-
taxial film." Thickness about 30Å,
$1/w \sim 1$. Prepared at same time as
"epitaxial" film. Bottom, transition of "epitaxial" film on one-
third monolayer structure. Thickness about 30Å and $1/w \sim 1$.

that such a film with nominal thickness of $\sim$25Å has near the bulk T_C.
I don't want to get ahead of things, but one might immediately wonder
why Al films on glass or other substrates with comparable $R_\square$ have T_C's
near 1.8K. In fact, when the present epitaxial films are oxidized
T_{C_1} rises: Why? Maybe some of the answer lies in recent work by
Šimanek[3] where he talks about enhancement of T_C due to surface disorder.

ULTRA THIN CRYOGENIC FILMS

Epitaxial films are extremely difficult to grow, and only special
cases are possible. Another more general approach to making ultra-
thin films is deposition onto cryogenic substrates.[4] In this case instead of achieving an equilibrium state, the motion of the deposited
atoms is restricted so that the metal does not agglomerate as much as
at higher temperatures and thus continuity can be attained for smaller
thicknesses.

Basically, high T_c's are obtained at moderate thicknesses in some cryogenic films[4] but as the thickness becomes near 20Å T_c decreases[5] in every material we have measured. Since we are looking for enhancements in T_c other than those usually found in Al and other similar materials, we have studied Pb in some detail since any enhancement would be unique in this material.

Even in cryogenic films there are essentially two cases.[5] On substrates where there is some motion and agglomeration, continuity does not occur until $\sim$75Å for Pb. On pre-deposited Ge or SiO continuity can be attained at $\sim$10Å. Both cases have very different superconducting properties.

In the agglomerated case when continuity first occurs[5,6] $\xi_{eff} < d$, the particle size. $\xi_{eff} \sim \sqrt{\ell_{eff}\xi_0}$ and $\ell_{eff} \sim dM$ where M is the transmission coefficient between grains. Hence when the coupling between grains is weak ξ_{eff} becomes much less than d. Note that there is also ξ_p, the coherence length of the material in the particle given by $\xi_p^2 \sim 0.7\ \xi_0\ell/\tau$, where $\ell \sim d$ and $\tau = (T-T_c)/T_c$. In figure 3 we show a film that has a transition in this regime.[5] Presumably the lead agglomerates and forms grains which retain a T_c near bulk Pb. Finally a transition occurs with a long tail due to critical fluctuations when $kT > E_J$.[6,7] Note that even though $R_\square \sim 30,000\ \Omega$--possibly the maximum metallic resistivity in a 2-D system[8]--and activated conduction is obtained, there is still a sharp transition down to a few % of R_N. The transition which is sharper than the Aslamozov Larkin[9] (AL) result, that the pair conductivity, $\sigma_p = \sigma_N \frac{\tau_0}{\tau}$ and $\tau_0 = 1.5 \times 10^{-5}\ R_\square$, is explained by putting a cutoff on the minimum fluctuation length. For a uniform material or one where $\xi_{eff} > d$ the minimum size for a fluctuation is ξ_{eff}, but in the case where $\xi_{eff} < d$ and $\xi_p > d$ we take the cutoff as the particle size. Then instead of the Al result we get[6]

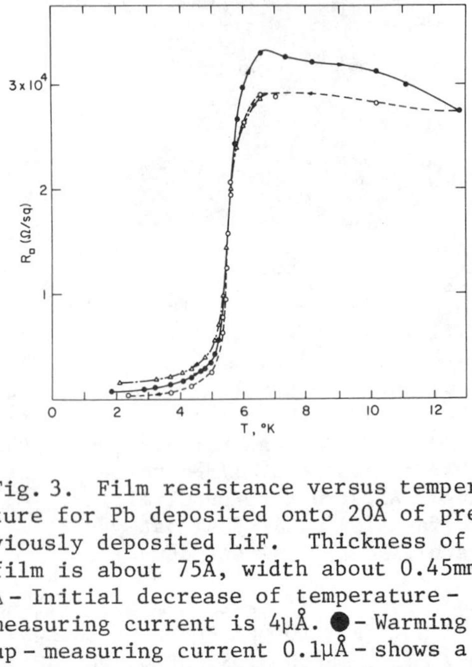

Fig. 3. Film resistance versus temperature for Pb deposited onto 20Å of previously deposited LiF. Thickness of film is about 75Å, width about 0.45mm. $\triangle$ – Initial decrease of temperature – measuring current is 4µA. ● – Warming up – measuring current 0.1µA – shows a change due to the decrease of current and then annealing starting near 7°K. ○ – cooling down again – measuring current 0.1Å.

$$\sigma_p/\sigma_N \sim [2\tau_0/\xi_{eff}^2(0)]\int_0^{1/d^2} k^2 dk^2/[k^2 + \xi_{eff}^{-2}(T)]^3 \qquad (1)$$

and finally $\sigma_p/\sigma_N = \tau_0/\tau \left(\frac{\xi_0 \ell_{eff}}{d^2\tau}\right)^2$, which leads to a much narrower transition than Al. Hence even though $R_\square \sim 30,000\ \Omega$, in special systems there can be a relatively sharp drop, which is then followed by a long tail as in figure 3.

The next case which is more interesting from T_c considerations is the ultra-thin film case.[5] In this case, films of Pb or Bi are put on previously deposited SiO or Ge and the results shown in figure 4 are obtained. At about 30,000 $\Omega/\square$ there is activated conduction and no trace of superconductivity. Finally as more metal is deposited a

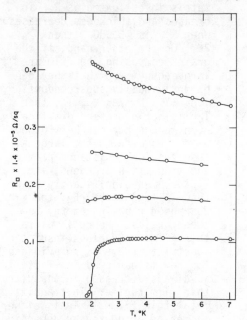

Fig. 4. Resistive behavior as Pb is built up. First stages show nonmetallic conduction where film resistance increases as temperature is decreased. As more metal is deposited the resistance decreases and metallic behavior and superconductivity appear. In the middle two curves there is nonmetallic conduction in the normal state and the beginning of a superconducting transition. When the full transition appears the film thickness, as determined by the Sloane thickness monitor, is usually from 10Å to 20Å.

partial transition is evident at $\sim$12,000 $\Omega/\square$ and then there is a transition to the superconducting state at 7,000 $\Omega/\square$, well below the $T_{c_{\frac{1}{2}}}$ of bulk lead. There has been much speculation about why $T_{c_{\frac{1}{2}}}$ decreases so dramatically in these films, and most explanations involve "dead layers"[10] or some kind of proximity effect.[5,11] There have also been some estimates of how the activated conduction effects T_c. If A is the activation energy, the BCS equation was solved with a gap 2A around E_F.[5] This yields that

$$\Delta^2 = \Delta_0(\Delta_0 - 2A). \tag{2}$$

Hence when the activation energy is about $\frac{1}{2}\Delta_0$, then $\Delta \to 0$. In our case when superconductivity disappeared, A was $\sim$2K and only a depression of 1K is accounted for. Another factor to be considered in this ultra-thin film case is that small particles <25A will not stay superconducting independently, due to quantization of energy levels in the particles,[5] and also because large fluctuations will exist since $kT > H_c^2/8\pi V_{part}$. Hence it is important for the particles to be connected, and clearly $R_\square$ is a measure of the connectivity and determines the fluctuation broadening of the tail. Next we mention that besides fluctuations broadening the transition, as $R_\square$ increases, there will also be a decrease in $T_{C\frac{1}{2}}$ due to fluctuations that is of the order of the transition width.[5] At $R_\square \sim 5,000\ \Omega$, this is of the order of 1K. I also should emphasize again that these are general considerations and that the very thinnest films of Al and Sn also have depressed T_C's in the thinnest cryogenic films; this is shown in figure 5.

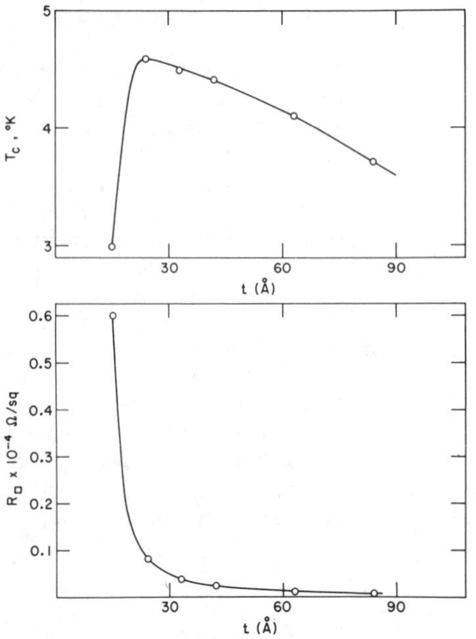

To summarize, T_C is depressed in ultra-thin films of all metals investigated as $R_\square$ increases and thickness decreases. When $R_\square$ is $\sim 5,000\ \Omega$ then $T_{C\frac{1}{2}} \sim$ 2K. On the other hand, if the grains composing the film are large enough, so that they can be individually superconducting, i.e. $kT < H_C^2/8\pi\ V_{grain}$, then $T_{C\frac{1}{2}}$ is not depressed drastically even though $R_\square$ can be $\sim 30,000$ Ω. However in the large $R_\square$ case the low resistance part of the transition broadens, i.e. T_{C_0} becomes significantly lower than $T_{C\frac{1}{2}}$ due to $kT > E_J$, the Josephson coupling energy between grains. Hence in ultra-thin films on various insulating substrates there is no evidence for new mechanisms. In fact, T_C is always decreased in the ultra-thin film regime. In transition metal thin films,[12] T_C is either increased or decreased depending on changes in the density of states and this more complicated case is not particularly relevant to the present discussion.

Fig. 5. T_C vs. thickness for Al films deposited on previously deposited SiO. Lower graph shows sharply increased resistance at small thicknesses.

LAYERED STRUCTURES AND MIXTURES

Perhaps the best evidence that something unique may happen in thin films is provided by layered structures, mixtures and by experiments where films are deposited on semiconductor surfaces. In figure 6 we show some results where Al and Ge layers[1] are deposited at cryogenic temperature. $T_{C\frac{1}{2}}$'s near 6K are possible here with Ge, and similar results can be obtained with SiO, oxygen, etc.[13] One might think that these results show there is some interaction mediated through the layers or even an excitonic mechanism. In other cases Al and Ge and other dielectrics[14] have been mixed in granular materials and increased T_C's are observed, again leading to speculation that some interaction involving the dielectric is involved. I don't think that these experiments conclusively show this. It can be seen from figure 7, where we have made

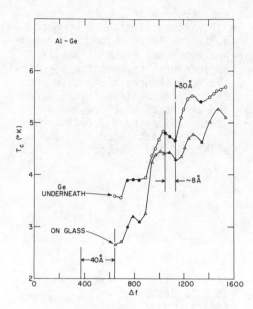

Fig. 6. Plot of T_C vs. thickness for alternate layers of Al and Ge. The thickness scale is in units of frequency change in a crystal oscillator thickness monitor. Some characteristic thicknesses are given in the figure.

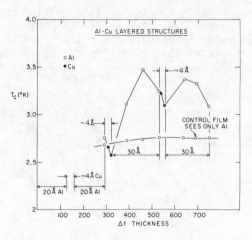

Fig. 7. Plot of T_C vs. thickness for alternate layers of Al and Cu. The thickness scale is in units of frequency change on a crystal-oscillator thickness monitor. Some characteristic thicknesses are given in the figure. On this run there was also a control film. Every time Al was deposited to make the Al-Cu layers, Al was deposited at the same time under the same conditions on the control film. It can be seen that the control on which only Al is deposited stays at about 2.7K, the T_C of thick Al films on cryogenic substrates.

layers of Al and Cu,[15] that every time the Al layers are interrupted by a Cu layer $T_{C\frac{1}{2}}$ goes down, as expected for an addition of Cu, but the next layers of Al actually raise $T_{C\frac{1}{2}}$ again, and to a T_C above the T_C before the Cu was deposited. Hence the important thing is to make an interface, it doesn't matter whether it's a metal, semiconductor, or an insulator. The common explanation for the effect of the interface was softening of phonon-modes.[15] My feeling about this, and I emphasize it's just a feeling, is that soft phonons don't account for everything and there is some other mechanism that remains to be understood which involves interfaces. I think that the suggestion of Simanek[3] of an interaction at disordered interfaces sounds attractive. In any case because the effect is observed even with metallic layers, the increased T_C is most likely <u>not</u> due to an excitonic mechanism or some interaction through a dielectric. Certainly, better experiments must be done to prove these effects, and the situation remains inconclusive because of our lack of knowledge of the exact nature of these systems.

In concluding this session on layered systems it should be mentioned that large effects in the T_c in ultra-thin films have been found when overlayers are put over ultra-thin films.[5,6] In figure 8 an example of this effect is shown. These experiments are especially difficult to interpret because the $R_\square$ of the film changes along with the changes at the interface. Hence the effect of coupling which is parameterized by $R_\square$ cannot be completely separated from the effect of the interface.

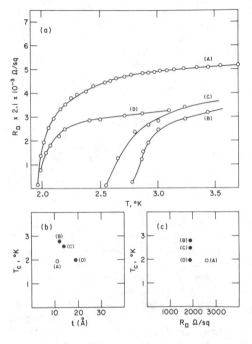

Fig. 8. Effect of Ge overlay on Pb film deposited on Ge. (A) Film as deposited; (B,C,D) Effects of different amounts of Ge. Note large T_c increase and decrease in $R_\square$ after initial deposition of Ge given by B.

EPITAXIAL LAYERS ON SEMI-CONDUCTORS

Experiments on metal-semiconductors interfaces have also shown phenomena that are not completely understood. In an experimental search for an excitonic mechanism we grew epitaxial films of Pb, In and Tl on PbTe and Te surfaces.[17,18] In figure 9 we show the (111) face of Pb on the (100) PbTe surface. In and Tl grow in a similar manner to Pb although the bulk crystal structure is different. One of the interesting results we found in these experiments was that the Pb films could be made electrically continuous and superconducting at thicknesses as small as 10Å. Since the film was probably not structurally continuous at these thicknesses, it implied to us that the substrate was intimately involved in the superconductivity and that some of the conduction was through the substrate. A further indication that this was the case, was that the critical field of the films actually decreased below about 25Å.[18] Of course in thin films the critical field should go as 1/d if there is no paramagnetic limiting, and decreasing critical field in the thinnest films implies that grains of superconductor must be weakly coupled through the PbTe where the critical field is low, and that the PbTe is part of the superconducting state. Experiments were also done where Pb was grown on single crystal Te[18] and also on single crystal Si.[19] A first look at the data shows that the depression in T_c as thickness decreases for epitaxial films on PbTe that

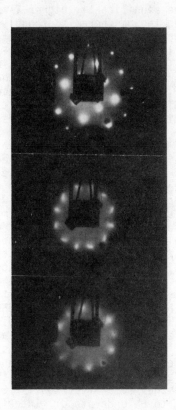

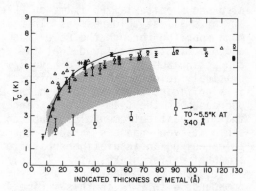

Fig. 10. Superconducting transition temperature, measured resistivity, as a function of the thickness of metal deposited, indicated by a calibrated quartz-crystal-oscillator-rate monitor. ● - Pb deposited on PbTe at 77K, measured in situ; ○, × ▽ - Pb deposited on Te at about 7K, measured in situ; Δ - Pb deposited on PbTe at 77K, warmed to room temperature and exposed to air before measurement; ▉ - In deposited on Te at about 7K, measured in situ; ◻ - In deposited on PbTe at about 7K, measured in situ. + - In deposited on PbTe and annealed to room temperature: dotted region are T_c s of cryogenic depositions on Ge and SiO.

Fig. 9. (a) LEED picture of a {100} PbTe face, at 98 eV. (b) LEED picture at 94 eV of the same PbTe crystal covered with 9-13Å Pb. The twelvefold rotational symmetry results from the superposition of two equivalent orientations of the sixfold pattern produced by the (111) plane of crystalline Pb. (c) LEED picture at 99 eV of an In layer, ∿30Å thick, on (100) PbTe face. A similar pattern is observed for Tl.

is not very different from the old cryogenic depositions onto disordered Ge or SiO surfaces discussed before,[5] or films made on crystalline Si or Te. In figure 10 some of this data is accumulated. The dotted region indicates the spread of the old data on Ge and SiO. However, note that the ordered films on PbTe discussed here define the high T_c border of the hatched region. The different microstructures in the cryogenic films clearly provide a large T_c variation with thickness; this is to be expected because of the variation in microstructure which shows up as a variation of $R_\square$. It is also important to mention that the data also shows epitaxial Pb films on PbTe have significantly higher T_c's at the smallest thicknesses. This is even though there is probably more coupling through the PbTe than through the insulating substrates and one might have argued that the proximity effect to a non-super-conducting substrate should have lowered T_c. In fact, the decreasing critical fields in the very thinnest Pb on PbTe films shows that there is significant coupling through the PbTe. Hence, even though T_c always decreases as the films become thinner, PbTe appears to be the substrate that is least detrimental to superconductivity. Actually it is pos-sible it even enhances T_c above the value it would have at the same thickness on an insulating substrate. The case of In on PbTe shows somewhat different results. In this case T_c for In on PbTe, or even In on Te, goes up to near 6K.[17,18] As far as I know there are no In-Te compounds with T_c's in this regime, and somehow the surface of the semi-conductor must be involved in the superconductivity. Again, we do not think this is an excitonic mechanism since T_c increases as more indium is deposited. In fact, for In deposited on PbTe held at 7K and measured in situ, T_c is increasing gradually to 5.5K for thicknesses near 300Å.[18] Other runs show T_c's over 6K for 30-50Å films deposited at 100K. We don't understand why such thick layers, especially those near 300Å, have such high T_c's. Possibly the indium agglomerates, and the high T_c is in the surface layer or inversion layer of the substrate. There are also reports of an impurity stabilized non-equilibrium phase of In with a T_c near 5.7K; however both LEED and Auger studies indicate an In surface without observable impurities. Tl on PbTe also has a T_c near 5.5K, while Al and Sn have T_c's near $\sim$2.5K and 3.5K which is simi-lar to their T_c's on other surfaces.[5] One can speculate that Al and Sn are expected to produce a less highly inverted inversion region[17] than Pb, Tl and In and it is possible that this has some effect on T_c. Clearly there are some problems here that deserve to be understood. Interface compounds of some sort may be involved, such as the 1/3 monolayer Al on Si structure. However such structures have not been observed in LEED measurements.

Other examples of interface phenomena in other kinds of systems may be found in the work of Ghosh and Douglass,[20] where T_c's near 16K are found at the NbGe$_2$--Ge interface and also the work of Tsuei and Johnson[21] where high T_c's were found in adjacent layers of metal and semiconduc-tors produced in bulk samples by metallurgical techniques.

SUMMARY

In this paper I have briefly discussed some aspects of the transi-tion temperature of thin film superconductors relevant to establishing whether there are unique interactions in film-substrate composites. Be-cause in this configuration fluctuations, disorder, and the substrate itself affect the transition temperature, it has been necessary to give some discussion of the nature of these effects so that any intrinsic phenomena due to interfaces or interactions through the substrate can be separated out. We have shown that when films are grown epitaxially on an insulating substrate, T_c's near the bulk T_c can be obtained. On the other hand in cryogenically deposited films large depressions in T_c occur as the thickness becomes less than about 30-50Å. How much of this depres-sion is due to fluctuations, activated conduction and localization, or proximity to the substrate is not completely understood.

Then there is the case of layered structures. Large rises in T_C can be obtained in such systems, but it is not clear how much is due to soft phonons, an interaction mediated in the dielectric, or how much is due to creating the interface itself.

Finally there is the case of films on semiconducting surfaces. In this case there is significant coupling through the semiconducting surface and there are effects in T_C that are not understood. I think that there are some unique phenomena here that are worthy of further study.

My feeling in looking back at our work and the work of others is that most empirical and exploratory types of things have been tried. Of course, there are always new ideas which may produce something surprising and interesting. However, as a general approach to ultra-thin films I think more emphasis should be placed on understanding the effect of the substrate and the metal-substrate interface. Difficult experiments must be done using modern surface analysis and vacuum techniques to characterize the structure of films on clean surfaces. With the more general availability of photoemission apparatus there is also hope of understanding how the electronic structure of both the metal and the substrate change when they are combined into the usual composite configuration. With these kinds of techniques there is also the possibility of investigating superconductivity in unique surface structures, such as the 1/3 monolayer Al structure on Si. I emphasize that these experiments require a significant investment in time and equipment and they are not worth doing without serious theoretical input about which systems are likely to provide interesting results. I hope such theoretical activity will be expanded.

ACKNOWLEDGMENTS

Many people have played a major role in the experiments discussed here and rather than risk leaving out someone, I would like to express my thanks to the people I have collaborated with over the years. Those pertinent to this work are easily identifiable in the references. My special thanks are due to O.F.Kammerer, my friend and colleague whose knowledge about materials made these experiments possible. This work is supported by the Dept. of Energy under contract EY-76-C-02-0016.

REFERENCES

1. M.Strongin, O.F.Kammerer, H.H.Farrell and D.L.Miller, Phys. Rev. Letters 30, 129 (1973).
2. J.J.Lander and J.Morrison, Surface Sci. 2, 553 (1964).
3. E.Simanek - preprint.
4. V.Buckel and R.Hilsch, Z. Physik 132, 420 (1952); N.V.Zavaritsky, Dokl. Akad. Nauk. SSSR 86, 501 (1952).
5. M.Strongin, R.S.Thompson, O.F.Kammerer and J.E.Crow, Phys. Rev. B 1, 1078 (1970).
6. R.S.Thompson, M.Strongin, O.F.Kammerer and J.E.Cros, Phys. Letters 29A, 194 (1969).
7. T.D.Clark and D.R.Tilley, Phys. Letters 28A, 62 (1968).
8. R.C.Dynes, J.P.Garno and J.M.Rowell, Phys. Rev. Letters 40, 479 (1978)
9. L.G.Aslamazov and A.I.Larkin, Phys. Letters 26A, 238 (1968).

226

10. C.G.Grandquist and T.Claeson, J. Phys. (Paris) 35, C4-301 (1974).
11. D.Miller, M.Strongin and O.F.Kammerer, Phys. Rev. B 13, 4834 (1976).
12. J.E.Crow, M.Strongin, R.S.Thompson and O.F.Kammerer, Phys. Letters 30A, 161 (1969); M.M.Collver and R.H.Hammond, Phys. Rev. Letters 30, 92 (1973).
13. M.Strongin, O.F.Kammerer, D.H.Douglass and M.H.Cohen, Phys. Rev. Letters 19, 121 (1967).
14. A.Fontaine and F.Meunier, Phys. Kondens, Mater. 14, 119 (1972); J.P.Hurault, J. Phys. Chem. Solids 29, 1765 (1968); M.Rappaport and G.Deutscher - unpublished.
15. M.Strongin, O.F.Kammerer, J.E.Crow, R.D.Parks, D.H.Douglass and M.A.Jensen, Phys. Rev. Letters 21, 1320 (1968).
16. D.G.Naugle, Phys. Letters 25A, 688 (1967); V.M.Golyanov, M.I. Mikheeva, N.B.Tsetlin, Sov. Phys. JETP 41, 365 (1975).
17. D.L.Miller, M.Strongin, O.F.Kammerer and B.G.Streetman, Phys. Rev. B 8, 4416 (1973).
18. D.L.Miller, M.Strongin, O.F.Kammerer and B.G.Streetman, Phys. Rev. B 13, 4834 (1976).
19. D.L.Miller, Phys. Rev. B 15, 4180 (1977).
20. A.K.Ghosh and D.H.Douglass, Phys. Rev. Letters 37, 32 (1976).
21. C.C.Tsuei and W.L.Johnson, Phys. Rev. B 9, 4742 (1974).

SUPERCONDUCTIVITY AT DISORDERED INTERFACES

E. Šimánek

University of California, Riverside, Ca. 92521

ABSTRACT

The contribution of the negative U-centers to the enhancement of T_C at a disordered metal-semiconductor contact is examined using an extended Anderson impurity model coupled, via tunneling, to the conduction electrons of the metal. The presence of a bipolaron interaction of electronic origin is found essential to produce ΔT_C of experimental significance.

INTRODUCTION

The problem of the interface between a normal metal and a disordered semiconductor has recently received a new impetus from the ideas advanced by Varma and Pandey.[1] These authors suggest that the metal-semiconductor bonds at the interface behave in a similar way as the negative U-bipolarons previously proposed by Anderson[2] for chalcogenide glasses. Tunneling of the metallic electrons into these bipolaron states has been shown recently[3] to lead to an enhancement of the superconducting transition temperature capable of explaining the experimental data on the coevaporated $A\ell$-Ge mixtures[4] and the eutectic $A\ell$-Ge and $A\ell$-Si alloys.[5] In our original calculation[3] we assumed a bipolaron interaction mediated by a local phonon, representing the displacements of rearranging bonds.[1,2] Recently Kastner[6] proposed an electronically induced negative U for chalcogenide glasses and Elliot[7] advocated similar ideas for tetrahedrally bonded semiconductors.

In the present paper we calculate the enhancement of superconductivity by bipolaron interface centers, including this electronically mediated interaction.

ENHANCEMENT OF T_C

We consider a single center-localized state coupled, via tunneling, to the conduction electrons of the metal, which also exhibits the usual BCS interaction.

The Hamiltonian of this system is

$$\mathcal{H} = \mathcal{H}_{BCS} + \sum_{k,s} \varepsilon_k a_{ks}^+ a_{ks} + E(n\uparrow + n\downarrow) + Un\uparrow n\downarrow$$
$$+ \sum_{k,s} V_k(a_{ks}^+ a_s + a_s^+ a_{ks}) + \sum_{i=1,2} [\frac{\lambda_i}{\sqrt{2\omega_i}}(n\uparrow + n\downarrow)(b_i^+ + b_i)$$
$$+ \omega_i(b_i^+ b_i + 1/2)] \tag{1}$$

where E, U and V_k are the one-electron energy, Coulomb energy and tunneling matrix element for the localized state. The last two terms in eq. (1) represent the coupling of the localized electron

228

to the phonon (i=1) and the electronic rearrangement (i=2). We
apply a canonical transformation

$$\tilde{\mathcal{H}} = e^{-iS}\,\tilde{\mathcal{H}}\,e^{iS} \tag{2}$$

where

$$S = \sum_{i=1,2} \frac{i\lambda_i}{\omega_i \sqrt{2\omega_i}} (n\!\uparrow+n\!\downarrow)(b_i^+ - b_i) \tag{3}$$

The transformed Hamiltonian $\tilde{\mathcal{H}}$ is of the form (1), except that
the linear terms in the b_i operators are eliminated, and E, U and
V_k are replaced by $E_{eff}= E - \sum_{i=1,2} i\lambda_i^2/2\omega_i^2$, $U_{eff}= U - \sum_{i=1,2}\lambda_i^2/2\omega_i^2$
and

$$\tilde{V}_k = V_k \exp\left[- \sum_{i=1,2} \frac{\lambda_i(b_i^+ - b_i)}{\omega_i \sqrt{2\omega_i}} \right] \tag{4}$$

respectively.

The increase of T_c due to the tunneling into a single localized state is calculated from the linearized gap equation[8]

$$1 = g \sum_{k,k'} \int_0^{1/T_c} d\tau <T_\tau \tilde{a}_{k\uparrow}^+(o)\tilde{a}_{-k}^+(o)\tilde{a}_{-k'\downarrow}(\tau)\tilde{a}_{k'\uparrow}(\tau)> \tag{5}$$

where the g is the BCS coupling strength and the two electron
Green's function is to be evaluated with the use of the normal part
of $\tilde{\mathcal{H}}$.

We use perturbation expansion in $\tilde{V}_k$ and adopt the Fermi liquid
expansion technique to treat U_{eff}. For an order of magnitude estimate we confine ourselves to the contribution which involves the inelastic scattering of the electrons via U_{eff}. The calculation of
this contribution to the two-electron Green's function in eq. (5)
is based on the method of Sakurai[8], modified to take into account
the presence of the boson operators in the tunneling term in
eq. (4). We obtain[3]

$$\frac{\Delta T_c}{T_c} = - \frac{1}{\rho}(\frac{N_i}{N})T_c^2 \sum_{\omega_m}^{\omega_D} \sum_{\omega_n}^{\omega_D} \sum_{k,k'} \sum_{\omega_\ell}^{\omega_2} \sum_{\omega_{\ell'}}^{\omega_2} G_k(\omega_m)G_{-k}(-\omega_m)$$

$$G_{k'}(\omega_n)G_{-k'}(-\omega_n)\Gamma_{\uparrow\downarrow}(\omega_m+\omega_{\ell'},\ \omega_n-\omega_{\ell'}) \tag{6}$$

$$G(\omega_m+\omega_\ell)G(-\omega_m-\omega_\ell)D_k(\omega_\ell)G(\omega_n-\omega_{\ell'})G(-\omega_n+\omega_{\ell'})D_{k'}(\omega_{\ell'})$$

where ρ is the conduction electron density of states at the Fermi
level of the metal and N_i/N is the relative concentration of the
centers. G is the Green's function of the localized electron fully

renormalized by U_{eff}, $\Gamma_{\uparrow\downarrow}$ is the vertex part due to the inelastic scattering of the up and down spin electron at the center.[8] The retarded nature of U_{eff} makes $\Gamma_{\uparrow\downarrow}$ vanish for ω_ℓ, $\omega_{\ell'} > \omega_2$. This produces an effective cutoff $\simeq \omega_2$ in the ω_ℓ and $\omega_{\ell'}$ summations. $D_k(\omega)$ is the Fourier transform of the correlation function $\langle \tilde{V}_k(\tau)\, \tilde{V}_{-k}(o)\rangle$. Noting that $\omega_2 \gg \omega_1$ we use, for $\omega_\ell < \omega_1$, the low ω - approximation:

$$D_k(\omega) \simeq 2\pi |V_k|^2 e^{-(\alpha_1+\alpha_2)} [\delta(\omega) + \alpha_1 \delta(\omega-\omega_1) + \ldots] \qquad (7)$$

where $\alpha_i = \lambda_i^2/2\omega_i^3$. Neglecting the weak k-dependence of V_k and using eq. (7) in eq. (6), we obtain

$$\frac{\Delta T_c}{T_c} \simeq -\frac{1}{\rho}(\frac{N_i}{N})(\pi\rho \ |V_k|^2 >_{T_c})^2 e^{-2(\alpha_1+\alpha_2)} \Gamma_{\uparrow\downarrow}^{(2)} \qquad (2)$$

$$\{\sum_{\omega_m}^{\omega_D} \frac{1}{|\omega_m|} [G^2(\omega_m)+\alpha_1 G^2(\omega_m+\omega_1) + \frac{\alpha_1^2}{2!} G^2(\omega_m+2\omega_1)+ \ldots\}^2 \qquad (8)$$

where $\Gamma_{\uparrow\downarrow}^{(2)}$ is the vertex part due to the "electronic" interaction $U_{eff}^{(2)} = U - \lambda_2^2/\omega_2^2$. We note that the α_1-expansion in (8) is limited to n terms where $n\omega_1 \lesssim \min(\omega_2, \omega_F)$.

In the case of a large width of the localized state, $\Gamma = \pi\rho<|v|^2> \gg \omega_1$, we have $G^2(\omega_m+n\omega_1) \simeq -\Gamma^{-2}$, valid up to $n\omega_1 \lesssim \Gamma$. This allows us to simplify the expression (8) to the following

$$\Delta T_c/T_c \simeq -\frac{1}{\rho}(\frac{N_i}{N})\frac{\Gamma_{\uparrow\downarrow}^{(2)} e^{-2\alpha_2}}{\pi^2 \Gamma^2}[\ell n(\frac{1.14\omega_D}{T_c})]^2 \qquad (9)$$

For eq. (9) to hold, the coupling to an electronic "boson", with $\omega_2 \gg \omega_1$, is necessary. We also see that the phonon overlap factor $e^{-2\alpha_1}$ cancels out in this limit. For an Aℓ-Ge interface we take $\omega_2 = 2eV$, $U_{eff} = -0.5eV$ and $U = 0.5eV$, which implies $\alpha_2 \simeq 0.25$. Taking $\Gamma = 0.3eV$ makes the many-body enhancement[8] of the vertex function negligible so that $\Gamma_{\uparrow\downarrow}^{(2)} \simeq U_{eff}$. Using these values, and letting $\rho = 0.39/eVat$ and $\omega_D = 400K$ we obtain from eq. (9) $\Delta T_c/T_c \simeq 30$ (Ni/N). The as-cast Aℓ$_{70}$ Ge$_{30}$ alloy[5] is characterized by Aℓ domains ranging from 400-3500A° and it shows $(\Delta T_c/T_c)exp \simeq 0.3$. The latter value can be explained by the present theory if Ni/N $\simeq 10^{-2}$, which can be supplied by the surface dangling bonds of an average 1000A° domain.

In the opposite limit of small Γ, the local Green's function develops a structure,[8] composed of the "central peak" of width $\tilde{\Gamma} \simeq \Gamma \exp\{-|U_{eff}|/8\Gamma\}$ and the "side bands" at energies $\pm U_{eff}/2$. For $T_c \ll \Gamma \ll \omega_0$ only the first term in the α_1-sum of eq. (8) contributes and we obtain for the "central peak" contribution

$$(\Delta T_c/T_c)_{c.p.} = - \frac{1}{\rho}(\frac{N_i}{N}) e^{-2(\alpha_1+\alpha_2)} \frac{\Gamma_{\uparrow\downarrow}^{(2)}}{\pi^2\Gamma^2}[\ln(\frac{0.42\tilde{\Gamma}}{T_c})]^2 \tag{10}$$

Although $\Gamma_{\uparrow\downarrow}^{(2)}$ is enhanced by the bipolaron interaction the expression (10) is greatly suppressed by the phonon-overlap factor $e^{-2\alpha_1}$. The side-band contribution is estimated by calculating $\Gamma_{\uparrow\downarrow}^{(2)}$ in the ladder approximation. For $U_{eff}^{(2)} \gg \omega_0$, we also have $G^2(\omega_m+n\omega_1) \simeq 4/U_{eff}^2$, allowing the cancellation of the phonon-overlap in eq. (8). The resulting side-band contribution to T_c is then

$$(\Delta T_c/T_c)_{s.b.} = - \frac{1}{\rho}(\frac{N_i}{N}) \frac{16\Gamma^2 e^{-2\alpha_2}}{\pi^2(1 + \frac{2}{\pi}\arctan\frac{2\omega_2}{\upsilon_{eff}^{(2)}})U_{eff}^{(2)3}} \tag{11}$$

Consistent with the condition $\Gamma \ll U_{eff}^{(2)}$, we take $\Gamma = 0.05$ eV, $U_{eff}^{(2)} = -0.5$eV and $\omega_2 = 2$eV for which eq. (11) predicts $\Delta T_c/T_c \simeq 0.6$ (Ni/N).

The above results indicate that large values of Γ and V_k are needed to produce experimentally significant enhancements of T_c. Since the matrix element V_k is proportional to the amplitude of the wave function penetrating into the semiconductor we have $\Gamma = \Gamma_0\exp(-y^{-1/2})$ where $y = E_F/ma^2Eg^2$, a being the distance of the center from the metal and Eg is the semiconductor gap.[9] Thus as E_F increases we pass from the limit of small $\tilde{\Gamma}$, for which eqs. (10) and (11) are valid, into the region of large $\tilde{\Gamma} \simeq \Gamma$, where eq. (9) is valid. This process is accompanied by a dynamical suppression of the phonon overlap factor, $e^{-2\alpha_1}$, since in the limit of large Γ the "fast" transitions of the electrons between the metal and the centers do not allow the "slow" lattice displacement to readjust. In ref. 3 we have suggested that the crossover between the static (small $\tilde{\Gamma}$) and dynamic (large $\tilde{\Gamma}$) limit is rapid enough to account for the experimentally observed[5] threshold below which there is no enhancement of T_c. We would like to point out here a few additional possibilities which may contribute to further sharpening of this crossover. The first one takes into account the static fluctuations of the one-electron energy E. When the width $\tilde{\Gamma}$ becomes comparable to the r·m·s value of ΔE we expect an effective wipe-out of the density of states of the centers at the Fermi level, leading to a suppression of the contributions (9) and (10) to ΔT_c. Another contribution to the variation of ΔT_c with E_F may be due to the dependence of U_{eff} on E_F. We note that the Coulomb integral U will be decreased by the image potential due to the nearby metal. If one takes into account the finite screening length $\lambda \propto E_F^{-1/4}$, the image potential given by[10] $V_{im} \propto (a+\lambda)^{-1}$ will itself become an increasing function of E_F leading to a decrease of U and increase of $|U_{eff}|$ with E_F.

Tsuei and Johnson[5] have considered the exciton mechanism of Allender et al[9] to account for their observations of ΔT_c in Aℓ-Si and Aℓ-Ge eutectic alloys. With the phonon mechanism turned-off, the exciton mechanism[9] alone yields a dependence of T_C on E_F very similar to that observed. Physically, what appears to cause this dependence is the removal of the states of the attracting electrons when E_F becomes smaller than the width of the exciton spectrum. We anticipate this dependence to weaken when the electron-phonon interaction in the metal is considered to act in parallel with the exciton mechanism.

The experiments of Strongin et al[11] on ultrathin films, grown epitaxially on Si, provide further guidance in the search of the superconductivity-enhancement mechanism. The fact that no increase of T_C is observed in the metal film is essential for the enhancement. Tsuei and Johnson,[5] on the other hand, have proposed that different Aℓ-atoms in the semiconductor enhance the tunneling and the relative time the electron pairs are exchanging excitons. Although diffusion can be expected in the eutectic alloys,[5] this is not probably so with the AℓGe alloys[4] coevaporated at low temperatures. The mechanism proposed in the present paper offers a natural explanation of the above observations. We suggest that samples[4,5] exhibiting large enhancements of T_C involve disordered interfaces. This allows for sizable electron and nuclear relaxations to take place around the metal-semiconductor bonds, making the electron-"boson" coupling constants λ_i to be large. We note that the topological constraints, hindering such relaxations in ordered structures, are reduced by the disorder. This is illustrated by the example of the three-coordinated defects T_3 intetrahedrally-bonded materials.[7] A negatively charged defect sp T_3^- is proposed to undergo a dehybridization sp $T_3^- \rightarrow$ p T_3^-, associated with sizable electron and smaller bond angle relaxations producing a negative correlation energy.[7] The electronic relaxation is a "localized" example of the exciton mechanism.[9] In fact, as emphasized by Allender et al[9], it is the "localized" valence valence bond polarization which is essential for the exciton-mediated attraction. The nuclear relaxation leads, as shown above, to a suppression of the resulting ΔT_C, due to the phonon overlap effects. Only in the limit of large Γ are these effects removed and there seems to be no essential distinction between the proposed and the exciton mechanism in this case.

It is also interesting to consider the role of the negative U-center for the superconductivity of an interface involving metals with vanishing electron-phonon interaction (g=o). This case is illustrated by the example of the Be-eutectic alloys,[5] showing large enhancements of T_C. In this case we can consider superconducting order which originates from the transfer of Cooper pairs between the cneters.[12] This transfer is presumably due to the indirect interaction mediated by the presence of the nearby metal surface.[13] For vanishing couplings ($\lambda_i = 0$) the one-electron transfer $t_{ij} a_i^+ a_j$ between the center i and j is of long range,[14] which suggests an interesting possibility of a two-dimension surface superconductivity without destruction of the long range order due to fluctuations. However the range of t_{ij} is affected by the phonon overlap effects. This is seen from the derivation of t_{ij} as a second order matrix element of $\tilde{v}_k a^+_k a$

$$t_{ij} \propto \sum_k \frac{e^{i\vec{k}(\vec{R}_i - \vec{R}_j)}}{E - \varepsilon_k} \langle \tilde{V}_{ki}\, \tilde{V}_{-kj} \rangle \tag{12}$$

Using the expression (4) with the "electronic bosons" neglected, we have

$$\langle \tilde{V}_{ki}\, \tilde{V}_{-kj} \rangle \simeq |V_k|^2 \exp\{-\alpha(1 - \langle b_i b_j^+ \rangle)\} \tag{13}$$

where $\alpha = \alpha_i = \alpha_j$ are the local phonon coupling constants. The correlation function $\langle b_i b_j^+ \rangle$ represents the phonon propagation between the sites $\vec{R}_i$ and $\vec{R}_j$. For a perfect crystal $\langle b_i b_j^+ \rangle$ is a slowly decaying function of R_{ij} and the long range character of t_{ij}, given by the k-sum in eq. (12), is preserved. The local bond displacements in a disordered interface may be, however, topologically decoupled so that $\langle b_i b_j^+ \rangle$ vanishes beyond nearest neighbor distance and the range t_{ij} is correspondingly diminished. This may be the reason for the broad and incomplete resistive transition observed in the Be-Si eutectic alloy.[5]

REFERENCES

1. C. M. Varma and K. C. Pandey, preprint, see also P. W. Anderson, J. de Physique 37, C-4, 339 (1976).
2. P. W. Anderson, Phys. Rev. Lett. 34, 953 (1975).
3. E. Šimánek, Solid State Commun. 32, 731 (1979).
4. K. Fontaine and R. Meunier, Phys. Kondens. Matter. 14, 119 (1972).
5. C. C. Tsuei and W. L. Johnson, Phys. Rev. B9, 4742 (1974).
6. M. Kastner, J. Noncryt. Solids 31, 223 (1978).
7. S. R. Elliot, Phil. Mag. B38, 325 (1978).
8. A. Sakurai, Phys. Rev. B17, 1195 (1978).
9. D. Allender, J. Bray and J. Bardeen, Phys. Rev. B7, 1020 (1973).
10. J. W. Gadzuk, J. K. Hartmann and T. N. Rhodin, Phys. Rev. B4, 241 (1971).
11. M. Strongin, O. F. Kammerer and H. H. Farrell, Phys. Rev. Lett. 30, 129 (1973).
12. P. Pincus, P. Chaikin, C. F. Coll, Solid State Commun. 12, 1265 (1973).
13. E. Abrahams, private communication.
14. E. Šimánek, to be published.

JOSEPHSON EFFECTS IN GRANULAR NbN MICROBRIDGES

E. J. Cukauskas, J. H. Claassen and M. Nisenoff
Naval Research Laboratory, Washington, DC 20375

C. H. Galfo, R. L. Steiner and B. S. Deaver, Jr.
University of Virginia*, Charlottesville, Va.

ABSTRACT

High resistance granular NbN microbridges with submicron dimensions have been fabricated and investigated. Devices with critical currents less than 5 microamps and bridge resistances of the order of 50 ohms have been studied as a function of temperature at both zero and finite voltages. The current-voltage characteristics were measured with various levels of applied radiation in the frequency range 11-40 GHz. For these frequencies, constant voltage-current steps were observed at the Josephson frequency, $2eV/h$ for low applied voltages, at higher voltages the radiation induced step spacing deviated from that of ideal Josephson behavior. Additional current steps were also observed at temperatures just above the bridge T_c where no finite critical current could be detected. These effects and other characteristics observed on the I-V curves will be reported and discussed.

INTRODUCTION

There is considerable interest in high T_c refractory superconducting materials for the fabrication of microwave radiation and magnetic field detectors.[1] The use of these materials should yield devices which are more rugged and durable than devices fabricated from soft materials or mechanical point contacts. Recently, we have reported that granular niobium nitride microbridges when fabricated in the rf SQUID geometry exhibit intrinsic noise characteristics and operate over a wide temperature range below the bridge T_c.[2,3] Because of their near ideal properties in the SQUID geometry, it was decided to evaluate similar devices as microwave radiation detectors. In this paper, we present preliminary results on the response of granular niobium nitride microbridges to applied microwave radiation with frequencies up to 40 GHz.

SAMPLE PREPARATION

The niobium nitride films were deposited onto quartz substrates in an oil free ultra high vacuum system by reactive rf sputtering in an argon-nitrogen atmosphere. Prior to sputtering the system was evacuated to a pressure of 1×10^{-9} torr after which the sputtering chamber was isolated from the pumping system and then back-filled to a pressure of 10 micrometers with 99.9995% purity Argon. During a

*Work at University of Virginia partially supported by O.N.R.

10-minute pre-sputtering period, the substrates were heated radiatively to approximately 600°C. With a 0.3 micrometer partial pressure of N_2 added to the sputtering atmosphere, the NbN films were then deposited at a rate of 100Å/min. A typical film prepared in this manner was 1200Å thick and had a transition temperature of approximately 15.6°K.

The as sputtered films were configured into the desired weak link geometry using photolithographic and ion milling techniques. The first step in the process resulted in a bridge of approximately one micrometer in width and several micrometers long. With additional photoresist masking and exposure using reverse projection through an optical microscope, a short strip less than one micrometer in length was exposed across the bridge region. This region was then thinned using ion milling until the critical current density dropped to the order of 10^5 amp/cm^2 from which we infer that the bridge material is granular.[4] Due to the tapering of the photoresist, this technique resulted in a bridge which was sub-micrometer in dimensions and 50 to 100Å in thickness. Figure 1 illustrates the geometry of the weak link region and an electron micrograph of a weak link fabricated using these techniques. The SEM picture suggests that the actual bridge dimensions are less than 0.5 micrometers. Typical bridge resistances were approximately 50 ohms.

EXPERIMENTAL DETAILS

The devices were mounted on a copper block and enclosed in a single vacuum can which was heat sunk to the helium bath. For temperatures above 4.2K, the temperature was maintained by controlling the current to a resistance heater embedded in the copper block. For lower temperatures, the vapor pressure of the helium bath was regulated. Four electrical contacts were made to indium pads which were ultrasonically soldered to the device prior to thinning. The twisted pair current and voltage leads were filtered at the top of the cryostat before connection to the measurement circuit. Because of the high resistance of the bridges, great care was taken to minimize noise pick up. All measurements were made in a screen room with the cryostat shielded by a superconducting shield and a pair of mu metal shields. Markedly different characteristics were obtained when measurements were taken with less precautions.

Systematic studies of the I-V curves and the derivatives as functions of temperature and applied microwave power were facilitated by use of a microcomputer controlled data acquisition system that permits simultaneous recording with high precision of all the pertinent parameters during each current scan. The system has an interactive graphics mode that permits monitoring of the data in real time as it is recorded and provides great versatility in studying the data once a data base of a large number of scans has been accumulated. This mode is extremely valuable for examining the detailed variation of structure on the I-V curves.

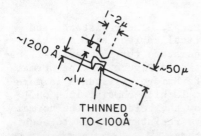

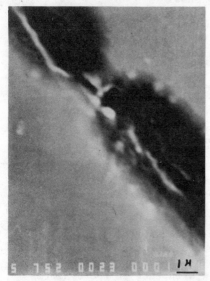

Figure 1. The geometry and an SEM picture of a granular microbridge. The bridge dimensions are less than 0.5 micrometers.

RESULTS

The data presented here (see Fig. 2) is for a device which has a transition temperature of 15.9°K for the banks and 3.3°K for the weak link. The bridge T_c is defined as the point at which the resistance goes to zero for vanishingly small measuring currents. The resistive transition and the critical current as a function of temperature for this device is illustrated in Fig. 2. The broad transition is probably due to the tapered film thickness of the bridge. Critical current values have been plotted up to a temperature of 5.2K even though the bridge resistance for temperatures above 3.3K is not zero. In this region the "critical current" was taken to be that current at which a definite break was observable in the current-voltage characteristics. This device also exhibited microwave induced current steps in this resistive region. The maximum measured critical current was approximately 5 micro-amps at 1.35°K, the lowest temperature for which measurements were taken. If the bridge width is taken as 0.5

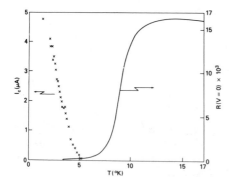

Figure 2. The resistance and critical current as a function of temperature for the device illustrated in Figure 1. The normal state bridge resistance is more than 15 kilo-ohms at $15°$K while below the bridge T_c, the normal state resistance drops to about 50 ohms.

micrometers and its thickness as 50Å, the apparent critical current density is of the order of 10^5 amps/cm^2. Critical current densities of this order are characteristic of granular niobium nitride films.[4]

The current-voltage characteristics as a function of the amplitude of the applied microwave radiation are illustrated in Fig. 3. This data was taken at a temperature of 3.2K with 16.84 GHz applied microwave radiation. For low power levels the induced current steps up to n = 4 are clearly observed at voltages which were multiples of the Josephson voltage hf/2e. As the power is increased, the steps become more rounded and wash out probably due to heating. However, there is enough range to observe the first minimum in what may be "Bessel-like" oscillations of step amplitude vs rf level. Figure 4 is the corresponding dynamic resistance for the set of curves illustrated in Figure 3. The step spacing is more evident in this set of curves. At higher voltages distinctive structure in the dynamic resistance appears for higher microwave drive levels. The nearly regular spacing of the minima are intriguing but are not related by the Josephson voltage-frequency equation. We have no simple explanation for this structure at present.

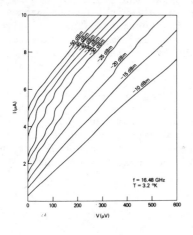

Figure 3. The current voltage characteristics as a function of 16.48 GHz microwave power for the device illustrated in Figure 1. The temperature is $3.2°$K and the current axis is offset 0.7 μa for each trace. The n = 1 step clearly shows oscillations in height.

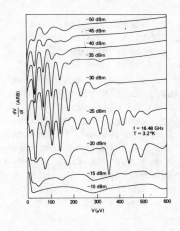

Figure 4. The dynamic resistance vs voltage for the set of traces illustrated in Figure 3. The Josephson step spacing is observed up to the n = 4 step, non-Josephson structure is also present particularly at the higher rf power levels.

A second bridge which was investigated had a higher T_c and a slightly higher bridge resistance. This device had a critical temperature approximately $6.5^\circ K$ and a maximum critical current of 2 microamps. The bridge resistance was about 60 ohms. Its small critical current and high resistance probably mask the true onset T_c. This device had little response to applied microwave radiation below about 25 GHz. Above this frequency microwave induced current steps were observed at temperatures up to approximately $6^\circ K$ in the dV/dI vs V trace, but were not as readily observable in the I-V characteristic due to noise rounding. At lower temperatures steps were observed out to n = 7 at the Josephson spacing with 25 GHz applied microwave radiation. The additional rf induced non-Josephson structure as observed in the previous sample was not present in this device. It also had a peak in the dynamic resistance at about 2.1 mv for temperatures below $2^\circ K$. This peak is probably related to the gap and moved to lower voltages with increasing temperatures as expected.

CONCLUSIONS

High resistance granular niobium nitride thin film microbridges with resistance of approximately 50 ohms have been fabricated and exhibit microwave induced current steps on the current-voltage characteristics. These steps have been observed at frequencies up to 40 GHz. The high resistance of these microbridges causes significant rounding of the steps on the I-V characteristics. Although these microbridges are sub-micrometer in dimensions they are large relative to the coherence length for NbN which is about $50\mathring{A}$. Thus the response to applied microwave radiation may be due to vortex motion synchronized by the applied radiation.[5,6] However, the evidence for oscillating steps does not agree with the vortex model.[7] In order to observe this repsonse, the film thickness must be reduced to a thickness less than the grain size which is less than $100\mathring{A}$.

The thickness of the bridge limits the T_c of the device to a maximum temperature of approximately $10^{\circ}K$ to obtain granular behavior for films prepared as described above. The granular nature of the weak link results in a critical current density of the order of 10^5 amps/cm^2 which is approximately 2 orders of magnitude less than that of the starting film. Once the bridge is sufficiently thin to become granular, the individual grains are believed to be electrically isolated but coupled by Josephson tunneling currents. Although the mechanism by which the microwave response of these devices is observed is not clear, these effects have only been observed in those devices which have granular microbridges. This then may suggest that somehow the phase of the individual grains are coupled perhaps by the microwave field and act as a single Josephson junction. Analogous effects have been observed in NbN SQUIDs with microbridges fabricated in the same manner.

REFERENCES

1. M.R. Beasley, Future Trends in Superconducting Electronics, AIP Conf. Proc. No. 44, Edited by B. S. Deaver, Jr., et al. (A.I.P. New York, 1978), pp. 389-396.
2. S.A. Wolf, E.J. Cukauskas, F.J. Rachford and M. Nisenoff, IEEE Trans. on Magnetics, MAG-15, 595 (1978).
3. F.J. Rachford and E.J. Cukauskas, Appl. Phys. Lett. (Dec. 1979) to be published.
4. S. Wolf and W.H. Lowrey, Phys. Rev. Lett., 39, 1038 (1977).
5. C.H. Galfo, PhD Dissertation, University of Virginia, unpublished.
6. Li-Kong Wang, Dae-Jin Hyun and B.S. Deaver, Jr., J. Appl. Phys. 49, 5602 (1978).
7. K.K. Likharev, Sov. Phys.-JETP 34 (1972).

SQUARE ARRAYS OF Au/In PROXIMITY EFFECT BRIDGES
PRELIMINARY RESULTS IN SMALL $H_\perp$

Daniel H. Sanchez & Jean Luc Berchier
DPMC - Geneva University - Geneva - Switzerland

ABSTRACT

These devices show two transition temperatures in their R(T) vs. T curve, one at about Tc(In) and another one at Tc*. There is evidence that some sort of phase transition is occurring at Tc* due to the Josephson type coupling between In squares. The recent calculation of Doniach and Huberman is in qualitative agreement with our preliminary results in small $H_\perp$ and permits to get some insight into the nature of the transition at Tc*.

INTRODUCTION

Recently interactions between junctions that individually show Josephson type effects have been studied extensively.
The group of Rosenblatt (1) worked on a possible collective interaction that may appear in a lattice of junctions made of spheres of superconducting materials (Nb and Ta) pressed together. They proposed that the weak Josephson coupling between spheres may produce a phase transition from a state of superconducting phase disorder to a state of superconducting phase coherence at a temperature Tc_J lower than the material Tc. Work done on granular films (2) may also be interpreted as evidence of a phase transition occurring well below TcG of each grain.

The main inconvenience with pressed spheres and granular films consist in the irregularity of the lattice formed by those systems.

With the aim of studying possible collective effects coming from Josephson coupling, we studied n x n 2D arrays of proximity effect bridges made of Au/In.

Here we will briefly review experimental work done at Geneva (3, 4, 5), and discuss preliminary results in small $H_\perp$.

THE SAMPLES AND GENERAL FEATURES

The arrays consist of n x n (n = 10, 20, 30 and 40) In squares separated by regions of Au/In. A photograph showing one of them is given in figure 1. Details on sample preparation are given in References 4, 5 and 6, and on measuring equipment in References 5 and 7.

FIGURE 1. - Photograph of a sample having ds(In) = 15 μm and dn(Au/In) = 11 μm, and film thicknesses 230Å of Au and 500Å of In, after repeated recycling between room and He temperatures. Array eR16G (20 x 20) of Reference 3.

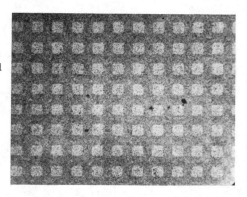

From the V-I characteristics of these devices we obtained the DC resistance at the origin R(T) vs. T. A typical curve is shown in figure 2, where it is also shown the normalized resistance of a control sample consisting of a square of Au of sides (20 ds + 19 dn) in contact with the In film. This control sample (aC 16 P) was made simultaneously with the array (aR 16 P 20 x 20).

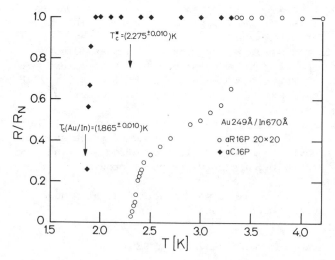

FIGURE 2. - Typical normalized resistance of an array and its control sample, as a function of temperature.

The array R vs. T curve shows two transition temperatures one at about Tc(In), and, another one at Tc* to a resistanceless state. The second transition at Tc* occurs at higher T's than Tc(Au/In) (as measured by the control sample) when the mean free path, ℓ, of the In film is ≳ 0.5 μm.

We have shown (3, 4) that between Tc* and Tc(Au/In), the arrays behave as SNS junctions with a Bardeen-Johnson type of critical current for T << Tc*, namely

$$Ic(array, T) = Ic(array) \ exp - (\ \beta \ (array) \ T)$$

EXPERIMENTAL EVIDENCE FOR A PHASE TRANSITION AT Tc*

At present it is difficult to prove beyond doubt from the experiments alone, that a phase transition occurs at Tc* (3). But there is evidence that that is the case.

The most interesting one is, that within 10 %, the arrays follow a formalism proposed by Wolf et al. (8), where an universal expression to describe the V = V(I,T) curves for T > Tc* is given. This formalism based on scaling laws of critical phenomena and analogies with a 2D Ising model, also predicts the behaviour of the critical current for T < Tc* when T → Tc* if universality holds.

Figure 3 shows an example on how this formalism is followed by these devices, and Table I gives typical "critical exponents" found for two series of two simultaneously made samples.

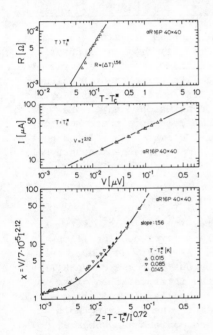
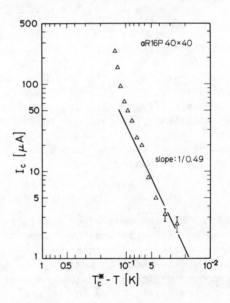

Figure 3. - Example on how the arrays follow Wolf et al.'s (8) formalism at Tc*.

From Table I we observe that: i) $x > 1$, and in consequence the condition "sine qua non" to apply this formalism is satisfied; ii) λ and Θ are about the same as proposed if universality holds; iii) we cannot understand why μ varies between 0.7 and 1.6 although there are at least three physical mechanisms that may give $\mu \sim 1$. One of them predicts a phase transition (Josephson coupling (9)), another does not (simple Bardeen Johnson coupling) and, the third (percolation) is not clear (see Ref. 3).

TABLE I

Typical "critical expo-
nents" found when Wolf
et al.'s formalism (8)
is applied to simul-
taneously made samples.

2D In squares in finite arrays of SNS junctions					
Samples	d_S(In (μm) d_N(Au/In)(μm)	μ	x	λ	θ
eR40G 20×20 230 Å Au 500Å In	6 4	0.77	1.31	0.40	0.54
eR16G 20×20 230 Å Au 500 Å In	15 11	0.87	1.86	0.98	0.92
aR16P 40×40 249 Å Au 670 Å In	12.5 5.2	1.56	1.80	0.51	0.42
aR16P 20×20 249 Å Au 670 Å In	11 5.8		2.12	0.72	0.49

Other evidence favouring the idea of a phase transition at Tc*
are the systematic deviations of Ic (array, T) from an exponential
behaviour in T, when T → Tc*. These deviations have been analyzed
(3, 5) using ideas that could be extrapolated from theoretical approaches (1, 9, 10) done for arrays of SIS junctions coupled by the
Josephson effect. Although no definite conclusions can be drawn from
this analysis, it could be said with some certitude that these devices show a sort of phase transition at Tc* which is related to the
existence of the Josephson type effect (SNS, Bardeen-Johnson type)
between In squares.

PRELIMINARY RESULTS IN SMALL $H_\perp$

The work of Beasley et. al (11) discussing the possibility of
binding of vortices-antivortices in thin superconducting films, and,
the calculation of Doniach and Huberman (12), motivated our preliminary measurements in small $H_\perp$. It is obvious that the curve R(T) vs.
T shown in figure 2 accepts naturally the interpretation given in
Reference (12), based in the Kosterlitz-Thouless (KT) (14) model. The
unexplained variations of the μ coefficient when applying Wolf et.
al.'s (8) formalism, are also avoided since Doniach and Huberman obtained, when pinning forces are negligible and $H_\perp = 0$, that for
$T > T_{KT}$

$$\ln (R/R_N) \approx (-\tilde{\mu}_o/k_B T) (1/t + x\ t^{\frac{1}{2}})$$

where $t = [(T/T_{KT}) - 1]$

This expression is slightly different in small $H_\perp$. Figure 4 shows
R(T, $H_\perp$) vs. T and the variation of Tc (In) and Tc* as a function of
small $H_\perp$.

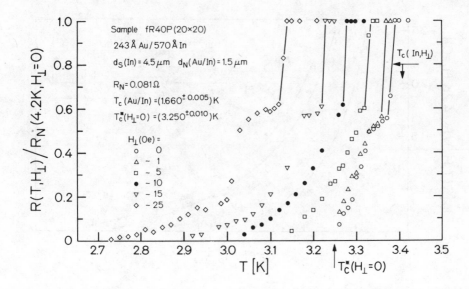

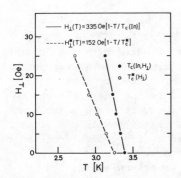

Figure 4. - R/R_N as a function of T and $H_\perp$, and, variation of Tc(In) and Tc* in small perpendicular fields

Figure 5 shows the experimental $\ln(R/R_N)$ vs. t, where it is seen that the experimental points have a tendency to fall into an hyperbola in agreement with Doniach and Huberman's calculation. It is difficult at present to say if they follow a $(1/t)$, a $(1/t^{\frac{1}{2}})$ or a $(1/t + x\ t^{\frac{1}{2}})$ dependence.

Pearl's vortices exist in the In squares, but simple estimations based on Beasley et. al.'s work give $T_{KT} \approx Tc(In)(3)$. We plan more precise measurements to determine the exact dependence in t, if we clarify first which are the vortices responsible for the transition at Tc*. Pearl's are excluded and the search should be directed to topological type of vortices produced by the particular geometry of our devices viewed as inhomogeneous superconductors. Two equally important conditions should be satisfied, a binding temperature Tc*, and, the possiblility of vortex motion to be observed in the resistance.

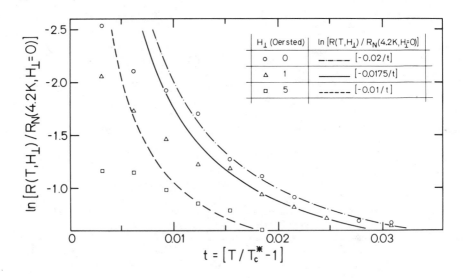

FIGURE 5. - Experimental $\ln(R/R_N)$ vs. t. measured in the fR 40P
(20 x 20) sample.

CONCLUSIONS

The second transition at Tc^* in the R vs. T curve of n x n 2D proximity effect bridges, accepts a natural interpretation as T_{KT} where binding of vortices-antivortices occurs as predicted by Kosterlitz and Thouless (14, 11). These devices seem to be the ideal systems to show its existence in thin films. Pearl's type vortices are excluded in this interpretation, and our work concentrates now in characterising a topological type of vortices allowed by the geometry of these devices viewed as inhomogeneous superconductors.

The technical support of Mr. R. Cartoni is acknowledged.

REFERENCES

1. Rosenblatt, Revue Phys. Appl. 9, 217 (1974)
2. Gubser & Wolf, J. Phys. Coll. 39, C6-579 (1978)
3. Sanchez & Berchier, To be published
4. Berchier & Sanchez, Revue Phys. Appl. 14, 757 (1979)
5. Berchier, Ph. D. Thesis (Geneva University, Sept. 1979)
6. Berchier & Sanchez, Rev. Sci. Instrum. 49, 1452 (1978)
7. Berchier & Sanchez, To be published
8. Wolf, Gubser & Imry, Phys. Rev. Lett. 42, 324 (1979)
9. Giovannini & Weiss, Sol. State Commun. 28, 1005 (1978)
10. Barnes, Phys. Lett. 66A, 422, (1978)
11. Beasley et. al., Phys. Rev. Lett. 42, 1165 (1979)
12. Doniach & Huberman, Phys, Rev. Lett. 42, 1169 (1979)
13. J. Pearl, LT9 (Plenum Press, NY, 1965) p. 566
14. Kosterlitz & Thouless, J. Phys. C 6, 1181 (1973)

VORTICES IN SUPERCONDUCTING FILMS

John R. Clem
Ames Laboratory-USDOE and Department of Physics
Iowa State University, Ames, Iowa 50011

ABSTRACT

The local magnetic flux density and electrical current density generated by a vortex in a superconducting film is calculated approximately using an extension of Pearl's method. The results apply to arbitrary ratios of the film thickness to the penetration depth and reduce to Pearl's thin-film and semi-infinite results in the appropriate limits. In addition, the vanishing of the order parameter on the vortex axis is accounted for by a simple model which removes the London-model divergences of the flux density and supercurrent density and leads to a physically correct description in the vortex core. The results are then applied to a calculation of the interaction energy of vortex-vortex and vortex-antivortex pairs.

INTRODUCTION

The suggestion that a logarithmic interaction energy between vortex-antivortex pairs in a thin superconducting film[1] might lead to a Kosterlitz-Thouless transition[2,3] has stimulated a considerable amount of recent experimental and theoretical work.[4-9] It is thus of interest to examine the conditions under which the interaction energy is indeed logarithmic. Towards this end, in this paper I first present a method by which the local magnetic flux density and electrical current density distribution generated by a vortex in a film of arbitrary thickness can be calculated to good approximation. I then use the results to derive an expression for the electromagnetic interaction energy of a vortex-antivortex pair.

ISOLATED VORTEX IN A FILM

Consider the local magnetic flux density and electrical current density generated by a singly quantized vortex in a superconducting film describable in terms of the Ginzburg-Landau equations.[10] Let the vortex, which carries magnetic flux $\vec{\phi}_0 = \phi_0 \hat{z} = (hc/2e)\hat{z}$, be centered on the z axis, and let the film of thickness d be centered on the x-y plane. Using cylindrical coordinates $\rho = (x^2+y^2)^{1/2}$, $\phi = \tan^{-1}(y/x)$, and z, with unit vectors $\hat{\rho} = \hat{x}\cos\phi + \hat{y}\sin\phi$, $\hat{\phi} = \hat{y}\cos\phi - \hat{x}\sin\phi$, and $\hat{z}$, and denoting by primes various dimensionless quantities[10] (lengths measured in units of the weak-field penetration depth λ, magnetic flux density in units of $\sqrt{2}\,H_c = \kappa\phi_0/2\pi\lambda^2$, vector potential in units of $\sqrt{2}\,H_c\lambda$, current density in units of $c\sqrt{2}\,H_c/4\pi\lambda$, and energy density in units of $H_c^2/4\pi$, where $\kappa = \lambda/\xi$), the Ginzburg-Landau equations for the superconductor (region 2, $|z'| < d'/2$) become

0094-243X/80/580245-06$1.50 Copyright 1980 American Institute of Physics

$$-\frac{1}{\kappa^2}\left[\frac{1}{\rho'}\frac{\partial}{\partial\rho'}\left(\rho'\frac{\partial f}{\partial\rho'}\right) + \frac{\partial^2 f}{\partial z'^2}\right] + (a'_\phi - \frac{1}{\kappa\rho'})^2 f = f - f^3 \quad , \tag{1}$$

$$\frac{\partial}{\partial\rho'}\left[\frac{1}{\rho'}\frac{\partial}{\partial\rho'}(\rho'a'_\phi)\right] + \frac{\partial^2 a'_\phi}{\partial z'^2} = (a'_\phi - \frac{1}{\kappa\rho'})f^2 \quad . \tag{2}$$

Here we have written the normalized order parameter in the form $\Psi(\vec{\rho}') = f(\rho',z')\exp(i\gamma)$, where $\gamma = -\phi$, and have used $\vec{j}' = j'_\phi\hat{\phi} = \vec{\nabla}'\times\vec{b}'$ and $\vec{b}' = b'_\rho\hat{\rho} + b'_z\hat{z} = \vec{\nabla}'\times\vec{a}'$, where $\vec{a}' = a'_\phi\hat{\phi}$ satisfies the Coulomb gauge condition $\vec{\nabla}'\cdot\vec{a}' = 0$. Introducing the reduced superfluid velocity

$$\vec{v}' = \vec{a}' + \kappa^{-1}\vec{\nabla}'\gamma \quad , \tag{3}$$

we find that the second Ginzburg-Landau equation (2) also can be written as

$$j'_\phi = -f^2 v'_\phi \quad . \tag{4}$$

Equations (1) and (2) should be solved, together with

$$\frac{\partial}{\partial\rho'}\left[\frac{1}{\rho'}\frac{\partial}{\partial\rho'}(\rho'a'_\phi)\right] + \frac{\partial^2 a'_\phi}{\partial z'^2} = 0 \tag{5}$$

in the space outside the superconductor ($|z'| > d'/2$), subject to the boundary conditions that $b'_\rho = -\partial a'_\phi/\partial z'$, $b'_z = \rho'^{-1}\partial(\rho'a'_\phi)/\partial\rho'$, and a'_ϕ be continuous and $\partial f/\partial z' = 0$ at the interfaces $z' = \pm d'/2$.

Although the boundary value problem posed above apparently cannot be solved exactly using analytical techniques, it can be solved approximately. One approach is first to note that $f = 0$ on the vortex axis, that $f \approx 1$ far from the axis, and that [see Eq. (1)] the characteristic reduced length over which f varies is $\xi' = \xi/\lambda = \kappa^{-1}$. If one is unconcerned about the behavior of $\vec{b}'$, $\vec{j}'$, and $\vec{a}'$ at distances $\rho' \lesssim \xi'$, one may solve Eqs. (2) and (5) approximately by assuming the London model,[10] in which the replacement $f = 1$ is made. Following this approach, Pearl obtained solutions for two cases: (a) a vacuum–semi-infinite superconductor interface,[11] which corresponds in the present geometry to the top surface of a very thick film ($d' \gg 1$), and (b) a thin film[1] ($d' \ll 1$). In the latter treatment, Pearl ignored the possibility of any spatial variation of j'_ϕ across the film and obtained results in which only a single length $2/d'$ (or $\lambda_\perp = 2\lambda^2/d$ in nonreduced units) appeared. This assumption leads to slightly incorrect results for the current density at reduced distances $\rho' \lesssim 1$ (or $\rho \lesssim \lambda$). In both cases (a) and (b), Pearl's London-model approach yields $j'_\phi \approx (\kappa\rho')^{-1}$ and $b'_z \approx \kappa^{-1}\ln(1/\rho')$ for small ρ'. In addition, the vortex self-energy diverges logarithmically unless a cutoff (at the reduced core radius $\xi' = \kappa^{-1}$) is introduced. In this paper I extend Pearl's calculations in two ways: First, I use the vortex-core model of Refs. 12-14 to more accurately account for vortex core effects in the region $\rho' \lesssim \xi'$, where $f \approx \rho'$. Second, I solve the resulting Eqs. (2) and (5) for arbitrary reduced film thickness d'.

To obtain the vector potential a'_ϕ throughout all space, first consider the film (region 2, $|z'| < d'/2$) and assume that f depends only upon ρ'. Then write

$$a'_{\phi 2}(\rho',z') = a'_{\phi 2b}(\rho') + a'_{\phi 2s}(\rho',z') \ , \tag{6}$$

where the first (bulk) term on the right-hand side obeys an inhomogeneous equation, as in a superconductor of infinite thickness,

$$\frac{\partial}{\partial \rho'}\left[\frac{1}{\rho'}\frac{\partial}{\partial \rho'}(\rho' a'_{\phi 2b})\right] - f^2 a'_{\phi 2b} = -f^2/\kappa\rho' \ . \tag{7}$$

If the order parameter is modeled by $f=\rho'/R'$, where $R'=(\rho'^2+\xi_v'^2)^{1/2}$, ξ_v' being a reduced variational core radius parameter determined as in Ref. 12, the exact solution of Eq. (7) is

$$a'_{\phi 2b}(\rho') = \frac{1}{\kappa\rho'}\left[1 - \frac{R'K_1(R')}{\xi_v'K_1(\xi_v')}\right] \ . \tag{8}$$

Associated with this bulk driving term are the bulk supercurrent density [see Eqs. (3) and (4)]

$$j'_{\phi 2b}(\rho') = \frac{\rho'}{\kappa R'}\frac{K_1(R')}{\xi_v'K_1(\xi_v')} \tag{9}$$

and the magnetic flux density

$$b'_{z2b}(\rho') = \frac{1}{\kappa}\frac{K_0(R')}{\xi_v'K_1(\xi_v')} \ . \tag{10}$$

In an infinite superconductor or far from the surface of a thick film $(d'\gg 1)$, Eqs. (8)–(10) realistically describe the currents and fields generated by a vortex and, in particular, are free from the London-model divergences on the vortex axis. (The present model reduces to the London model in the limit $\xi_v'\to 0$.)

Next consider the surface correction term, $a'_{\phi 2s}(\rho',z')$, which is necessary to satisfy the boundary conditions at $z'=\pm d'/2$. Note that $a'_{\phi 2s}$ describes the surface response of the superconductor to the magnetic field that spreads out into the space above and below the film. At either surface, $a'_{\phi 2s}$ varies only as $(\kappa\rho'^2)^{-1}$ at large ρ', but, as a function of z', $a'_{\phi 2s}$ decays exponentially within a penetration depth of either surface. Having accounted for the main effects of the vortex core via the term $a'_{\phi 2b}$ and noting that the contribution of $a'_{\phi 2s}$ is most important at distances $\rho'\gg\xi_v'$, we solve for $a'_{\phi 2s}$ by making the replacement $f=1$ in the homogeneous equation for $a'_{\phi 2s}$ that results from combining Eqs. (2), (6), and (7), which yields

$$\frac{\partial}{\partial \rho'}\left[\frac{1}{\rho'}\frac{\partial}{\partial \rho'}(\rho' a'_{\phi 2s})\right] + \frac{\partial^2 a'_{\phi 2s}}{\partial z'^2} - a'_{\phi 2s} = 0 \tag{11}$$

Using a method similar to that of Ref. 11, we obtain the following solutions in regions 1 $(z'<-d'/2)$, 2 $(|z'|<d'/2)$, and 3 $(z'>d'/2)$, respectively,

$$a'_{\phi 1}(\rho',z') = \kappa^{-1}\int_0^\infty dq' J_1(q'\rho')f_1(q')f_2(q')f_4(q')\exp[q'(z'+d'/2)] \tag{12}$$

$$a'_{\phi 2b}(\rho') = \kappa^{-1} \int_0^\infty dq' J_1(q'\rho') f_1(q') f_4(q') \qquad (13a)$$

$$a'_{\phi 2s}(\rho',z') = -\kappa^{-1} \int_0^\infty dq' J_1(q'\rho') f_1(q') f_2(q') f_4(q')$$

$$\cdot [q'\cosh(Q'z')]/[Q'\sinh(Q'd'/2)] \qquad (13b)$$

$$a'_{\phi 3}(\rho',z') = \kappa^{-1} \int_0^\infty dq' J_1(q'\rho') f_1(q') f_2(q') f_4(q') \exp[-q'(z'-d'/2)] \quad ,$$
$$\qquad (14)$$

where $q'=q\lambda$, $Q'=(q'^2+1)^{1/2}$, and

$$f_1(q') = 1/Q'^2 \qquad (15)$$

$$f_2(q') = [1 + (q'/Q')\coth(Q'd'/2)]^{-1} \qquad (16)$$

$$f_4(q') = [Q'\xi'_v K_1(Q'\xi'_v)]/[\xi'_v K_1(\xi'_v)] \quad . \qquad (17)$$

Corresponding expressions for b'_ρ and b'_z in the three regions can be obtained from $b'_\rho = -\partial a'_\phi/\partial z'$ and $b'_z = \rho'^{-1}\partial(\rho'a'_\phi)/\partial\rho'$. The total current density in the film is $j'_{\phi 2}=j'_{\phi 2b}+j'_{\phi 2s}$, where $j'_{\phi 2b}$ is given by Eq. (9) and $j'_{\phi 2s} = -a'_{\phi 2s}$.

VORTEX–ANTIVORTEX INTERACTION ENERGY

In the Ginzburg-Landau theory the total reduced free energy of a vortex-antivortex pair of separation s', relative to the energy of the Meissner state, is

$$F' = F'_c + F'_{kg} + F'_{em} \quad , \qquad (18)$$

where the three terms are the costs in condensation energy

$$F'_c = (1/2) \int_{film} d^3r' \, (1 - f^2)^2 \quad , \qquad (19)$$

kinetic energy from the gradient of the magnitude of the order parameter

$$F'_{kg} = \kappa^{-2} \int_{film} d^3r' \, (\vec{\nabla}'f)^2 \quad , \qquad (20)$$

and electromagnetic energy

$$F'_{em} = -\kappa^{-1} \int_{film} d^3r' \, \vec{j}' \cdot \vec{\nabla}'\gamma \quad . \qquad (21)$$

Here, $\Psi=fe^{i\gamma}$ is the order parameter, $\vec{v}'=\vec{a}'+\kappa^{-1}\vec{\nabla}'\gamma$ the superfluid velocity, and $\vec{j}'=-f^2\vec{v}'$ the supercurrent density. Eq. (21) is obtained by applying the divergence theorem to the sum of the integral of the field energy b'^2 over all space and the integral of the supercurrent kinetic energy $f^2v'^2$ over the film volume. We expect F'_c and F'_{kg} to vary with s' on the scale of $\xi'=\kappa^{-1}$; for $s'=0$, $F'_c=F'_{kg}=0$, and for $s'\gtrsim 2\xi'$ we expect F'_c and F'_{kg} to be nearly equal to their saturation values at $s'=\infty$. We evaluate Eq. (21) with the help of the divergence theorem and $\vec{\nabla}\cdot\vec{j}'=0$, noting that γ is a multiple-valued function changing by 2π (-2π) as one makes a complete circuit around a vortex (antivortex) in the clockwise direction. The result is

$$F'_{em} = (2\pi/\kappa)(I'_+ - I'_-) \quad , \tag{22}$$

where I'_+ and I'_- are the total currents flowing in the counterclockwise sense around the vortex (+) and the antivortex (−). To evaluate Eq. (22) we use linear superposition to approximate $\vec{j}'$ by $\vec{j}'=\vec{j}'_++\vec{j}'_-$, where $\vec{j}'_+$ and $\vec{j}'_-$ are the current densities that would be generated by an isolated vortex (+) or antivortex (−). The result is

$$F'_{em}(s') = (4\pi/\kappa)\int_{-d'/2}^{d'/2} dz' \int_0^{s'} d\rho' j'^2_{\phi 2}(\rho',z') \quad . \tag{23}$$

Writing $U'_{em}(s')=F'_{em}(s')-F'_{em}(\infty)=U'_{emb}(s')+U'_{ems}(s')$ and $S'=(s'^2+\xi_v'^2)^{1/2}=S/\lambda$, we obtain

$$U'_{emb}(s') = -\frac{4\pi}{\kappa^2} d' \frac{K_0(S')}{\xi'_v K_1(\xi'_v)} \tag{24}$$

$$U'_{ems}(s') = -\frac{8\pi}{\kappa^2} \int_0^\infty dq' J_0(q's') f_1^2(q') f_2(q') f_4(q') \tag{25}$$

or, in nonreduced units,

$$U_{emb}(s) = -\left(\frac{\phi_0}{2\pi}\right)^2 \frac{1}{\lambda_\perp} \frac{K_0(S/\lambda)}{(\xi_v/\lambda)K_1(\xi_v/\lambda)} \tag{26}$$

$$U_{ems}(s) = -\left(\frac{\phi_0}{2\pi}\right)^2 \int_0^\infty dq J_0(qs) f_1^2(q\lambda) f_2(q\lambda) f_4(q\lambda) \quad , \tag{27}$$

where $\lambda_\perp=2\lambda^2/d$. For a vortex-vortex pair the only change is a reversal of the signs of Eqs. (24)–(27).

To evaluate $U_{em}(s)$ from Eqs. (26) and (27) for arbitrary values of ξ, λ, and d, a numerical integration of Eq. (27) is required. In the thin-film limit, when $d\ll\lambda$ and $s\gg\lambda$ or ξ, however, $U_{emb}(s)$ is negligibly small and the dominant contribution to the integral of Eq. (27) arises from q's satisfying $q\lesssim s^{-1}\ll\lambda^{-1}$ or ξ^{-1}. Then, to good approximation,

$$U_{em}(s) = -\left(\frac{\phi_0}{2\pi}\right)^2 \int_0^\infty dq J_0(qs)/(1 + q\lambda_\perp) \tag{28a}$$

$$= -\left(\frac{\phi_0}{2\pi}\right)^2 \left(\frac{\pi}{2\lambda_\perp}\right) [H_0(s/\lambda_\perp) - Y_0(s/\lambda_\perp)] \quad , \tag{28b}$$

where $H_0(s/\lambda_\perp)$ is the Struve function and Y_0 the Bessel function of the second kind. When ξ, $\lambda \ll s \ll \lambda_\perp$,

$$U_{em}(s) \approx -(\frac{\phi_0}{2\pi})^2 \frac{1}{\lambda_\perp} \ell n(\lambda_\perp/s) \quad , \tag{29}$$

and when ξ, $\lambda \ll \lambda_\perp \ll s$,

$$U_{em}(s) \approx -(\frac{\phi_0}{2\pi})^2 \frac{1}{s} \quad , \tag{30}$$

as found by Pearl.[1]

ACKNOWLEDGMENTS

This work was supported by the U.S. Department of Energy, contract No. W-7405-Eng-82, Division of Materials Sciences, budget code AK-01-02-02-3. I am grateful to Dr. P. Martinoli, Dr. A. T. Fiory, and Dr. A. M. Goldman for stimulating discussions and correspondence.

REFERENCES

1. J. Pearl, in Proceedings of the Ninth International Conference on Low Temperature Physics, J. G. Daunt, D. V. Edwards, F. J. Milford, and M. Yaqub, eds. (Plenum Press, New York, 1965), Part A, p. 566; J. Pearl, Appl. Phys. Lett. 5, 65 (1964).
2. J. M. Kosterlitz and D. J. Thouless, J. Phys. C 6, 1181 (1973).
3. M. R. Beasley, J. E. Mooij, and T. P. Orlando, Phys. Rev. Lett. 42, 1165 (1979).
4. S. Doniach and B. A. Huberman, Phys. Rev. Lett. 42, 1169 (1979).
5. B. I. Halperin and D. R. Nelson, J. Low Temp. Phys., to be published.
6. L. A. Turkevich, J. Phys. C 12, L385 (1979).
7. B. A. Huberman and S. Doniach, Phys. Rev. Lett. 43, 950 (1979).
8. N. A. H. K. Rao, E. D. Dahlberg, A. M. Goldman, C. Umbach, and L. E. Toth, to be published.
9. D. U. Gubser and S. A. Wolf, to be published.
10. A. L. Fetter and P. C. Hohenberg, in Superconductivity, R. D. Parks, ed. (Marcel Dekker, New York, 1969), Vol. 2, p. 817.
11. J. Pearl, J. Appl. Phys. 37, 4139 (1966).
12. J. R. Clem, J. Low Temp. Phys. 18, 427 (1975).
13. J. R. Clem, Phys. Rev. B 12, 1742 (1975).
14. J. R. Clem, in Low Temperature Physics-LT14, M. Krusius and M. Vuorio, eds. (North-Holland, Amsterdam, 1975), Vol. 2, p. 285.
15. Handbook of Mathematical Functions, M. Abramowitz and I. A. Stegun, eds. (National Bureau of Standards, Washington, 1967).

MAGNETIC FIELD-INDUCED DISSIPATION IN GRANULAR SUPERCONDUCTING COMPOSITES

J.C. Garland and D.J. Resnick
Dept. of Physics, The Ohio State University, Columbus, Ohio 43210

R.S. Newrock
Dept. of Physics, University of Cincinnati, Cincinnati, Ohio 45231

ABSTRACT

The resistivity of a granular composite of NbTi particles embedded in a normal In host has been measured in magnetic fields to 6T. The volume fraction of superconducting particles varied from 0.01 to 0.14. In strong fields, the resistivity of the composite was found to be much larger than the resistivity of the homogeneous normal metal. The field induced dissipation is attributed to long range distortion of the current flow in the normal metal arising from a polarization charge on the surface of the superconducting particles.

INTRODUCTION

A class of inhomogeneous superconductors which exhibits very interesting physical properties is a random composite of super-conducting and normal metal (S/N) particles. The most important parameter which characterizes an S/N composite is the superconducting volume fraction p; if p exceeds the "percolation concentration" p_c, the resistance of the composite is zero. Conversely, if p is well below p_c, the composite exhibits a "remanant" resistance, inasmuch as no connected cluster of superconducting particles links the boundaries of the material. (Actually, this view of the percolation fraction as a quantity which delineates two regimes of conduction is oversimplified. Because of the superconducting proximity effect, an S/N composite will generally have zero resistance somewhat below the percolation concentration.)[1,2]

If we model an S/N composite as a classical two-component random system, the remanant resistance can be easily computed using Effective Medium Theory (EMT).[3] As expected, the resistance of the composite is found to decrease smoothly with increasing volume fraction, reaching zero as $p \to p_c$. Although the EMT has serious shortcomings near p_c, it correctly predicts the remanant resistance in the dilute regime, characterized by $p << p_c$.

For our purposes, it is useful to look beyond the EMT equations and to inquire about the physical processes associated with conduction in a dilute S/N system. There are really two mechanisms which influence the resistivity when superconducting particles are randomly added to a normal metal. The first is a simple volume exclusion effect; as p is increased, particles having zero resistance displace material having finite resistance. The second, more

interesting mechanism is associated with polarization of the superconducting particles. In an electric field, polarization charge is
induced on the surface of each particle, weakening the electrostatic
field in the surrounding normal region; in effect, current is drawn
away from the normal metal into the particle, reducing the average
Joule dissipation in the composite. Both the volume exclusion
effect and the polarization effect act cooperatively to reduce the
resistivity, so that the addition of one percent of superconductor
to a normal metal lowers the resistivity about three percent.

The situation is quite different if the S/N composite is subjected to a strong magnetic field (but not so strong as to drive the
superconducting particles into the normal state!). In a strong
field, there is a competition between the volume exclusion effect
and the polarization effect, the latter tending to increase the
dissipation. Of course, the volume effect ultimately wins the
competition because the resistance of the composite must vanish
when $p=p_c$. As we shall see, however, the polarization effect is
overwhelmingly stronger at lower values of p. Thus we have the
peculiar notion that the resistance of a normal metal can be increased by adding superconducting particles to the metal!

EXPERIMENTAL RESULTS

The N/S system we have studied consists of a pure indium normal
host containing a random distribution of small NbTi particles. The
material was prepared by adding NbTi powder in small increments to
molten In until the desired volume fraction of superconductor was
reached. During this process, the molten mixture was continuously
stirred in order to minimize clumping of the particles. Once the
proper concentration was reached, the mixture was quench-cooled to
prevent settling. After cooling, the ingot was rolled into strips,
which were then annealed at 95°C for 12 hours to relieve strains
introduced by the rolling process. Table I summarizes the relevant
physical parameters of the material. In all, seven samples were

TABLE I Sample Properties

Symbol	Description	Quantity
D	NbTi particle diameters	25–120µm
ξ_o	NbTi coherence length	50Å
λ	In mean-free-path	10µm
RRR	In residual resistance ratio	8000
p_c	percolation concentration	~0.30

prepared, with superconducting volume fractions ranging from 0.01 to 0.14.

Electrical resistance measurements of these specimens were made at 4.2K using a SQUID voltmeter with a resolution of about 10^{-13}V at the maximum magnetic field strength. This resolution was limited by flux noise induced into the SQUID circuit by residual vibration of the superconducting magnet. To keep this vibration to a minimum, the entire magnet and dewar assembly was mounted on a damped air suspension platform, and the magnet was operated in the persistent current mode. Typical sample currents were about 10mA, resulting in voltages of about 10^{-10}–10^{-11}V. In no case was the critical field H_{c2} of the superconducting particles reached. (Note that the superconducting coherence length was much smaller than the particle diameter, so that the NbTi particles behaved like bulk superconductor, with H_{c2} well in excess of 10T.)

Figure 1 shows the magnetic field dependence of the fractional resistivity of four S/N samples. In the figure, the magnetic field is expressed in reduced form $h=\omega_c\tau$, where ω_c is the cyclotron frequency of the indium and τ is the the zero-field relaxation time for elastic scattering. In a two-component system such as this one, the relaxation time τ is not directly related to the zero field resistivity $\rho(p,0)$; interested readers are referred to an earlier publication for details of our procedure for estimating τ.[4]

It is clear from Figure 1 that the addition of superconducting grains to the normal host induces large fractional increases in the resistivity at strong magnetic fields. In the high field regime, ordinarily defined as $h\gg1$, the resistivity is seen to increase as a linear function of h up to the highest fields attained in the experiment. (The rapid increase in resistivity observed at low fields, $h\lesssim1$, can be attributed to magnetoresistance of pure indium and not to the presence of the superconducting particles.[5])

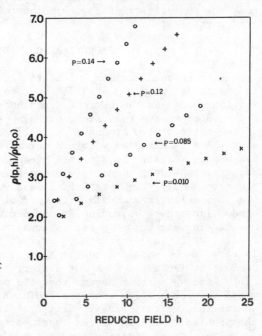

Figure 1. The fractional resistivity $\rho(p,h)/\rho(p,0)$ as a function of reduced magnetic field h of NbTi-In granular composites. The data illustrate the linear increase of resistivity with magnetic field.

The slope of the high field linear resistance S(p) increases with the volume fraction of superconductor and may be described approximately by the expression S(p) $\approx$ 2p.

It is natural to inquire how one reconciles the large field-dependent increase in the fractional resistivity of the composites at large p with the requirement that the resistance of the composites vanish at p = p_c. There is no conceptual difficulty, of course, in having the fractional resistivity of the specimens become quite large even while the absolute resistivity is tending to zero. In fact, if we assume that the zero-field resistivity of the composites varies with p according to Effective Medium Theory, then our results[4] suggest that the absolute resistivity of the composite will reach a maximum at a volume fraction of approximate $p_c/2$. At larger values of p, the absolute resistivity will drop, reaching zero at p=p_c, even though the fractional resistivity may continue to increase. It is interesting to note that the absolute resistivity of the composite at moderate field strengths (h$\approx$10) may be significantly greater than the resistivity of the normal metal containing no superconducting particles.

THEORETICAL CONSIDERATIONS

As mentioned earlier, we attribute the field-induced increase in the resistivity of our S/N composites to the influence of polarization charge on the current distribution in the material. In order to elucidate this idea, we have performed a model calculation of the current flow around a perfectly conducting spherical inclusion which is embedded within a normal metal. Our calculation does not produce easily the explicit field dependence of the composite resistivity, but it does provide some insight into the physical processes underlying the field-induced resistivity.

Our calculation deals with current flow past a single superconducting sphere of radius R embedded within a free-electron normal metal. The direction of the external magnetic field $\hat{H}$ defines the $\hat{Z}$-axis, while the direction of current injection into the composite is taken to be parallel to the $\hat{X}$-axis. We assume that the superconducting inclusion does not distort the uniform external magnetic field, and we further assume that the mean-free-path λ of the normal metal is much smaller than the radius R of the sphere. This latter assumption, which is easily satisfied in our experiment, reduces the problem to one involving local potentials and fields.

The current distribution in the vicinity of the superconducting inclusion is obtained by solving a boundary value equation for the electrostatic potential $\Phi(\vec{r})$ and by invoking the constitutive equation for the current density $\vec{J}(\vec{r})$:

$$\vec{J}(\vec{r}) = - \overleftrightarrow{\sigma}(h)\vec{\nabla}\Phi(\vec{r}). \tag{1}$$

The boundary value equation is obtained by setting $\vec{\nabla}\cdot\vec{J}(\vec{r})=0$. In equation 1, $\overleftrightarrow{\sigma}(h)$ is the magnetic field-dependent conductivity tensor of the normal metal,[6] given by

$$\overset{\leftrightarrow}{\sigma}(h) = \sigma_o \begin{pmatrix} \gamma & h\gamma & 0 \\ -h\gamma & \gamma & 0 \\ 0 & 0 & 1 \end{pmatrix} \qquad (2)$$

where $h=\omega_c\tau$ and where $\gamma\equiv(1 + h^2)^{-1}$. It is interesting to note that the unusual features of the solution to this problem arise directly from the anisotropy of the conductivity in strong fields. In the limit $h=\infty$, the normal metal becomes a one dimensional conductor, unable to support a current (at finite electric field) in any direction except parallel to the magnetic field.

The method for solving the boundary value problem is straight-forward, though tedious.[7] Basically, it involves making a scale transformation which reduces the differential equation for $\Phi(\vec{r})$ into a form of Laplace's Equation. The scale transformation changes the spherical boundary of the superconducting inclusion into an oblate spheroid, so that the solutions are expressed in oblate spheroidal coordinates. In this paper we will not attempt to give the details of the calculation, which are of no particular interest, but will simply cite the answer. The potential function $\Phi(\vec{r})$ outside the inclusion is given exactly by

$$\Phi(\eta,\theta,\phi) = \frac{Rh\gamma^{\frac{1}{2}}J_o}{\sigma_o} \left(\cos\phi + h\sin\phi \right) \left(\frac{\cosh \eta_o}{Q_1^1(i\sinh \eta_o)} - \cosh \eta \right). \qquad (3)$$

In the above expression η_o is the surface of the inclusion in spheroidal coordinates and $Q_1^1(z)=(z^2-1)dQ_1(z)/dz$, where $Q_1(z)$ is the Associated Legendre function of the second kind.

Figure 2 shows the computer-generated trajectory of two lines of electric current flowing above the sphere, at a magnetic field strength $h=100$. The trajectories were obtained by combining Equations 1 and 3. In the plotting algorithm, the current vector was computed at a starting point near the sphere (in this case, Z=4R, X=3R, and Y=±0.3R). A short line segment was then drawn from the starting point in the direction of the current vector. At the end of this line segment, the current vector was recomputed, and another line segment was drawn. This process was repeated until the trajectory was finished.

Figure 2a shows the current trajectory projected onto the X-Z plane (i.e., a "side view" of the current) while Figure 2b shows the X-Y projection ("top view") of the same current lines. These trajectories illustrate several general features of the current flow at all fields above $h\approx10$. First, the current tends to avoid the "shadow" region of normal metal immediately above and below the superconducting sphere. Second, in contrast to the zero-field situation, the region over which the current distortion extends is much larger than a sphere diameter. Although the figure illustrates current injection at Z=4R, a noticeable distortion could be discerned for current injected at Z=50R. Third, there is a distinct asymmetry to the current flow, with current moving over one hemisphere veering upward, away from the sphere, while current moving over the other hemisphere veers down toward the sphere. Current lines which pass sufficiently close to the sphere are pulled into it on one side, although in the limit of infinitely strong magnetic field current enters the sphere only at the equator. Finally, the current which is excluded from the shadow region above and below the sphere is compressed within a thin cylindrical shell which defines the perimeter of the shadow. We believe it is the Joule dissipation associated with this shell of compressed current which is ultimately responsible for the large field-dependent resistance observed in our measurements.

This last point is illustrated by Figure 3, which shows an isometric map of the Joule dissipation in planes of various distances above the sphere. The vertical axis in each of the countour diagrams is the volume power density $\vec{J}\cdot\vec{E}$, whereas the two horizontal axes specify an X-Y plane at fixed distance Z above the sphere. In all the drawings, the magnetic field is h=100. It is clear from the diagrams that the Joule heating induced by the superconducting particle can be quite pronounced, even at moderate magnetic field strength (a value of h=100 is readily attainable in pure metals at low temperatures).

This localized heating may be significant in certain commercial applications of S/N composites. For example, in the manufacture of wire for high field

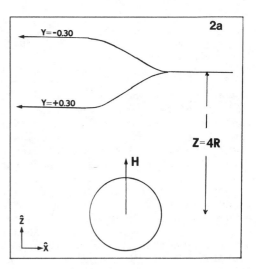

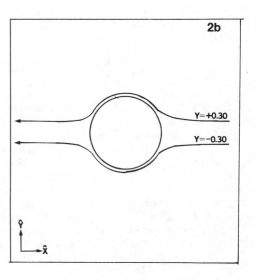

Figure 2: (a) An X-Z projection of two lines of electric current at a field h=100. The current lines were injected into the metal at Z=4R, X=3R, and Y= 0.3R and -0.3R. (b) An X-Y projection of the same current lines as in (a).

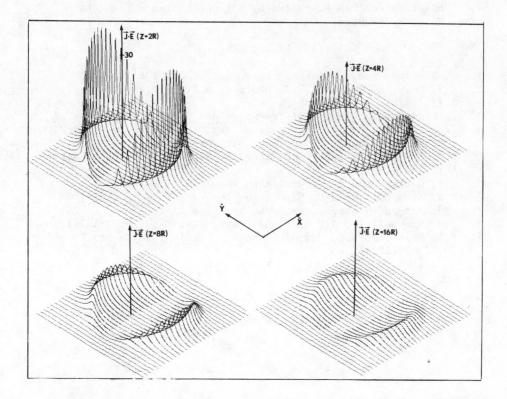

Figure 3. Contour maps of the Joule dissipation $\vec{J} \cdot \vec{E}$ in planes of fixed height above the superconducting sphere.

superconducting magnets, it is common practice to surround small filaments of type II superconductor with a normal metal medium having a high thermal conductivity. The purpose of this normal metal is to stabilize the filaments against temperature fluctuations resulting from vortex motion. In some types of wire, there is a small remnant resistance which results from currrent spreading out from one filament to the next through the normal medium. Our analysis suggest that if h>1, the current will not fan out uniformly between filaments but will instead be focused into thin current sheets. The localized Joule heating associated with these current sheets could ultimately have a destabilizing effect on the filaments at fields near the upper critical field of the superconductor. This effect will be exacerbated by the anisotropic thermal conductivity of the normal metal, which functionally resembles the electrical conductivity tensor in strong magnetic fields.[8]

This research was supported by National Science Foundation Grant No. DMR 78-09428.

REFERENCES

1. A. Davidson and M. Tinkham, Phys. Rev. B 13, 3261 (1976).
2. C.J. Lobb, M. Tinkham, W.J. Skocpol, Solid State Commun. 27, 1273 (1978).
3. R. Landauer in Electrical Transport and Optical Properties of Inhomogeneous Media, J.C. Garland and D.B. Tanner, eds.(American Institute of Physics, New York, N.Y., 1978), p.2.
4. D.J. Resnick, J.C. Garland, and R.S. Newrock, Phys. Rev. Lett. 43, 1192 (1979).
5. J.C. Garland and R. Bowers, Phys. Rev. 188, 1121 (1969).
6. N.W. Ashcroft and N.D. Mermin, Solid State Physics (Holt, Rinehart and Winston, New York, 1976), p 234.
7. J.B. Sampsell and J.C. Garland, Phys. Rev. B 13, 583 (1976).
8. F.P. Esposito, R.S. Newrock, and K. Loeffler, Phys. Rev. B 20, 2348 (1979).

EFFECT OF PROXIMITY OF A NORMAL LAYER ON THE ANISOTROPY OF THE SUPERCONDUCTING ENERGY GAP

Kurt Scharnberg
Abteilung für Theoretische Festkörperphysik der Universität Hamburg
Jungiusstrasse 11, D - 2000 Hamburg 36, W. Germany

ABSTRACT

To investigate the effect of a normal layer in close contact with an anisotropic superconductor on the observable anisotropy, a simplified description of gap anisotropy in terms of a two-band model is used. Within McMillan's tunneling model of the proximity effect, tunneling into the normal layer provides a mechanism for interband scattering, which serves to smear the gap structure. It is suggested that this mechanism is responsible for the failure to observe gap anisotropy in tunneling experiments on single crystal Nb.

INTRODUCTION

In view of the anisotropy of normal state properties (Fermi surface, phonon dispersion relations, electron-phonon matrix elements) present in almost all metals it seems reasonable to expect that the superconducting state will also show some anisotropy, which would manifest itself in a wavevector dependent order parameter. This expectation, however, is not fully borne out by the experimental results[1]. Tunneling experiments on clean single crystals, which should be best suited for an investigation of anisotropy effects because in any particular junction only quasiparticles within a narrow range of wavevectors $\vec{k}$ contribute to the tunnel current, did indeed reveal anisotropic and/or multiple energy gaps in several s-p metals (Al, Pb, Sn, Ga; see Ref. 1 for references).

However, the results are not very consistent and seem to depend on details of junction fabrication, so that an alternative explanation for the observation of anisotropic and/or multiple gaps has been advanced which is based on non-ideal features of "real world" junctions[1] and not on intrinsic physical properties of the materials involved.

In transition metals, where one would expect anisotropy effects to be even more pronounced than in simple metals, tunneling experiments seem to give perfectly isotropic energy gaps[2,3].

Detailed and careful microscopic calculations, based on pseudopotential theory, for Al[4], Pb[5], and Zn[6] predict considerable anisotropy. Similarly extensive studies for transition metals have only been performed for Nb. Because of the presence of the d-bands, local field effects have to be included in the screening of the electron - phonon interaction so that the theory becomes much more involved and recourse is taken to a variety of approximation schemes.

Peter et al.[7], using a tight binding formulation, predicted a sizable anisotropy while Butler and Allen[8], using band theory and the rigid muffin-tin approximation, found very little anisotropy. However, Butler and Allen did not include the anisotropy of the phonon dispersion relations, so that the predictions of Peter et al. appear to be more significant.

We would like to point out that the calculations on the s-p metals are done in the extended zone scheme since the Fermi surface is nearly free electron like. In this scheme an anisotropic single energy gap is predicted which, however, is only defined for certain directions of the electron wavevector $\vec{k}$. For some directions of $\vec{k}$ the Fermi surface does not exist and tunneling through a plane perpendicular to these directions should be impossible. It seems to be more reasonable, though, to use the selection rule that the wavevector in the reduced zone has to be perpendicular to the tunnel barrier. Folding the Fermi surface back into the first zone leads to the appearance of multiple gaps, one for each sheet of the Fermi surface, each of which will in general be anisotropic with respect to a variation of $\vec{k}$ over this particular sheet of the Fermi surface.

For Nb the calculations are performed in the reduced zone scheme and multiple gaps appear in a natural way. These will be observed in those directions only, though, for which parallel $\vec{k}$-vectors on different sheets of the Fermi surface can be found. For example, when tunneling parallel to the <100> direction only states on the jack can contribute to the tunneling current so that a single gap would be observed. When tunneling parallel to the <110> direction, all three sheets of the Nb Fermi surface will contribute so that three gaps should be observed.

Unfortunately, a careful tunneling study of single crystal Nb did not provide any evidence for anisotropic or multiple gaps[2]. I find the theoretical studies sufficiently convincing to believe that the anisotropy observed in s-p metals is real, even though the fabrication of good junctions presents some difficulty. I am, therefore, faced with the problem of explaining the absence of anisotropy effects in tunneling experiments on Nb.

The explanation proposed here is based on the assumption that between superconductor and tunnel barrier a thin normal layer is interposed. In the experiments done by E. L. Wolf et al.[9] such a normal layer is produced deliberately by depositing an Al-film on the superconductor and oxidizing only part of it to form the tunnel barrier. The data are analyzed in terms of a generalization of the isotropic strong coupling theory which takes into account the presence of the normal layer[10]. The same theory has been used to re-analyze data taken on Nb tunnel junctions in which the tunnel barrier was formed by the native oxide[11]. In this case one may expect that a thin layer of metallic NbO separates the Nb from the insulating Nb_2O_5. Assuming the presence of such a normal layer of NbO with a thickness of about 10Å lead to satisfactory values for the electron-phonon parameter λ and the Coulomb pseudopotential $\mu*$[11].

We contend that the proximity of a normal layer, having a band

structure different from that of the superconductor, provides a mechanism for interband scattering which will reduce or even eliminate
any band structure effects in the superconductor.

To analyze this contention in a more quantitative fashion we
shall use an isotropic two-band model for the superconductor[12]. In
this model the Fermi surface in the reduced zone is simplified to
two concentric spheres and all physical properties are assumed to be
isotropic with respect to variations of the wavevector within one
of the two spheres. This model emphasizes the anisotropy with respect to different sheets of the Fermi surface. de Haas – van Alphen
experiments on Nb[13] have indeed shown that there is little variation
of the mass enhancement within one sheet of the Fermi surface whereas considerable changes are observed as one goes from one sheet to
another. The calculated order parameter also shows considerable anisotropy within individual sheets of the Fermi surface[7].

The model used is, therefore, by no means an accurate representation of the anisotropy in Nb, but it can still provide some
valuable information on the effect which a close contact between
two metals will have on their band structure related properties.

The quasiparticles in the normal metal are assumed to be free.
The proximity effect is described by McMillan's tunneling model[14].
This model is not really applicable to almost transparent interfaces
which appear to be present in the experiments[9]. To treat transparent
interfaces one needs to use a real space representation including
boundary conditions at the various interfaces of the proximity
tunnel junction. Such theories have only been worked out under the
assumption that the two metals involved are identical (same Fermi
energy, same Fermi momentum) free electron metals, which differ only
in the interaction that leads to superconductivity[10]. It is not obvious how this kind of theory can be generalized to include band
structure effects, but attempts at such a generalization are
presently undertaken.

McMillan's tunneling model[14], however, is readily applied to
the situation under consideration and it is hoped that it describes
at least qualitatively the effect of proximity on superconducting
gap anisotropy.

THEORY

We describe pairing in the superconductor by the two-band
Hamiltonian first introduced by Suhl et al.[12]. We allow for a finite
pairing interaction in the normal metal and use the tunneling
Hamiltonian of Cohen et al.[15] to describe the coupling between the
two metals. For the time being we use wavevectors $\vec{q}$ and $\vec{k}$ to label
states in the normal metal and the superconductor respectively.
We do not consider interband scattering in the superconductor, which
would reduce anisotropy[16], because we want to focus on the extent to
which anisotropy effects are removed by the presence of a proximity
layer.

In the absence of tunneling the temperature Green function of the superconductor is diagonal with respect to band indices. Including tunneling leads to nondiagonal elements, but these can be neglected just as in the case of interband impurity scattering[16]. Since we do not consider spin-dependent forces it is sufficient to introduce three 2 x 2 Nambu matrix Green functions[14]. In second order, self-consistent perturbation theory we obtain the following self-energies:

$$\hat{\Sigma}_\nu(\vec{k},\omega_n) = \sum_q \hat{T}^\nu_{kq} \hat{G}(\vec{q},\omega_n) \hat{T}^\nu_{qk} \qquad \nu = 1, 2 \qquad (1)$$

$$\hat{\Sigma}(\vec{q},\omega_n) = \sum_{\nu=1,2} \sum_k \hat{T}^\nu_{qk} \hat{G}_\nu(\vec{k},\omega_n) \hat{T}^\nu_{kq} \qquad (2)$$

with

$$\hat{T}^\nu_{kq} = \begin{pmatrix} T^\nu_{kq} & 0 \\ 0 & -T^\nu_{-q,-k} \end{pmatrix} \qquad (3)$$

Following McMillan[14] we shall assume that $T^\nu_{kq}T^\nu_{qk} = |T^\nu_{kq}|^2$ is independent of $\vec{k}$ and $\vec{q}$ and also of the band index ν. This last assumption could easily be dropped at the expense of introducing another parameter.

With these assumptions the self-energies (1) and (2) are independent of $\vec{k}$, $\vec{q}$, and ν so that we have to introduce labels s and n to distinguish the self-energies of the superconductor and the normal metal. Writing the matrix self-energies (1) and (2) in the form[14]

$$\Sigma_{s(n)} = i\Sigma^G_{s(n)} \tau_o - \Sigma^F_{s(n)} \tau_1 \qquad (4)$$

where τ_o and τ_1 are Pauli matrices, the three matrix equations (1) and (2) can be reduced to 4 scalar equations. Introducing the quantities

$$u_{s\nu} = \frac{\omega_n + \Sigma^G_s}{\Delta_{s\nu} + \Sigma^F_s} \qquad u_n = \frac{\omega_n + \Sigma^G_n}{\Delta_n + \Sigma^F_n} \qquad \nu = 1, 2 \qquad (5)$$

this system of equations can be further reduced to

$$u_{s\nu}\Delta_{s\nu} = \omega + \frac{i}{\tau_n} \frac{u_n - u_{s\nu}}{\sqrt{u_n^2 - 1}} \qquad \nu = 1, 2 \qquad (6)$$

$$u_n\Delta_n = \omega + \sum_{\nu=1,2} \frac{i}{\tau_{s\nu}} \frac{u_{s\nu} - u_n}{\sqrt{u_{s\nu}^2 - 1}} \qquad (7)$$

so that we are left with three coupled equations instead of two, which are usually encountered in this type of problem. In (6) and (7) the analytic continuation $i\omega_n \to \omega + i\delta$ has been performed and the scattering times have been defined in accordance with McMillan[14].

The order parameters have to fulfill the self-sonsistency equations

$$\Delta_{s\nu} = \sum_{\nu'=1,2} N_{\nu'}(0)V_{\nu\nu'} \int_{o}^{\omega_c^s} d\omega \tanh\frac{\omega}{2T} \text{ Re } \frac{1}{\sqrt{u_{s\nu'}^2(\omega) - 1}} \tag{8}$$

$$\Delta_n = N_n(0)V_n \int_{o}^{\omega_c^n} d\omega \tanh\frac{\omega}{2T} \text{ Re } \frac{1}{\sqrt{u_n^2(\omega) - 1}} \tag{9}$$

These three equations together with (6) and (7) have to be solved numerically to obtain the density of states

$$N_n(\omega) = N_n(0) \text{ Re } \frac{u_n(\omega)}{\sqrt{u_n^2(\omega) - 1}} \text{ sgn } u_n(\omega) \tag{10}$$

at the tunnel barrier, which is measured in a tunneling experiment[10].

The necessary numerical calculations are under way, but unfortunately are not yet completed.

However, we can get some idea of the coupling induced between bands by studying the transition temperature. Near T_c the quantities u become very large so that (6) and (7) can be solved:

$$\frac{1}{u_{s\nu}} = \frac{\Delta_{s\nu}}{\omega} + \frac{i}{\tau_n} \frac{\Delta_n - \Delta_{s\nu}}{\omega(\omega+i\rho)} + \frac{i}{\tau_n} \frac{i}{\tau_{s\nu'}} \frac{\Delta_{s\nu'} - \Delta_{s\nu}}{\omega(\omega+i/\tau_n)(\omega+i\rho)} \tag{11}$$

$$\frac{1}{u_n} = \frac{\Delta_n}{\omega} + \frac{i}{\tau_s} \frac{\frac{1}{2}(\Delta_{s1} + \Delta_{s2}) - \Delta_n}{\omega(\omega+i\rho)} + \frac{1}{2}(\frac{i}{\tau_{s1}} - \frac{i}{\tau_{s2}})\frac{\Delta_{s1} - \Delta_{s2}}{\omega(\omega+i\rho)} \tag{12}$$

Here, the definitions

$$1/\tau_s = 1/\tau_{s1} + 1/\tau_{s2} \qquad \rho = 1/\tau_s + 1/\tau_n \tag{13}$$

have been introduced. The first two terms in both equations are usually encountered in this treatment of the proximity effect. They describe the depression of T_c in the superconductor due to the weaker superconductivity in the normal layer.

Inserting these expressions into the properly expanded self-consistency equations (8) and (9) and performing the frequency integrals[16] leads to a set of three homogeneous equations for the order parameters. The corresponding secular equation determines T_c.

When the interband coupling parameters V_{12} and V_{21} vanish, the two bands have distinct transition temperatures. If $V_n \neq 0$, then the two order parameters Δ_{s1} and Δ_{s2} are coupled through (12) in 1. order with respect to $|T|^2$ so that the two bands undergo a superconducting transition at the same temperature. If there is no pairing interaction at all in the normal metal we need the third term in (11), which is of 2. order in $|T|^2$, to couple the two bands. We can, therefore, conclude that the presence of a film, which itself becomes

superconducting at some temperature (like Al or NbO), reduces anisotropy more readily than a normal metal.

SUMMARY

We have developed a formalism for calculating the density of
states observed in a tunneling experiment when a thin, normal or
weakly superconducting film is interposed between a two-band superconductor and the potential barrier. From the formulas presented it
is clear that the presence of such a film will reduce the observable
gap anisotropy. Numerical results for the density of states will be
presented elsewhere.

ACKNOWLEDGMENT

Stimulating discussions with Drs. J. L. Bostock, J. P. Carbotte,
J. Clem, K. Gärtner, D. G. Walmsley and E. L. Wolf are gratefully
acknowledged. I am also very grateful for the kind hospitality extended to me by the members of the Ames Laboratory at Iowa State
University, where part of this work was performed. I am indebted to
the Deutsche Forschungsgemeinschaft for providing a travel grant.

REFERENCES

1. J. L. Bostock and M. L. A. MacVicar, Anisotropy Effects in
   Superconductors, ed. H. W. Weber (Plenum, N. Y., 1977), p. 213
2. J. L. Bostock, K. Agyeman, M. H. Frommer and M. L. A. MacVicar,
   J. Appl. Phys. $\underline{44}$, 5567 (1973)
3. K. Gärtner and A. Hahn, Z. Naturforschung $\underline{31a}$, 861 (1976)
   B. Schöneich, D. Elefant, P. Otschik and J. Schumann,
   phys. stat. sol. (b) $\underline{91}$, 99 (1979)
4. H. K. Leung, J. P. Carbotte and C. R. Leavens,
   J. Low Temp. Phys. $\underline{24}$, 25 (1976)
5. P. G. Tomlinson and J. P. Carbotte, Phys. Rev. $\underline{B13}$, 4738 (1976)
6. P. G. Tomlinson and J. C. Swihart, Phys. Rev. $\underline{B19}$, 1867 (1979)
7. M. Peter, J. Ashkenazi and M. Dacorogna,
   Helv. Phys. Acta $\underline{50}$, 267 (1977)
8. W. H. Butler and P. B. Allen, Superconductivity in d- and f-Band
   Metals, ed. D. H. Douglass (Plenum, N. Y., 1976) p. 73
9. E. L. Wolf and J. Zasadzinski, Solid State Commun. $\underline{31}$, 32, (1979).
   and J. Low Temp. Phys. (to be published)
10. G. B. Arnold, Phys. Rev. $\underline{B18}$, 1076 (1978)
11. J. L. Bostock, M. L. A. MacVicar, G. B. Arnold, J. Zasadzinski
    and E. L. Wolf, Proceedings of the 3. Conference on Supercon-
    ductivity in d- and f-Band Metals, La Jolla, 1979
12. H. Suhl, B. Matthias, L. Walker, Phys. Rev. Lett. $\underline{3}$, 552 (1959)
13. G. W. Crabtree, D. H. Dye, D. P. Karim, D. D. Koelling and
    J. B. Ketterson, Phys. Rev. Lett. $\underline{42}$, 393 (1979)
14. W. L. McMillan, Phys. Rev. $\underline{175}$, 537 (1968)
15. M. Cohen, L. Falicov, J. Phillips, Phys. Rev. Lett. $\underline{8}$, 316 (1962)
16. N. Schopohl and K. Scharnberg, Solid State Commun. $\underline{22}$, 371 (1977)

CURRENT-VOLTAGE CHARACTERISTICS OF INTERACTING JOSEPHSON JUNCTIONS*

A.K. Jain, J.E. Lukens, Kin Li, R.D. Sandell** and C. Varmazis***
State University of New York, Stony Brook, N.Y. 11794

ABSTRACT

Results of model calculations for the current voltage characteristic of coupled Josephson junctions are presented. It is shown that the junctions can lock to a common voltage over a range of bias currents. The details of the I-V characteristic in the locked region can provide information on the coupling mechanism.

COUPLED JUNCTIONS

One class of inhomogeneous superconductors consist of small superconducting elements with Josephson coupling between them, e.g. granular films. An example of such inhomogeneous superconductors is a long superconducting strip interrupted by a series of Josephson junctions.[1,2] Such an array can provide a model for a number of these inhomogeneous systems. While such a model is rather idealized, there are pronounced effects due to the coupling of the junctions, such as voltage or phase locking between the junctions. Since this model can be quantitatively analyzed to obtain such information from the I-V curves as coupling strengths and phase shifts between the junctions, it may provide a useful guide to some aspects of the behavior of more complex systems.

In this paper we will develop a model for calculating the characteristics of coupled junctions. The basic approach assumes that the oscillating voltage at the Josephson frequency in one junction induces an oscillating current in another and thus phase -locks the two junctions. Of course the effect is reciprocal. For concreteness we will consider junctions coupled by a lumped inductor and resistor as shown in Fig. 1a. The results however just depend on the coupling strength and phase shifts due to the coupling. Thus they can be used to describe coupling due to non-equilibrium quasiparticle currents in the superconductor between the junctions or to radiation fields in a cavity.

This paper will concentrate on the effects of coupling in two junctions, however the method can easily be used for large arrays. Figure 1b shows a typical I-V for one junction of a coupled pair. As can be seen there is a region of bias currents over which the junction locks to a common voltage. We will be concerned only with this common voltage region where the two

---

*Work supported by the Office of Naval Research
**Present address: Aerospace Corp., Box 2957, Los Angeles, CA.
***Present address: University of Crete, Irakliou, Greece

266

junctions are phase-locked. In particular we wish to relate the locking range and the voltage and phase variation in the phase-locked region to the parameters of the coupling circuit.

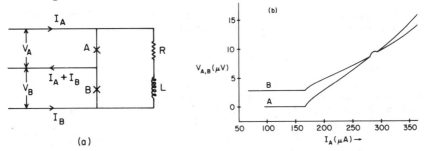

(a)

Fig. 1 (a). Equivalent circuit for biasing and coupling two resistively shunted junctions (RSJ). RSJs are indicated by X. (b) Voltage variation across junctions A and B as I_A is varied at constant I_B.

At high frequencies $V \gg I_c R_J$ where supercurrent oscillations are nearly sinusoidal, i.e., the phase of supercurrent is

$$\phi(t) = 2\pi \, Vt/\phi_0 + \delta \tag{1}$$

Forder[3] has shown the rf properties of the junction can be modelled by an rf current generator, $\tilde{I}_G = I_c \sin(\omega t + \delta)$, where $\omega = 2\pi \, V/\phi_0$, in parallel with a resistance R_J as shown in Fig. 2a. Thus if an rf current $\tilde{I}_x = I_\omega \sin \omega t$ with $I_\omega \ll I_c$ is applied to the junction, the rf voltage will be

$$\tilde{V} = R_J I_\omega \sin(\omega t) - R_J I_c \sin(\omega t + \delta) \tag{2}$$

i.e. the applied rf current does not change the amplitude of the rf current generated by the junction. It does, however, cause a change in the dc supercurrent $\bar{I}_s$ carried by the junction. This change is given by Forder as

$$\Delta \bar{I}_s = -\frac{1}{2} I_c \frac{R_J I_\omega}{V} \cos \delta \tag{3}$$

If the junction has a dc current bias $I_B = V/R_J + \bar{I}_s$, Eq. 3 shows that the junction will remain phase locked to the external rf over a range of bias currents $\Delta I_B = I_c R_J I_\omega/V$ giving the usual current step at constant voltage. In reduced units (currents, voltages, impedance, inductance and frequency in units of I_c, $I_c R_J$, R_J, $L_J = \phi_0/2\pi I_c$ and $I_c R_J/\phi_0$ respectively) the change in the supercurrent caused by the external radiation is

$$\Delta \bar{i}_s = -\frac{1}{2} \frac{i_\omega}{v} \cos \delta \tag{4}$$

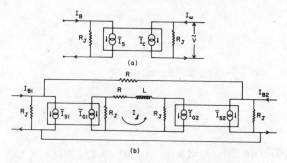

Fig. 2 (a). Forder's equivalent circuit model for an RSJ with v>1 having an applied dc current I_B and rf current $I\omega$. (b) Equivalent circuit for two coupled RSJs.

Equations 2 and 3 also allow us to calculate the change in the junction I-V curve due to a passive external load with impedance z_ℓ. Since the junction impedance R_J is known, the amplitude and phase of the current i_ℓ induced in the load by the junction can be calculated. The junction, of course, can not tell the difference between this induced current and an identical current from an external generator. Thus, Eq. 3 can be used to calculate the change in $\bar{I}_S$ produced by i_ℓ and thus the change in the bias current needed to produce a given voltage when the load is placed across the junction. Of course if the load has a finite dc resistance $z_\ell(0)$ the bias current must also be increased by an amount $v/z_\ell(0)$ to make up for the increased normal current. An important feature of these results is that the dc response of the junction depends linearly on i_ω. Thus, the effects of different perturbations on the junction can be considered separately. Thus, if a second junction is placed in the circuit, the change in $\bar{I}_{S1}$, the average supercurrent of the first junction will be the sum of the changes due to the changing load seen by junction one plus the change due to the rf current induced in junction one by two.

We will use Forder's model to examine the effect of coupling one junction to another junction on the current-voltage characteristics of the junctions. The equivalent circuit is shown in Fig. 2b, where for simplicity the two junctions have been taken to be identical. In general, if the two bias currents are close enough, i.e., $i_{B2} - i_{B1} \equiv \Delta i_B$ is small, the junction will phase lock and have a common dc voltage. We start by assuming the junctions to be phase locked with a phase difference δ. To find the change in $\bar{I}_{S1}$ due to i_{G2} we must find the induced current i_ℓ due to i_{G2}. Note that i_{G1} will also produce a contribution to i_ℓ which will change i_{S1}. This just produces a frequency change for a given $i_T \equiv i_{B1} + i_{B2}$ and does not contribute to the locking, so we will neglect it for now. For the case where z_ℓ is an inductor and resistor in series, $z_\ell = r + jv\ell$, i_ℓ due to i_{G2} is

$$\tilde{i}_{\ell 1} = \frac{-\tilde{i}_{G1}}{[(2+r)^2 + (v\ell)^2]^{\frac{1}{2}}} \; e^{j(\theta-\delta)} \quad , \qquad (5)$$

where $\theta = \tan^{-1} \left(\frac{v\ell}{2+r} \right)$, so from Eq. 3

$$\Delta \bar{i}_{s1} = \frac{1}{2} \frac{\cos(\theta-\delta)}{v[(2+r)^2+(v\ell)^2]^{\frac{1}{2}}} \quad , \qquad (6)$$

or $\Delta \bar{i}_{s1} = \Delta \bar{i}_s(0) \cos (\theta-\delta)$ where $\Delta \bar{i}_s(0) \equiv 1/(2v[(2 + r)^2 + (v\ell)^2]^{\frac{1}{2}})$ is just the amplitude of the constant voltage step which would be induced in the junction by an external r.f. current with amplitude i_ℓ at a frequency v. Similarly, $\Delta \bar{i}_{s2} = \Delta i_s(0) \cos (\theta+\delta)$. If i_T is kept constant as Δi_B is changed, then $\Delta \bar{i}_B = \Delta \bar{i}_{s1} - \Delta \bar{i}_{s2}$ and so

$$\Delta i_B = -2 \Delta \bar{i}_s(0) \sin\theta \sin\delta \quad . \qquad (7)$$

This relation between Δi_B and δ is not purely sinusoidal since v and thus $\Delta \bar{i}_s(0)$ are also a function of δ for constant i_T. This can most easily be seen by calculating the change in i_T with δ needed to keep v constant throughout the locking range. We define $\Delta i_T \equiv i_T(\delta)-i_T(0)$. For $\delta = 0$, v will be the same as for a coupled RSJ biased at $i_T(0)/2$, since $\delta = 0$ implies $\tilde{i}_\ell = 0$ and thus the circuit has no effect on the junction. For constant v, $\Delta i_T = \Delta \bar{i}_{s1} + \Delta \bar{i}_{s2}$. Thus:

$$\Delta i_T = 2 \Delta \bar{i}_s(0) \cos\theta(1-\cos\delta)] \qquad (8)$$

where we have included the effect of the loop current generated by a junction on that same junction. This is given by Eq. 6 with $\delta = 0$, since δ is now the phase shift between the junction and itself.

Thus:

$$\Delta i_B = \frac{\ell}{[(2+r)^2+(v\ell)^2]} \sin \delta \qquad (9)$$

$$\Delta i_T = \frac{2+r}{[(2+r)^2+(v\ell)^2]} (1-\cos\delta) \qquad (10)$$

It is usually a good approximation, if v is not too small, to assume that v is independent of δ when using Eq. 9. However it is simple to solve Eqs. 9 and 10 self-consistently on a calculator if the variation in v is significant.

When the coupling between junctions is weak, i.e. $|Z_\ell| \gg R_J$ it is possible to obtain generalizations of Eqs. 9 and 10 which are valid at all frequencies.[4,5] To do this we select the amplitude of the rf current source $\tilde{i}_G$ to give the correct

value of the fundamental rf voltage calculated from the RSJ
model in the absence of external circuits. Namely

$$\overset{\text{2v}}{i}_G = 2v[(1+v^2)^{\frac{1}{2}} - v] \sin (2\pi vt) \qquad . \qquad (11)$$

Also Eq. 3 is replaced by the more general result[4]

$$\Delta \bar{i}_S = - \frac{i_\omega}{2(1+v^2)^{\frac{1}{2}}} \cos \delta \qquad . \qquad (12)$$

Thus Eqs. 9 and 10 become

$$\Delta i_B = \frac{2v^2 \ell [(1+v^2)^{\frac{1}{2}} - v]}{(1+v^2)^{\frac{1}{2}}[(2+r)^2+(v\ell)^2]} \sin \delta \qquad , \qquad (13)$$

$$\Delta i_T = \frac{2(2+r)v[(1+v^2)^{\frac{1}{2}} - v]}{(1+v^2)^{\frac{1}{2}}[(2+r)^2+(v\ell)^2]} (1-\cos \delta) \qquad . \qquad (14)$$

These results can also be obtained directly by a perturbation
analysis[6,7,8] of the coupled equations describing the circuit in
Fig. 2.

We now investigate the manner in which Δi_B and Δi_T depend
on the circuit parameters ℓ and v. Equations 13 and 14 show that
there must be a phase shift in the coupling loop, i.e. $\ell \neq 0$,
in order for there to be a finite locking range with identical
junctions. This is just a consequence of a single junction
locked to external radiation being in the center of its current
step when the junction phase leads that of the applied current
by 90°. For locked junctions if the 90° phase shift is
supplied by the coupling loop, both junctions are in the center
of their "step" for equal bias currents and will thus stay
locked for a relatively large change in the bias currents. If
the coupling loop is purely resistive, the junctions will
again oscillate in phase for equal bias currents, but now each
is at the bottom of its "step." Thus any attempt to increase
Δi_B will decrease the current through one junction and unlock
the pair.

In Fig. 3a we use Eqs. 13 and 14 to calculate the variation
in Δi_B and v for constant i_T in the locked region. As can be seen
the shape of the curve depends strongly on θ and thus serves
as a measure of the phase shift produced by whatever mechanism
couples the junctions. For $v>1$ the ratio of the maximum voltage
variation to maximum current variation is just $R_J \cot\theta$. As can
be seen from the data[9] in Fig. 3b the variation of voltage in
the locked range which is predicted is in fact observed
experimentally in our coupled junctions.

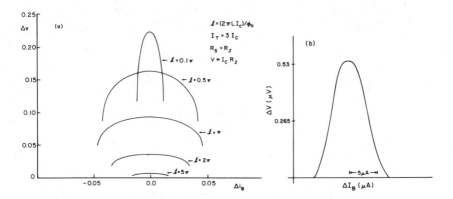

Fig. 3 (a). Predicted voltage variation of coupled junctions in locked region from Eqs. 13 and 14. (b) Observed voltage variation of junctions coupled by resistive-inductive shunt.

When r=0 the coupled junctions are just the familiar dc SQUID magnetometer with Δi_B being circulating dc current in the SQUID. Thus Fig. 3a along with the dc fluxoid quantization condition gives the variation of SQUID voltage with magnetic field. Figure 4a shows the variation with voltage of the predicted locking range for several coupling parameters. Our microbridge junctions differ enough from RSJs that a quantitative

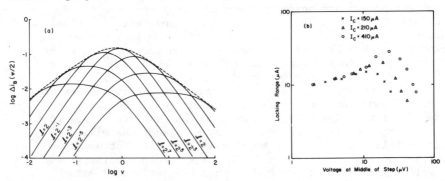

Fig. 4 (a). Predicted locking range $\Delta i_B(\Pi/2)$ vs locking voltage for various coupling inductances ℓ and r = 0 (solid lines). Dashed line shows the maximum locking range at any voltage with ℓ optimized for that voltage. (b) Observed locking range of microbridge junctions for several values of I_c.

comparison of the observed locking range with theory is not possible. The data in Fig. 4b, however, still show qualitatively the predicted behavior.

CONCLUSION

A simple method has been outlined here for solving circuits involving Josephson Junctions. The model gives results which are in qualitative agreement with experiment done on junctions coupled by different mechanisms[1,9] It should be possible to get information about the mechanism of coupling between coupled junctions by observing the current-voltage characteristic in the locked region. Finally, this approach gives the same results as obtained from perturbation theory.[5,6,7,8] Because of its simplicity, this analysis should be helpful in designing larger arrays of Josephson Junctions.

We would also like to acknowledge helpful discussions with V.Ambegaokar, A. Feingold, D. Fox, D. Jillie and E. Siggia. We would also like to thank P. Mankiewich for fabricating the coupled junctions.

REFERENCES

1. D.W. Jillie, J.E. Lukens, Y.H. Kao and G.J. Dolan, Phys. Lett. 55A, 381 (1976).
2. R.D. Sandell, C. Varmazis, A.K. Jain and J.E. Lukens, IEEE Trans. Mag-15, 462 (1979).
3. P.W. Forder, J. Phys. D 10, 1413 (1977).
4. L.G. Aslamazov and A.I. Larkin, J.E.T.P. Lett. 9, 87 (1979).
5. E.D. Thompson, J. Appl. Phys. 44, 5587 (1973).
6. E. Siggia and V. Ambegaokar, Private Communcation.
7. A. Feingold, Private Communication.
8. D. Jillie, M.A.H. Nerenberg, J.A. Blackburn, Private Communication.
9. R.D. Sandell, C. Varmazis, A.K. Jain and J.E. Lukens, Future Trends in Superconductive Electronics. AIP Conf. Proc. No. 44, edited by B.S. Deaver, C.M. Falco, J.H. Harris, S.A. Wolf (AIP, New York, 1979), pp 327-334.

CRITICAL CURRENTS AND PENETRATION DEPTH OF A RANDOMLY
ORIENTED THREE-DIMENSIONAL ASSEMBLY OF POINT CONTACTS

A. Raboutou, P. Peyral and J. Rosenblatt
Institut National des Sciences Appliquées
B.P. 14A, 35043 Rennes Cedex   France

ABSTRACT

Critical currents and the penetration depth of an assembly
of $\sim 10^6$ superconducting grains linked by Josephson contacts have
been measured as a function of applied magnetic field. Our experimental results are compared with a model based on the assumptions
of phase coherence and random orientation of the junctions in the
system. The main features of the data are well reproduced by the
model, particularly the critical current peak at H = 0.

INTRODUCTION

Experimental results on the temperature dependence of resistivity of an assembly of weakly coupled superconducting grains have
led us to suggest[1,2] that a phase transition to overall coherence in
the system could take place at a temperature lower than the superconducting critical temperature of individual grains. Characteristic
features of this transition, in the case of bulk grains of diameter
a $>> \lambda(T)$, $\xi(T)$ are described elsewhere in this Conference[3], hereafter
referred to as I. We just point out here that by averaging a free
energy similar to Josephson's over the random orientation of individual junctions with respect to an applied field or current, a non
linear differential equation

$$\nabla^2 \vec{\gamma} = \frac{3}{\lambda_c^2} \frac{\vec{\gamma}}{\gamma} \frac{d}{d\gamma}(1 - \frac{\sin\gamma}{\gamma}) \tag{1}$$

is obtained for the pseudophase $\vec{\gamma} = a(\nabla\tilde{\phi} - 2\pi\vec{A}/\Phi_o)|\Psi|$, where
$\Psi = <e^{i\phi}> = |\Psi| e^{i\tilde{\phi}}$ is the order parameter describing correlations
in the phases ϕ of individual grains. The field in the sample
$\vec{B}(\vec{r}) = \nabla \times \vec{A}$ results from an average over a small volume element
containing many grains, of the actual field penetrating into the
sample. The coherent penetration depth

$$\lambda_c = \left(3c\Phi_o a/(4\pi^2 \mu z I_J |\Psi|^2)\right)^{1/2} , \tag{2}$$

where z is the number of first neighbors of a grain and I_J the
critical current of individual contacts, is a cooperative effect
of Josephson interactions between grains.
    Another cooperative effect one may expect to observe is the
critical supercurrent, and more particularly its modulation by an
applied magnetic field H. This can again be calculated from Eq.(1).
One obtains, when $H >> H_1$

$$I_c(H)/I_c(0) = 0.82 \ (1 - \gamma_s^{-1} \ sin\gamma_s)^{1/2} \ H_1/H, \qquad (3)$$

where H_1 is the maximum field for the existence of the Meissner effect in a semiinfinite sample and γ_s, the value of γ at the surface, may be estimated as $\gamma_s \simeq 2.7(R/\lambda_c)(H/H_1)$, where R is a characteristic dimension of the sample (half the thickness in the case of a slab). Finally, we have discussed in I a percolation contribution to the current, with characteristic oscillations around a non zero average, which is relatively important when $H >> H_1$.

After describing the procedure for fabricating our samples, we present here results on their coherent penetration depth and dependence of critical current upon the applied field. We compare the data with the model developed in I and discuss the validity of the latter.

SAMPLES

Our samples are made by compacting commercially available Nb powder with an epoxy resin. Grains of size a $\lesssim$ 50 μm are chemically etched, dried and mixed with the resin and hardener to be moulded to a cylindrical shape. While hardening, resistance can be monitored and pressure adjusted so as to keep the former within a desired range. Current and voltage leads are attached to the sample allowing true four-point measurements to be performed. A typical system contains $\sim 10^6$ junctions and has normal resistivity in the range 0.1 - 1 Ω-cm. Differential contraction of the resin upon cooling brings about a hydraulic pressure on the grains which hopefully eliminates possible anisotropies in the distribution of contact properties. The samples can stand a few thermal cycles without degradation of their qualities.

PENETRATION DEPTH

If there were no Josephson coupling between grains the diamagnetic response of the latter to an applied field H would give a magnetic permeability $\mu \simeq 1 - f$ where f is the filling factor of the grains, simply because the field is excluded from their volume. In the next approximation one should consider effects due to the finite superconducting penetration depth λ_s in the grains and its possible dependence on temperature. Finally, λ_c produces a partial Meissner effect in a finite sample. The relative importance of these effects can be estimated by taking into account that flux exclusion from the grains depends on the parameter $a/2\lambda_s \simeq 10^3$, while that due to Josephson coupling depends on $R/\lambda_c \simeq 0.3 \stackrel{-}{=} 3$, R being the radius of the sample. The corresponding parameter in a cyclindrical thin film is $Rd/2\lambda^2 \simeq 10 - 10^2$ from experimental results on granular Al[4].

274

As pointed out in I, the apparent coherent penetration depth is expected to be extremely sensitive to fields of a few mOe. This precludes the use of a resonant frequency shift method[5], where the amplitude is difficult to control. We have therefore chosen to measure the signal induced by an external ac field on a pick-up coil closely wound around the sample. The field H is kept so small (H < 2 Oe) that it has no effect on λ_s, even when it is large enough to suppress the Josephson effect. For very small fields γ is also small and we may linearise Eq.(1). In cylindrical coordinates the solution is $\gamma_\phi = KI_1(R/\lambda_c)$ where I_1 is the modified Bessel function of the first kind of order one and K is a constant of proportionality adjusted to satisfy the boundary condition B(R) = μH. The flux across the sample is then given by

$$\Phi_c = 2\pi R\lambda_c \left(I_1(R/\lambda_c)/I_0(R/\lambda_c)\right) \mu H \qquad (4)$$

for H → 0 and
$$\Phi_s = \pi R^2 \mu H \qquad (5)$$

when the Josephson effect is suppressed. In a preliminary experiment we tried to measure the differential permeability by superimposing a dc field and a constant amplitude ac field. We had evidence of flux pinning and hysteresis, which had to be expected from the irregular structure of the granular sample. In order to get rid of flux pinning effects, we applied only an ac field of varying amplitude H_m. The ac voltage V across the pick-up coil should then be linear in H_m for small values of H_m (Eq.(4)) and approximately so for large values (Eq.(5)). Typical results are shown in Fig.1. The quantities $v_c = V/H_m$ ($H_m \to 0$) and $v_s = V/H_m$ ($H_m \to \infty$), allow us to obtain λ_c from the transcendental equation

$$\frac{\lambda_c}{R} \frac{I_1(R/\lambda_c)}{I_0(R/\lambda_c)} = \frac{1}{2} \frac{v_c}{v_s} \qquad (6)$$

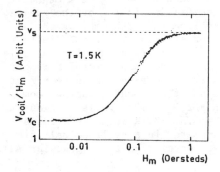

Fig. 1

Typical experimental data in a measurement of penetration depth.

If our interpretation is correct v_s should provide a measurement of the purely superconducting permeability. Therefore, it should have a practically constant value with temperature in the range explored ($T \ll T_c(Nb)$), which it does. A typical plot of $\lambda_c(T)$ is shown in Fig.2, together with a fit to a law $\lambda_c \sim (T_0 - T)^{-\beta}$.

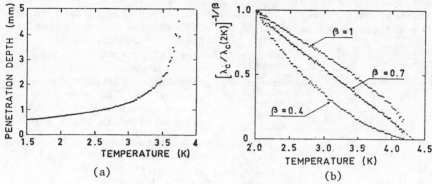

Fig.2 (a) Experimental values of λ_c vs T for a typical sample.
   (b) Critical behavior of λ_c. The exponent $1/\beta$ is varied until the data points fall on a straight line.

The value $\beta \simeq 0.7$ found here should be considered with caution. Analysis of quite a few samples, with a wide range of coherence temperatures T_0 is necessary before definite assertions on the value of β may be made. In any case, we may point out here that our data cannot be fitted by a law of the type $\lambda_c^{-2} \propto 1 - (T/T_0)^4$, contrary to the case of granular $Al - Al_2O_3$ films[4]. This is not surprising, since the coherence- to-paracoherence transition, being due to nearest neighbor interactions, need not be of the same type as the superconducting one.

QUANTUM INTERFERENCE EFFECTS

As indicated in I, a magnetic field should modulate the critical current in two ways : through a single peak in the total current centered at $H = 0$ and by creating percolation paths among the randomly oriented junctions, which should give a finite contribution to the current at high fields. From the experimental point of view the determination of the critical current I_c is not unambiguous. In fact, the V(I) characteristics of our samples display a smeared transition to the resistive state. This ought to be expected from Eq.(1), where the potential for phase slip is $1 - \gamma^{-1}\sin\gamma$, in contrast with the cosine potential for a single junction. Barriers opposing phase slip are lower in the former. Taking this into account, we have defined I_c experimentally through a fixed detectable value of the dynamical resistance R_d rather than voltage, as is usually done. This takes advantage of the large gain obtainable from a lock-in detector and of the $R_d(I)$ characteristic, somewhat steeper than V(I). The sample is then mounted in a feedback loop (Fig.3) where the output of a lock-in detector measuring R_d goes into a microcomputer which commands a summing circuit feeding current to the sample. The current is made to increase (decrease) by finite steps whenever R_d is smaller (greater) than a fixed value R_{ds}. Once the desired value of R_d is attained, the microcomputer stores the corresponding values of current and field and commands a current generator to increase the field by a finite step to proceed to a new measurement. A single point in the $I_c(H)$ curve typically takes about 3-6 seconds to be measured, depending on resolution. For the data of Fig.4 R_{ds} = 20 mΩ , about 3×10^{-3} the normal resistance of the sample. In (b) we have also shown the theoretical predictions of the model described in I.

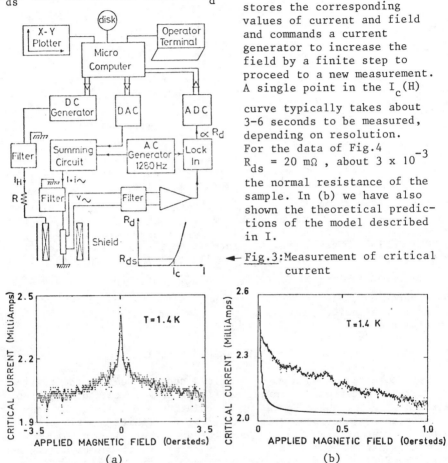

Fig.3:Measurement of critical current

Fig.4 : Critical current as a function of applied field of a granular Nb sample of normal resistance 6Ω. The temperature is 1.4K.
(a) Current resolution δI = 10μA. The full curve shows oscillations left after smoothing the data through a low-pass numerical filter.
(b) Data taken with a current resolution δI = 4μA. The full line is the theoretical prediction from the model developped in I.

DISCUSSION

Our experimental results on $\lambda_c(T)$ and its critical behavior shown in Fig. 2 give further support to the idea that a coherent-paracoherent phase transition takes place at the temperature T_c, which in this example is obviously smaller than T_c for Nb. The model described in I gives no indication of what the temperature dependence of λ_c should be, but beyond the very existence of a coherent penetration depth, allows an estimate of its order of magnitude at $T = 0$. This is verified by our data. On the other hand, predictions concerning magnetic field effects on the critical current are more precise. The model describes well the most relevant features of the data, namely a peak at $H = 0$, followed by a long tail with many oscillations in the $I_c(H)$ curve. However its fails to give a quantitative account of the width of the peak, or the period and amplitude of the oscillations. A more refined description is needed, in particular to take into account possible percolation processes along paths where short range order exists in contacts with a high critical current.

REFERENCES

1 - J. Rosenblatt, H. Cortès and P. Pellan, Phys. Lett. A33, 143(1970).
2 - P. Pellan, G. Dousselin, H. Cortès and J. Rosenblatt, Solid State Commun. 11, 427 (1972).
3 - J. Rosenblatt, P. Peyral and A. Raboutou, Proceedings of this Conference.
4 - D. Abraham, G. Deutscher, R. Rosenbaum and S. Wolf, Proceedings of LT15, J. Phys. C6, 586(1978).
5 - A.L. Schawlow and G.E. Devlin, Phys. Rev. 113, 120(1959).

RATIO OF SUPERCONDUCTING TRANSITION TEMPERATURES IN GRANULAR Nb FILMS

R. Laibowitz and A. Broers
IBM Thomas J. Watson Research Center
Yorktown Heights, New York 10598

and

D. Stroud[†] and Bruce R. Patton[†]
Dept. of Physics, Ohio State Univ., Columbus, Ohio 43210

ABSTRACT

Experimental results on the resistive transition of superconducting granular Nb thin film bridges are reported which show a two part transition. The data are analyzed to extract a single grain transition temperature, T_{co}, and the long-range phase-ordering temperature T_c. The data are then compared to a recent theoretical model which predicts $T_{co}/T_c = 1 + R_{ij}/R_o$ where R_{ij} is the average intergrain resistance, $R_o \sim z\hbar/e^2 \sim z \cdot 4500 \; \Omega$ and z is the average number of nearest neighbor grains.

It has been well known for a number of years that granular superconductors in the form of thin films with grain dimensions $L_o \approx 30\text{-}200$ Å frequently show a step structure in the resistance in the transition to a superconducting state.[1,2] The experimental data indicate that the transition occurs in two distinct parts, and the size of the low T_c, foot structure seems to vary from sample to sample. In the present note we compare the experimental data for thin granular Nb films with a theoretical equation emerging from a microscopic theory of a granular superconducting system.[3] The theory predicts that the individual grains become superconducting at a temperature T_{co} which, for grains not too small compared to the coherence length ξ, will be close to the bulk superconducting temperature. The whole material, however, does not show long-range superconducting behavior until a lower temperature T_c where the resistance goes to zero. T_c will depend on the magnitude of the intergrain Josephson coupling energy, which from the microscopic theory is related to the inverse of the intergrain resistance.[3,4,5] With certain simplifying assumptions, the theory predicts that the ratio of the two transition temperatures T_c and T_{co}, for a sample with all three dimensions large compared to L_o, is given by the equation[3]

$$T_c/T_{co} = R_o/(R_o + R_{ij}) \tag{1}$$

where

$$R_o = \left[\frac{\pi^2}{7\zeta(3)} z \frac{\hbar}{e^2} \right]$$

$$\approx 1.17 z \frac{\hbar}{e^2} \approx z \cdot 4500 \Omega \tag{2}$$

and R_{ij} is the average intergrain resistance, z being the average number of nearest

[†]Work at Ohio State supported by NSF Grants DMR 78-11770 and DMR 77-22829

neighbors seen by a given grain.

The granular Nb films were formed by vapor deposition from an electron-beam heated source and were generally around 300 Å thick. The films were deposited on window substrates which facilitated detailed examination by transmission electron microscopy (TEM). While details of the sample preparation can be found elsewhere[6,7] we show in Fig. 1 a micrograph of the 300 Å thick film, The granularity is apparent with grain sizes varying from 30 Å to greater than 200 Å.

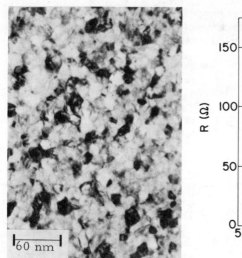

Fig. 1 Micrograph of 300 Å thick Nb film

Fig. 2 Resistance vs temperature for a Nb fine line (3rd row in Table 1)

Ultra-narrow thin film wires were then fabricated from the granular Nb films.[8,9] Typical conductor dimensions were length 0.12 to 1μm, width 25 to 75 nm, thickness 30 nm as shown in Table 1. The resistive transition for such a stripe is shown in Fig. 2. The two transitions are clearly visible, however the detailed shape of such curves generally can vary from sample to sample. The bridge fabrication process does contaminate the samples and in a few cases, the sample remains resistive even to temperatures as low as 1.5 K. The fabrication process also leaves a protective layer of carbon on the bridge which often makes it difficult to obtain clear micrographs of the final grain structure.

To apply Eq. (1) to the data, the average intergrain resistance must be extracted from the measured resistivity. If the films are assumed to consist of high-conductivity grains coated with a high-resistivity skin, then the effective resistivity ρ of the film is best calculated by means of the Clausius-Mossotti-Maxwell-Garnett[10] approximation, which gives in this limit

$$\rho = \frac{1}{3}f\rho_s = \frac{1}{3}fR_{ij}\frac{A}{t} \tag{3}$$

280

where ρ_s is the resistivity of the skin, A the area of contact between grains, t the skin thickness and f the volume fraction of film composed of insulator. If the grains are assumed cubical then

$$f = 3t/[\sqrt{A} + 3t] \tag{4}$$

which gives

$$R_{ij} = \rho(\sqrt{A} + 3t)/A. \tag{5}$$

The transmission electron microscopy studies indicate the grain size varies from $\sim$ 30-200 Å. We take A = (30 Å)^2 and the thickness of the tunneling barrier t=10 Å. The resulting values of R_{ij} are given along with other sample properties in Table I.

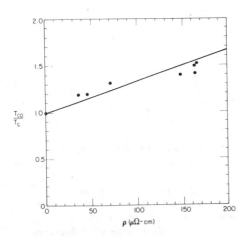

Figure 3 shows the observed ratio of transition temperature T_{co}/T_c plotted against resistivity. The straight line is based on Eq. (2) and (5) with $z_{eff} = 1.34$. While this value might seem low for a three-dimensional sample, we note that in high resistance materials near the percolation threshold,[11] the number of nearest neighbors is in the range 1-2. The agreement between theory and experiment as seen in Fig. 3 appears to be quite satisfactory and represents the first time this type of data has been systematically compared to a microscopic theory. Data on samples with larger ratios of T_{co}/T_c and from different materials would be desirable to further test the theoretical model.

The authors gratefully acknowledge discussions with W. Lamb, E. Alessandrini and J. Viggiano.

Fig. 3 Ratio of transition temperature in granular Nb films plotted against measured film resistivity. Resistivity can be converted to intergrain resistance with the help of Eq. (5). Straight line corresponds to $z_{eff} = 1.34$, as described in text.

R(Ω)	l(μm)	w(nm)	t(nm)	$\rho(\mu\Omega cm)$	$R_{ij}(\Omega)$	T_c(K)	T_c/T_{co}
137	0.28	110	30	164	1090	5.9	1.49
138	0.28	110	30	164	1100	5.8	1.52
146	0.33	110	30	148	990	6.3	1.40
595	1.0	40	30	71	470	6.7	1.31
306	1.0	50	30	46	310	7.4	1.19
19	0.35	300	100	165	1100	6.6	1.41
245	1.0	60	27	36	240	6.3	1.19

REFERENCES

1. R. B. Laibowitz, Appl. Phys. Lett. 23, 407 (1973).
2. G. Deutscher and M. L. Rappaport, J. dePhysique, C-6, 581 (1978).
3. B. R. Patton, D. Stroud and W. Lamb, Bull. Am. Phys. Soc. 24, 356 (1979); see also this proceedings.
4. G. Deutscher, Y. Imry and L. Gunther, Phys. Rev. B. 10, 4598 (1974).
5. V. Ambegaokar and A. Baratoff, Phys. Rev. Lett. 10, 486 (1963).
6. A. N. Broers, W. Molzen, J. Cuomo and N. Wittels, Appl. Phys. Lett. 15, 98 (1976).
7. W. W. Molzen, A. N. Broers, J. J. Cuomo, J. M. Harper and R. B. Laibowitz, J. Vac. Sci. Technol. 16, 269 (1979).
8. A. N. Broers and R. B. Laibowitz, AIP Conf. Proc. 44, 289 (1978).
9. R. B. Laibowitz, A. N. Broers, J. T. C. Yen and J. M. Viggiano, to be published, Appl. Phys. Lett.
10. See for example, R. Landauer, AIP Conf. Proc. 40, 2 (1978).
11. V. K. S. Shante and S. Kirkpatrick, Advan. Phys. 20, 325 (1971).

POLYSULFUR NITRIDE: A FIBROUS SUPERCONDUCTOR

P. Barrett, E.Z. da Silva, B.L. Gyorffy,
W.G. Herrenden-Harker and M.G. Priestley
H.H. Wills Physics Laboratory
University of Bristol, Bristol, U.K.

ABSTRACT

In this note we present experimental evidence and theoretical analysis which supports earlier suggestions that the superconducting properties of (SN)$_x$ are dominated by the fibrous morphology.

INTRODUCTION

In contrast to its behaviour in the normal state, the superconducting properties of (SN)$_x$ display effects of reduced dimensionality[1,2,3,4]. Provisionally, these have been attributed to the fact that all samples studied consist of tangles of more or less parallel metallic (SN)$_x$ fibers with diameters ranging from 50 to 1000 Å.

In this contribution we present further experimental evidence and theoretical analysis in support of this interpretation. Moreover, we suggest that in a magnetic field parallel to the fibers, and close to or above the upper critical field H$_{C_2}$, only the thinnest fibers are superconducting and they behave quite independently. At lower or perpendicular fields, when many nearest neighbour fibers are superconducting we expect the interactions to play an important role. Though we are unable to study this regime in detail it might be of considerable interest from the point of view of understanding inhomogeneous superconductors.

THE FLUCTUATION CONDUCTIVITY σ_f IN AN EXTERNAL FIELD

It was shown by da Silva and Gyorffy (dG) that the fluctuation conductivity of an independent anisotropic fiber can be written (apart from small correction terms) as

$$\left[\frac{\sigma_n}{\sigma_f(H,T,\theta)} \right]^{2/3} = B\ f(H,\theta)\ (T - T_c), \tag{1}$$

where

$$B = \left(\frac{16}{e^2} \right)^{2/3} \left(\frac{8\hbar k}{\pi} \right)^{1/3} \left(\frac{r_0^{4/3}}{D_{\parallel}^{1/3}} \right) \sigma_n^{2/3},$$

θ is the angle between the magnetic field and the fiber axis, r_0 is the fiber radius, and $D_{\parallel}$ the electronic diffusion constant parallel to the fibers. The function $f(H,\theta)$ takes the following two limiting forms: at low fields

0094-243X/80/580282-06$1.50

$$f \equiv f_\ell = [T_c(H)]^{-2/3}, \text{ valid for } r_o < \xi_\perp(0) < r_c,$$

with $r_c = (\hbar c/2eH)^{1/2}$, while at high fields, $r_o < r_c < \xi_\perp(0)$, we have

$$f \equiv f_h = \pi^{4/3}/(24\rho[T_c(H)]^{2/3}),$$

where ρ is the pair breaker that determines $T_c(H)$. The angular variation of the fluctuations is thus implicit in that of $T_c(H)$ and ρ. For the fiber model the temperature dependence is independent of the field direction, in contrast to the model of a bulk anisotropic conductor, where it is predicted that $\sigma_f \propto (T - T_c)^{-1/2}$ for $\theta = 90°$, but that $\sigma_f \propto (T - T_c)^{-3/2}$ for $\theta = 0$ (see dG for details).

We have measured the superconducting fluctuations in the conductivity of $(SN)_x$ for magnetic fields both perpendicular and parallel to the fiber. The perpendicular field data[3] show clearly that σ_f is proportional to $(T - T_c)^{-3/2}$, in agreement with Eq.(1) and unambiguously supporting the fiber model; when fitted to the theory in the high-field limit at a single point (386 G) the data give $r_o^4/D_{\parallel} = 1.59 \times 10^{-32}$ m^2.s.

The results of preliminary measurements on sample 7D (T_c = 279 mK; $\rho_{300}/\rho_{4.2}$ = 73) in parallel fields are given in Fig. 1. It is seen that $\sigma_f \propto (T - T_c)^{-3/2}$, which is consistent with either bulk or fiber model, but we note that when the bulk model is used the numerical value of the predicted slope (e.g. for curve a) is too small by almost two orders of magnitude. On the other hand, the measured slope in curve a is in good agreement with that calculated from the fiber model, using the parameters deduced from the perpendicular field data in the high field limit[3]. Hence, the fluctuations observed in both parallel and perpendicular fields give conclusive evidence for the fiber model. The remaining uncertainty is whether the dG theory, which neglects interactions between the fiber, accounts for the field dependence of the fluctuation conductivity. The relevant data is presented in Fig. 2, where the curves for f_ℓ and f_h are plotted using the data of Barrett et al.[3], while the circles show the normalized experimental slopes for several magnetic fields perpendicular to the fibers. It is clear that the dG model does not account satisfactorily for the low magnetic field variation of the fluctuation conductivity. In particular, there is no sign of the predicted low field region represented by f_ℓ.

However, we are able to use the parallel field fluctuation measurements to show that the dG fibre theory gives a good description of the angular dependence of σ_f, provided that measurements are compared at constant ρ, as in the implicit dependence in Eq. (1).

284

The + symbols in Fig. 2 show the normalized slopes of the temperature dependence of the fluctuation conductivity at different parallel fields, with the x-axis scaled to give values of ρ (and $T_c(H)$) equal to those for $H_\perp$. This normalization introduces no further adjustable parameters. The observation that the fluctuations in both parallel and perpendicular fields then give slopes that have the same field dependence enables us to conclude that the angular dependence of the fluctuations implicit in Eq. (1) is correct, but that the interfiber coupling, which has so far been neglected, leads to an additional field dependence of σ_f.

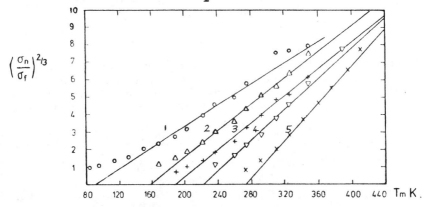

Fig. 1. Temperature dependence of the fluctuation conductivity σ_f of sample 7D at various magnetic fields parallel to the fibers. σ_n is the conductivity in the normal state. H (G): 1) 7710; 2) 6430; 3) 5140; 4) 3890; 5) 0.

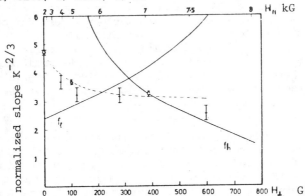

Fig. 2. Magnetic-field dependence of the slopes g of the curves in Fig. 1, normalized by dividing by the parameter B. f_ℓ is the prediction of the dG theory for low fields; f_h its prediction for high fields. o is $H_\perp$ (lower scale); + is $H_\parallel$ (upper scale). The dashed curve is a freehand fit to the data.

THE TEMPERATURE DEPENDENCE OF $H_{C_2}(T)$

Earlier[3,4] we have analyzed the experimental data on $H_{C_2}(T)$ using an anisotropic independent-fiber model based on the appropriate generalization of the Maki-de Gennes theory. The model gave a good fit for the full temperature range. Since Pauli paramagnetism was not taken into account and the pair breaker was given by $\rho = (e^2 H^2/4 \pi \hbar k T_{CO}) D_\perp r_0^2$, where $D_\perp$ is the perpendicular electronic diffusion constant and the other symbols have the usual meaning, it was easy to find small enough fiber radius r_0 to explain the large values of $H_{C_2}^{//}(T)$, which at low temperatures exceeded the paramagnetic limit $H_P = 5400$ G by a considerable margin $(H_{C_2}(T = 0) \simeq 8200$ G$)$. To render the theory meaningful we have now included both the Pauli term and an isotropic spin-orbit scattering term into our starting Hamiltonian. Following the argument of Maki we find that the gap equation which determines $H_{C_2||}(T)$ is given by the usual expression[5] with the orbital contribution to the pair breaker given by the fiber theory. For $D_\perp r_0^2 = 6.171 \times 10^{-12}$ cm^2 sec^{-1} for sample 7A $(6.061 \times 10^{-12}$ cm^2 sec^{-1} for sample 7D$)$ and a spin-orbit scattering time $\tau_{SO} = 2.3 \times 10^{-12}$ sec for 7A $(1.2 \times 10^{-12}$ sec for 7D$)$ we compare the predictions of the model with our own experimental values[3] for $H_{C_2}^{//}(T)$ in Fig. 3. The agreement is gratifying, though it must be stressed that the shape of the curve is not sufficiently sensitive to individual variations in $D_\perp r_0^2$ and τ_{SO} to fix their relative values to better than a factor of 2. Note that $h/\tau_{SO} \ll h/\tau$, the total scattering rate (for this sample we estimated $\tau \sim 10^{-14}$ sec). Hence the large values of $H_{C_2}^{//}$ can consistently be explained as a size effect.

INTERACTIONS BETWEEN FIBERS

Taking $D_{//}/r_0^4$ from the fit to σ_f and $D_\perp r_0^2$ from the discussion above we find $(D_\perp/D_{//}) r_0^6 = 9.44 \times 10^{-37}$ cm^6 for sample 7A and 7.69×10^{-37} cm^6 for 7D. From $D = (1/3) v_F^2 \tau$, using $v_F^{//2}/v_F^{\perp2} \sim 100$ (from band calculations[6]) and $\tau^{//}/\tau^{\perp} \sim 4$ (from optical measurements[7]) we estimate $D_{//}/D_\perp \sim 40$. However, this estimate is rather uncertain. We take advantage of this and choose $D_{//}/D_\perp = 55$ since with this value the dG theory gives $H_{C_2}^{\perp}(0)$ in good agreement with experiments[3].

286

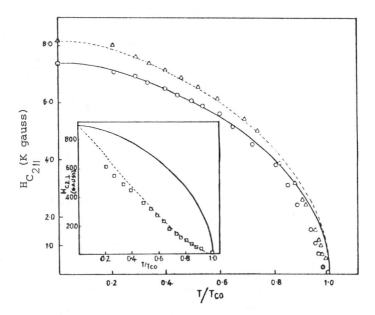

Fig. 3. Parallel critical fields. Δ sample 7D; O - 7A. The full (dashed) line shows the theoretical curve for sample 7A (7D). The inset shows $H_{C_{2\perp}}$; □ - 7A. The full (dashed) line is explained in the text.

This gives r_0 = 193 Å for 7A and 186 Å for 7D. We next estimate $D_{\parallel} r_0^2 = (D_{\parallel}/D_{\perp})(D_{\perp} r_0^2) = 3.39 \times 10^{-10} cm^4 sec^{-1}$ for 7A and then use the model (without the Pauli term and spin-orbit coupling, since $H_{C_2}^{\perp}$ is small) to predict $H_{C_2}^{\perp}(T)$. The result is compared with experiment in the inset in Fig. 3 (full curve). Although the independent-fiber model is relatively successful, it clearly does not account for $H_{C_2}^{\perp}(T)$. We note as a possibly significant fact that if the pair breaker for perpendicular fields is taken to be ρ (single fiber). $.[(T - T_{c0})/T_{c0}]^2$ we obtain a very good fit to the measured values of $H_{C_2}^{\perp}(T)$, as shown by the dashed line in the inset to Fig. 3.

We would like to suggest that the success of the independent-fiber model in explaining certain properties, together with its failure to account for others, is a consequence of a distribution in fiber diameters.

Consider the case of $H_{C_2}^{//}(T)$. According to the pair breaker given above for the fiber model, small r_0 means large H_{C_2}. Consequently, if a sample consists of fibers with differing radii, as H increases at a given T, many of the thick ones will go normal. Hence, near the experimental $H_{C_2}^{//}$ there will be only a few thin fibers still superconducting. As these will be far apart they will not interact strongly and it is reasonable to expect that H_{C_2}'' is then correctly predicted by a theory based on independent fibers. Without a proper theory of interactions it is not easy to see why this argument should not hold for $H_{C_2}^{\perp}$ (T) as well. The theory of interacting chains ($r_0 = 0$) developed by Manneville[8] and Klemm[9] is not helpful in this context, since they suggest that the interaction decreases with decreasing T and H. Nevertheless, it appears to be the case that the interactions are more important at low fields.

Interactions will first enter our formulae for σ_f by modifying the pair breaker ρ as a function of H. Near H_{C_2} the fibres are still independent but for lower fields, interactions will modify ρ and the field dependence of σ_f will change. These features are consistent with our observations above.

If the above general picture is correct, magnetization measurements at low fields ($\sim H_{C_1}$) should show striking deviations from the independent fiber behaviour.

We are grateful to the Science Research Council for financial support for the experimental work. One of us (E.Z. da Silva) was supported by FAPESP .

REFERENCES

1. R.I. Civiak, C. Elbaum, L.F. Nichols, H.I. Kao, and M.M. Labes, Phys. Rev. B 14, 5413 (1976).
2. L.J. Azevedo, W.C. Clark, G. Deutscher, R.L. Greene, G.B. Street, and L.J. Suter, Solid State Commun. 19, 197 (1976).
3. P. Barrett, R.G. Chambers, P. Feenan, W.G. Herrenden-Harker, M. G. Priestley, R.W. Trinder and S.F.J. Read. Submitted to J.Phys. F.
4. E.Z. da Silva and B.L. Gyorffy, Phys. Rev. B 20, 147 (1979).
5. K. Maki, Phys. Rev. 148, 362 (1966).
6. W.E. Rudge and P.M. Grant, Phys. Rev. Lett.35, 1799 (1975).
7. H. P. Geserich, W. Möller, G. Scheiber and L. Pintschovius. Phys. Status Solidi B 80, 119 (1977).
8. P. Manneville. J. Phys. (Paris) 36, 701 (1975).
9. L.A. Turkevich and R.A. Klemm, Phys. Rev. B 19, 2520 (1979).

288

FAR INFRARED ABSORPTION IN GRANULAR SUPERCONDUCTORS*

G.L. Carr, J.C. Garland and D.B. Tanner
Dept. of Physics, The Ohio State University, Columbus, Ohio 43210

ABSTRACT

Measurements of far infrared transmission and reflection have
been done on composites consisting of small tin particles (approximately 250Å radius) embedded randomly in an insulating matrix of
KCl, with volume fraction of tin ranging from 0.001 to 0.03. These
experiments measure the optical properties from 3 cm^{-1} to 50 cm^{-1}
and at temperatures from 1.7K to 27K, thus covering the energy gap
frequency and the transition temperature of the tin. The results
of these experiments show an enhanced absorption around the gap
frequency at superconducting temperatures.

INTRODUCTION

In this paper we present the results of far infrared absorption measurements on superconducting-insulator composites. Previous
work by Tanner et al[1] indicated no change in the absorption
spectrum, $\alpha(\omega)$, for very small (radius 70Å) Sn particles imbedded
in KCl at temperatures below T_c(bulk). Patton[2] has considered the
effect of particle size on superconductivity and finds that for
small particles of diameter less than the coherence length (ξ),
fluctuations exist which smooth out the energy gap structure in a
fairly wide temperature region about T_c. This smoothing would
account for the lack of structure in $\alpha(\omega)$ for such small particles.
However, for particles whose diameter approaches the coherence
length ($\xi \sim 1000$Å) we would expect a reasonably well defined gap to
emerge with corresponding structure in $\alpha(\omega)$. We have therefore
chosen to study larger particles with mean radii on the the order
of 250Å.

EXPERIMENT

Because we wish to observe the composite at temperatures well
below T_c, we have chosen Sn with T_c(bulk)=3.7K since temperatures
of ~1.7K can easily be reached with pumped helium. Also, the gap
frequency (2Δ) is 9.7 cm^{-1}, which falls within the range of our
instrumentation.

The small Sn particles were made by smoke evaporation, as described by Granqvist and Buhrman[3]. Sn was evaporated from an
alumina coated molybdenum boat in an atmosphere of 75% argon and
25% oxygen. The gas pressure ranged from 0.1 to 1 Torr. The
oxygen formed an insulating layer of tin oxide on the outer surface
to help avoid cold welding between particles. The particles
collected on a glass surface surrounding the boat. By varying the
gas pressure, mean particle radii ranging from 250Å to 400Å were

produced. The particle size distribution was measured with a transmission electron micro- scope (see Fig. 1).

The Sn particles were thoroughly mixed with finely ground (1μm≤ d< 10μm) KCl powder and then pressed under vacuum (10 kbar) into a solid disk. The sample was reground and repressed 3 to 5 times to help achieve uniformity. X-ray mappings (using a scanning elec- tron microscope) of the surface of a typical metal-insulator composite showed a reasonably uniform distribution of metal with little evidence of clus- tering.

Transmission and reflec- tion measurements of these samples were made on a lamellar grating interferometer[4] with a mercury arc lamp as a source and a germanium bolometer operating at 1.2K as a detector. The composite under study was anchored to a copper block which housed a heater and several carbon resistors for thermo- metry. Measurements were made at 1.7K, 3.3K, 4.2K and 27K.

An expression for the absorption coefficient $\alpha(\omega)$,

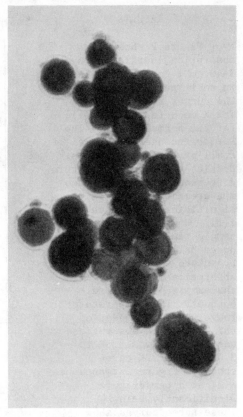

Fig. 1. Transmission electron micrograph of Sn particles. The mean particle radius is 250Å.

of a material can be easily derived in terms of the transmittance of the disc-shaped sample, $T(\omega)$. The expression, which allows for multiple internal reflections of the light, is:

$$\alpha(\omega) = - \frac{\ln T(\omega)}{x} - \frac{2\ln(1-R)}{x} \tag{1}$$

where x is the sample thickness and R is the reflectance. We have estimated the reflectance from $R = (n-1)^2/(n+1)^2$ with n = 2.2 being the refractive index of KCl. Note that in our low resolution measurements the interference pattern produced by the multiple internal reflections is averaged out and that the internally re- flected power is small enough to allow discarding all but its lowest order contributions to $\alpha(\omega)$.

RESULTS

Figure 2 shows the absorption coefficient over 3-40 cm^{-1} for 250Å radius Sn small particles in KCl. The curves for T=4.2K and T=27K each represent $\alpha(\omega)$ for the normal state. The ~ω^2 dependence is typical of small-particle composites.[5] Despite the wide temperature difference between the two measurements, there is no significant difference in $\alpha(\omega)$. However, when the sample temperature was reduced below 4.2K, the broadband far infrared absorption increased (i.e. the sample became more opaque). The temperature range where the onset of this increased absorption was observed was 3.5K to 3.0K. The 1.7K curve shown in Figure 2 represents $\alpha(\omega)$ at a temperature significantly below T_c. These three curves show clearly that $\alpha(\omega)$ is unaffected by the superconducting transition for $\hbar\omega >> 2\Delta$. However, for $\hbar\omega \sim 2\Delta$, there is a significant absorption associated with the transition to the superconducting state. This point is illustrated more clearly in Figure 3, where we have plotted the difference between the superconducting and normal state absorption coefficients.

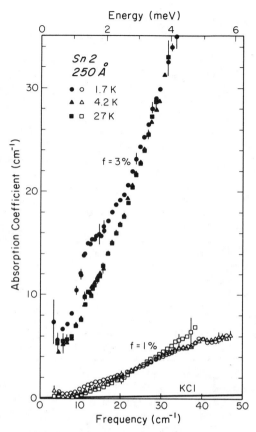

Figure 2. Far infrared absorption in Sn-KCl composite systems. Data are shown for two concentrations and three temperatures.

DISCUSSION

The effect described in the preceeding section - an enhanced absorption in the superconducting state - is not predicted by the commonly used theories for inhomogeneous media. The two models[6-9] commonly applied to the problem of infrared absorption in composites are the Maxwell-Garnett theory (MGT) and the effective medium (or self-consistent) theory (EMT). For metal volume fraction, f, on the order of 1% and for particle radii small compared to the skin depth, the two theories do not yield significantly different results. The far infrared abosrption in these limits is[1]

$$\alpha(\omega) = \frac{f\omega^2}{c}\left(\frac{9}{4\pi\sigma_1} + \frac{2\pi a^2 \sigma_1}{5c^2}\right), \quad (2)$$

where $\sigma_1(\omega)$ is the real part of the complex conductivity of the metal and a is the particle radius. The first term in brackets arises from electric dipole absorption while the second arises from eddy currents induced in the particle. For metallic values of the conductivity (i.e. $\sigma_1 \sim 10^5 \Omega^{-1} cm^{-1}$) the second term dominates the far infrared absorption for particle radii greater than 25Å. This theory gives the correct shape of $\alpha(\omega)$ for the normal state absorption, even though it falls short in magnitude by more than a factor of ten.[1,5,10]

We have calculated the far infared absorption in superconducting composites using the BCS expressions for $\sigma_1(\omega)$ in the superconducting state[11] within

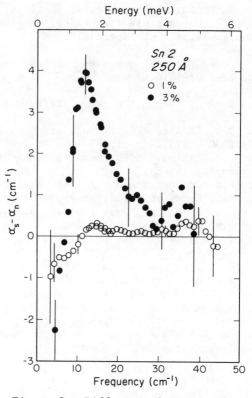

Figure 3. Difference between the absorption in the superconducting state and in the normal state in Sn-KCl composites. Data are shown for two concentrations.

both the MGT and EMT. The results of these simple theories give an absorption coefficient which is zero for $\hbar\omega < 2\Delta$, where 2Δ, is the full energy gap of the superconductor, and then rises, with an initially non-zero slope, approaching the normal state result for $\hbar\omega >> 2\Delta$. This result is the expected one, since the spheres, behaving much as in a bulk specimen, are not absorbing below 2Δ because no electronic excitations are possible. Such a simple theory is not capable of explaining the enhanced absorption which is experimentally observed.

CONCLUSIONS

These experiments have found an enhanced far infared absorption in composite superconductors at frequencies near the superconducting energy gap. A simple model for composites using BCS values for the frequency dependent conductivity does not explain the observed infrared absorption spectrum. Possible explanations may be based on size effects, electron hopping mechanisms from particle to particle (tunneling) or clustering of particles into a (non-spherical) macroparticle.

*Research supported by the U.S. Department of Energy, Contract No. ER-S-02-4914.

REFERENCES

1. D.B. Tanner, A.J. Sievers and R.A. Buhrman, Phys. Rev. B 11, 1330 (1975).
2. B.R. Patton, Ph.D. dissertation (Cornell University, 1973) (unpublished).
3. C.G. Granqvist and R.A. Buhrman, J. Appl. Phys. 47, 2200 (1976).
4. R.L. Henry and D.B. Tanner, Infrared Phys. 19, 163 (1979).
5. C.G. Granqvist, R.A. Buhrman, J. Wyns and A.J. Sievers, Phys. Rev. Lett. 37, 625 (1976).
6. J.C. Maxwell Garnett, Philos. Trans. Roy. Soc. London 203, 385 (1904); 205, 237 (1906).
7. D.A.G. Bruggeman, Ann. Phys. (leipz.) 24, 636 (1935).
8. D.B. Wood and N.W. Ashcroft, Phil. Mag. 35, 269 (1977).
9. D. Stroud and F.P. Pan, Phys. Rev. B 17, 1602 (1978).
10. N.E. Russell, G.L. Carr and D.B. Tanner in Electrical Transport and Optical Properties of Inhomogeneous Media, J.C. Garland and D.B. Tanner, eds. (AIP, New York, 1978), p. 263.
11. D.C. Mattis and J. Bardeen, Phys. Rev. 111, 412 (1958).

RADIO-FREQUENCY COMPLEX-IMPEDANCE MEASUREMENTS
ON THIN FILM TWO-DIMENSIONAL SUPERCONDUCTORS

A. T. Fiory and A. F. Hebard

Bell Laboratories, Murray Hill NJ 07974

Abstract

An experimental technique has been developed which enables us to measure directly the complex impedance of thin film two-dimensional superconductors at radio frequencies. The sample is placed between two coaxial coils and a signal proportional to the film sheet conductance is obtained by modulating the sample between the superconducting and normal states with an externally-applied transport current. We illustrate the technique with a presentation of field-dependent data taken on a 100-Å thick oxygen-doped aluminum film with a normal-state resistance at 4.2 K of 4130 $\Omega/\square$. The data, taken well below the temperature at which d.c. resistance disappears, is discussed in terms of a dynamic pinning model in which the dissipation arises from the flux-flow resistance of the moving vortices and the inductance from pinning and acceleration of the background superfluid.

Introduction

Recent suggestions[1-4] that the Kosterlitz-Thouless[5] theory of topological order and phase transitions in two dimensions is applicable to thin-film superconductors with high normal state sheet resistance have motivated us to develop a new experimental technique which is sensitive to the change in the relevant transport properties of the superconductor near this transition. Specifically, the theory predicts a phase transition in which vortex-antivortex pairs dissociate at a temperature T_{KT}, the Kosterlitz-Thouless transition temperature. For temperatures $T > T_{KT}$ the plasma of unbound thermally excited vortices contributes to the d.c. resistance and broadens the resistive transition in proportion to the normal-state sheet resistance R_N [1]. Because there are alternative and more mundane explanations for the resistance transition broadening[1,6] actually observed in thin-film superconductors, it is desirable to test the unusual frequency-dependent predictions of the theory[4,7,8] which should become uniquely manifest in the a.c. response of the superfluid. Accordingly, and with this end in mind, we shall discuss in this paper our experimental method for the measurement of the a.c. response of the superfluid. We also present preliminary data on the low-temperature complex field-dependent impedance of a granular aluminum film sample. The results are in good agreement with the predictions of a simple pinning model, in anticipation of an eventual understanding of the superfluid dynamics at all relevant temperatures and frequencies in these very interesting thin-film systems[9].

0094-243X/80/580293-06$1.50 Copyright 1980 American Institute of Physics

Experimental Procedure

Granular aluminum films, approximately 100Å thick, were prepared by eva-
porating aluminum onto fire-polished glass substrates at room temperature in the
presence of oxygen. These films were squares 3 mm on a side with normal-state
sheet resistances which could be varied between 10 and 5000 $\Omega/\square$ by adjusting the
oxygen pressure and/or rate of deposition during the evaporation. Small area contacts were positioned at each of the four corners so that the resistive transition
could be measured using the van der Pauw technique [10]. These same contacts
were used to pass sufficient transport current through the sample to drive it into
the normal state, a procedure used for the r.f. measurements.

The thin-film sample was mounted in a transverse plane between two
closely-spaced coaxial coils as shown schematically in Fig. 1. The drive coil,
approximately 1 mm in diameter, was wound with 9 turns of #50 copper wire and
positioned on the reverse side of the 1 mm-thick substrate directly at the center of
the square. The 100-turn receive coil, also approximately 1 mm in diameter, was
mounted directly on the sample which was protected by a varnish overcoat.

We now turn our attention to the response of a thin-film superconductor in
an external magnetic field. Following Pearl[11] we can write the two-dimensional
Fourier transform of the vector potential $A(r)$ in the form

$$A(q_t, z=0) = \frac{1}{2\pi} \int A(q) \, dq_z \quad , \tag{1}$$

where the three-dimensional Fourier transform satisfies:

$$A(q) = \int A(r) e^{-q \cdot r} dr = \frac{4\pi}{cq^2} [J_e(q) + dJ_s(q_t)] \quad . \tag{2}$$

The current $J_e(q)$ is the applied external drive coil current, $dJ_s(q_t)$ is the sheet
current in the film of thickness d and q_t is a two-dimensional transverse wave vector. The plane of the film is determined by $z=0$. With these relations it is a
straightforward matter to show that

$$A(q_t, z=0) - A_e(q_t, z=0) = \frac{2\pi d}{cq_t} J_s(q_t) \quad , \tag{3}$$

where $A_e(q) = 4\pi J_e(q)/cq^2$ is the vector potential source term. If we now assume
that screening currents which satisfy the fluxoid equation [12] are negligible and
$J_s(q_t) = \sigma E = -i\omega\sigma A(q_t)/c$, where σ is a complex conductivity, it is easy to
demonstrate that

$$A(q_t, z) - A_e(q_t, z) = \frac{i\omega A_e(q_t, z=0) e^{-q_z z}}{q_t c^2/2\pi\sigma d - i\omega} \quad . \tag{4}$$

By integrating Eq. (4) around the turns of the receive coil, we can compute the
magnetic flux threading the receive coil which is due *solely* to the currents flowing
in the sample. In the limit that these induced currents are weak, corresponding to
$\omega \ll q_t c^2/2\pi\sigma d$, we see from Eq. (4) that this flux is proportional to $G = \sigma d$, the

sheet conductance of the film. For thin superconducting films with high R_N this condition is always satisfied for our geometry. As discussed below, the film is a perfect inductor at low temperatures (in zero magnetic field) so that

$$G = 1/i\omega L_K = c^2/2\pi i\omega\Lambda \ , \tag{5}$$

where Λ is the magnetic screening length in thin films and is proportional to R_N [1]. Thus the vector potential difference of Eq. (4) is proportional to G when $q_t\Lambda \gg 1$.

Transforming back to real space and taking an additional time derivative to convert flux to voltage, we are able to write the receive-coil voltage $\Delta V_{receive}$ as

$$\Delta V_{receive} = K\omega^2 GI_{drive} \ , \tag{6}$$

where I_{drive} is the amplitude of the r.f. drive current and K is a computed constant depending on the configuration of the coils, number of turns, sample dimensions, *etc.* As G is a complex quantity, it is important to keep track of the relative phase shift of $\Delta V_{receive}$ with respect to I_{drive} .

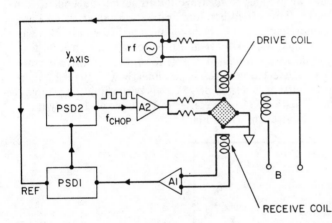

Fig. 1. Circuit diagram for r.f. impedance measurements on thin films.

Our method of detecting the amplitude and phase of $\Delta V_{receive}$ is depicted schematically in the circuit diagram of Fig. 1. The r.f. signal from the receive coil is preamplified by the amplifier A1 and fed to the input of a phase-sensitive detector PSD1. The correct phase settings were obtained by adjusting the phase shift in PSD1 to null the mutual coupling signal between the two coils with the sample in the normal state. This is the zero-degree phase setting and is used for measuring the in-phase or real part of G (Re$[G]$). The 90° setting of PSD1 gave a maximum in the mutual coupling signal and was used during measurements of the quadrature or imaginary part of G (Im$[G]$). With the sample in the superconducting state at a temperature well below the transition temperature this component is decreased by typically a few percent due to Meissner screening currents.

The 90° voltage reading at the output of PSD1 with the sample in the normal state can be written as

$$V_{out}^N (90°) = -A\omega M I_{drive} \ , \tag{7}$$

where A is the combined gain of the A1 and PSD1 and M is the mutual inductance between the drive and receive coils. The calculated value $M = 0.029\,\mu H$ was in good agreement with the measured value of $0.024\,\mu H$. As both $\Delta V_{receive}$ and V_{out}^N involve the gain factor A, we find it convenient to use Eq. (7) to eliminate A in solving for the calibration factors which determine the magnitude of G.

In order to discriminate against sample independent pick-up, we used a second phase-sensitive detector PSD2 to detect the modulation in the r.f. signal obtained by cycling the sample in and out of the superconducting state with an applied transport current at a frequency f_{chop} of the order of 3-10 Hz. As the normal state conductance is negligible compared to that of the superconductor, the output of PSD2 is still proportional to G as in Eq. (6).

Results and Discussion

Using these techniques we are able to measure the frequency-dependent complex sheet conductance as functions of temperature and external field B. In Fig. 2 we show the real and imaginary parts of the sheet conductance taken at 10 kHz as a function of field. For this sample $R_N = 4130\,\Omega$ and the mean-field transition temperature is 1.85 K [9]. These data were obtained at 1.21 K with an r.f. drive current amplitude of $50\,\mu A$ rms. The detected voltages scaled linearly with the r.f. amplitude at these levels. At this current level the drive coil is perturbing the sample with a magnetic field which is 0.45 mG at the center of the film, well below the charactertistic linewidths of the data shown in Fig. 2.

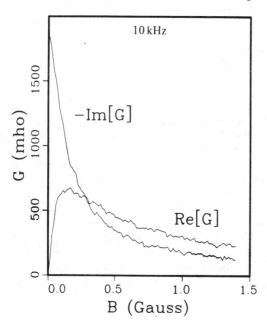

Fig. 2. Real and imaginary parts of the complex film sheet conductance as functions of the transverse magnetic field.

An important feature of the data in Fig. 2 is that at $B = 0$ there is no dissipation, $\text{Re}[G] = 0$, and the response of the film is purely inductive. As B is increased and vortices are introduced into the sample the most rapid change in both components occurs in the field region $B < 0.5\,\text{G}$. Greater physical insight into this field-dependent behavior is obtained by taking the inverse of G to derive the complex impedance, which can be written as the sum of two terms:

$$G^{-1} = R + i\omega L \;,$$

(8)

where R and L are the sheet resistance and inductance, respectively. These two impedance components, which have been plotted in Fig. 3, reveal a remarkably linear dependence on B which we shall now show might be expected from a straightforward consideration of vortex dissipation in a simple pinning model[13].

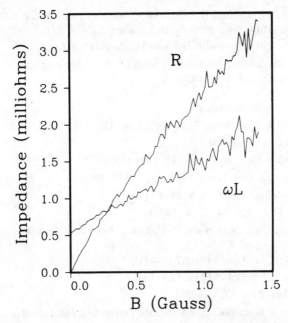

Fig. 3. Real and imaginary parts of the complex film sheet impedance as functions of the transverse magnetic field.

We start by writing the equation of motion for the displacement x of a single vortex in the form

$$\eta\dot{x} + kx = J\phi_o d/c \;,$$

(9)

where η is the viscosity coefficient, k the restoring force constant, J the applied current density and ϕ_o the flux quantum. The justification for using such an equation of motion for a single vortex is that in high R_N thin-film superconductors the vortices are most likely to be in a fluid state, in which correlations in the vortex motion can be ignored[14]. The only other investigated situations in which such a single vortex description is applicable is the case of a vortex lattice in a commensurate spatially periodic pinning potential[15,16].

Combining Eq. (9) with the relation $E = -\dot{x}B/c$ derived from Maxwell's equations one can show that the vortex pinning impedance is

$$Z_v = \frac{E}{Jd} = \frac{\phi_0 B}{c^2 \eta} \left[\frac{i\omega\tau}{1 + i\omega\tau} \right] , \tag{10}$$

where $\tau = \eta/k$ is a relaxation time [17]. Adding the kinetic inductance of the background superfluid, we arrive at

$$R + i\omega L = Z_v + i\omega L_K . \tag{11}$$

Equation (10) predicts that both R and L increase linearly with B in accordance with the behavior shown in Fig. 3. The zero-field intercept is the kinetic inductance L_K, given in Eq. (5).

In terms of circuit elements we see that the total impedance can be written as a parallel combination — see Eq. (10) — of a pinning inductance $L_P = \phi_0 B/kc^2$ and flux-flow resistance $R_f = \phi_0 B/\eta c^2$ in series with the kinetic inductance L_K.

The authors acknowledge stimulating discussions with D. S. Fisher and the technical assitance of R. P. Minnich and A. L. Bullock.

References

1. M. R. Beasley, J. E. Mooij and T. P. Orlando, Phys. Rev. Lett. **42**, 1165 (1979).

2. L. A. Turkevich, J. Phys. C **12**, L385 (1979).

3. S. Doniach and B. A. Huberman, Phys. Rev. Lett. **42**, 1169 (1979).

4. B. I. Halperin and D. R. Nelson, J. Low Temp. Phys. **35**, 599 (1979).

5. J. M. Kosterlitz and D. J. Thouless, J. Phys. C **6**, 1181 (1973).

6. P. M. Horn and R. D. Parks, Phys. Rev. **4**, 2178 (1971).

7. V. Ambegaokar, B. I. Halperin, D. R. Nelson and E. D. Siggia, Phys. Rev. Lett. **40**, 783 (1978).

8. V. Ambegaokar and S. Teitel, Phys. Rev. **19**, 1667 (1979).

9. A. F. Hebard and A. T. Fiory, submitted to Phys. Rev. Lett.

10. L. J. van der Pauw, Phillips Res. Rpts. **13**, 1 (1958).

11. J. Pearl, Thesis: *Vortex Theory of Superconductive Memories,* Polytechnic Institute of Brooklyn, New York (1965), unpublished.

12. P. G. De Gennes, *Superconductivity of Metals and Alloys,* (Benjamin, New York, 1966), page 60.

13. G. Possin and K. W. Shepard, Phys. Rev. **171**, 458 (1968).

14. B. A. Huberman and S. Doniach, Phys. Rev. Lett. **42**, 950 (1979); D. S. Fisher, private communication.

15. O. Daldini, P. Martinoli, J. L. Olsen, and G. Berner, Phys. Rev. Lett. **32**, 218 (1974).

16. A. T. Fiory and A. F. Hebard, J. de Phys. C **6**, 633 (1978).

17. We find that $\omega\tau \approx 1$ over the frequency range 1kHz to 2MHz for this $4130-\Omega/\square$ film.

CRITICAL CURRENT ANISOTROPY IN IN SITU FORMED MULTIFILAMENTARY Cu-Nb$_3$Sn TAPES

F. Habbal and J. Bevk
Division of Applied Sciences
Harvard University, Cambridge, MA   02138

ABSTRACT

Angular dependence studies of the superconducting properties (J_C and H_{C2}) of in situ formed multifilamentary Cu-Nb$_3$Sn tapes reveal a pronounced anisotropy in their critical current density. The observed behavior is linked to the presence of a large number of parallel, closely spaced matrix-filament interfaces. Studies of flux flow and H_{C2} angular dependence in these tapes show resemblance with superconducting behavior of multilayered and thin film superconductors.

INTRODUCTION

In situ formed multifilamentary superconducting composites are of considerable interest, both as practical conductors and as model systems, representing a broad class of microscopically inhomogeneous materials. A number of recent investigations have demonstrated their excellent mechanical and transport properties, often surpassing those of the best conventional composites.[1] The coupling mechanisms, which lead to a vanishingly small resistance in these composites with discontinuous filaments, are not yet fully understood and they continue to stimulate new theoretical and experimental studies.[2] There is sufficient evidence, however, that in composites with sufficiently large area-reduction-ratio (R $\gtrsim$ 1000), J_C is not limited by the coupling mechanism(s) but rather by the flux-pinning characteristics of the filamentary material itself. Thus, it should be of particular interest to study the critical properties of in situ formed multifilamentary tapes where the ribbon-like filaments are all aligned in the rolling plane. The resulting microstructure, characterized by a large number of closely spaced, parallel interfaces, would suggest strongly anisotropic behavior in an applied magnetic field.

In this paper, we present preliminary results of the angular dependence study of J_C(H) and H_{C2} in Cu-Nb$_3$Sn in situ tapes and point out various similarities between these tapes and layered superconductors.

EXPERIMENTAL

The samples used in the present study were prepared by induction melting high-purity copper and niobium in a water-cooled crucible.[3] The cast ingot, about 10 mm in diameter, with nominal composition Cu-18 vol.% Nb was then swaged and cold-drawn to a wire, 0.25 mm in diameter, and finally rolled to tape with aspect ratio 8:1. Shorter pieces of tape were then plated with tin and annealed at 560° C for 132 hours.

Critical currents (1 μV/cm criterion) were measured by a standard four-probe technique in a Bitter-type magnet, capable of producing fields up to 20 T. The samples were mounted in a cryostat equipped with a variable-angle sample holder; their orientation with respect to the applied magnetic field could be varied during the measurement with precision of ± 1°. The applied field was perpendicular to the axis of the tape and the measuring current; Figure 1 shows schematically the experimental configuration.

a) H // to the surface of the filaments; $\theta = 0°$

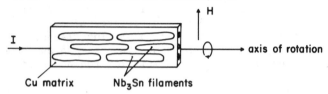

b) H ⊥ to the surface of the filaments ; $\theta = 90°$

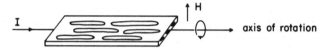

Fig. 1. Schematics of the experimental configuration. H is perpendicular to the tape (or filaments) axis while the surface of the tape (or filaments) can make different angle θ with the field. The situations θ= 0° and 90° are shown here.

The upper critical field, H_{c2}, was determined from a resistive transition (J = 3.4 A cm^{-2}) induced by sweeping the field in a Bitter-type solenoid rated at 23.6 T. H_{c2} is taken as the value of the field at which V(H) becomes independent of H.

RESULTS AND DISCUSSIONS

The filamentary structure of Cu–Nb$_3$Sn tapes can be seen clearly in Figure 2, which shows one of the samples with the matrix etched away. The filaments are reasonably well aligned in the rolling plane of the tape (Fig. 2b); their distribution along the direction normal to this plane is, however, random. The aspect ratio of many filaments is greater than that of the tape itself and reflects the fact that the filaments deform in the plane strain during composite formation.[3]

The angular dependence of the critical current was obtained, at each fixed field, from a series of V-I curves. Figure 3 shows an example of the experimental data taken at 16 T. As θ increases from 0° to 90°, the critical depinning current decreases and the flux-flow characteristics gradually change. The strongest pinning occurs when the fluxoids are parallel to the filament surfaces; furthermore, the decrease of J_c is most pronounced within 30° of this orientation. This is shown in Figure 4 where the experimental values of

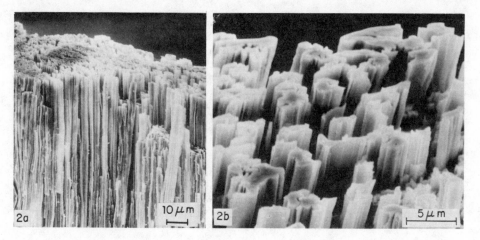

Fig. 2. Scanning electron micrographs of X-6. Notice the dense and uniform distribution of filaments.

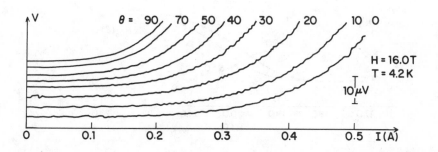

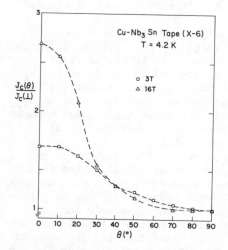

↑ Fig. 3. Typical V-I curves obtained at a constant field but at different angles.

← Fig. 4. Normalized critical current density versus θ for two values of applied field, H = 3 and 16 T.

$J_c(\theta)/J_c(\perp)$ are plotted versus θ for two different fields, H = 3 and 16 T.

From Figure 4, it can be also seen that the anisotropy in J_c, $\Delta(H) \equiv [J_c(||)/J_c(\perp)]_H$, depends strongly on the magnitude of the applied field. The maximum Δ values were measured close to H_{c2}, and as H decreases Δ gradually decreases to one at zero applied field. In the present samples, Δ reached values of about 4 at H = 0.9 H_{c2}. In tapes with high aspect ratio (R = 27) and smaller filament spacing (0.1 µm), the critical currents at H = 0.9 H_{c2} differed by almost an order of magnitude.[4]

The variation of H_{c2} with θ was found to be rather small, but measurable. From the traces of V(H) curves, shown in Figure 5, the ratio $H_{c2}(||)/H_{c2}(\perp)$ turns out to be about 1.01. The relative insensitivity of H_{c2} with respect to the sample orientation should not be surprising; in the dirty limit, the electron mean free path

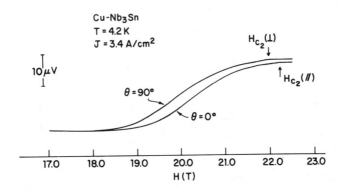

Fig. 5. V(H) curves obtained for two different tape orientations, θ = 0° and 90°.

becomes comparable to the coherence length which, in turn, is much smaller than the average grain size. However, in the smallest filaments, the size of Nb_3Sn grains is limited in one direction by the filament thickness, leading to a possible small anisotropy in the effective coherence length. Thus, it appears that variation of H_{c2} with orientation is like that expected for three-dimensional though highly anisotropic superconductor rather than manifestation of a two-dimensional character of these materials.

Grain boundaries are the prime source of flux pinning in bulk Nb_3Sn and the observed small grain size (about 400 Å) in the filaments is responsible for the high J_c values in these tapes. On the other hand, the large increase in J_c with decreasing θ can be interpreted as due to an additional pinning mechanism, namely surface pinning.[5] Although the vortex dynamics in in situ materials has not been studied in sufficient detail, it is clear that the presence of many parallel internal surfaces can effectively inhibit flux flow in the direction normal to the filament surface. As θ increases, the pinning strength of these internal surfaces decreases and reduces, in our tapes, to less than 1% of its maximum value for $\theta \gtrsim 50°$.

The effect of internal surfaces on J_c has been also observed in multilayered thin films where J_c was found to increase with the number-density of interfaces.[6] Qualitatively similar behavior has been observed in in situ tapes with different filament spacings.[7] Furthermore, in aligned laminar composites the highest values of J_c were obtained for flux flow perpendicular to the laminae, due to strong surface pinning.[8]

In summary, we conclude that in in situ formed Cu-Nb$_3$Sn tapes with sufficiently small filaments, surface pinning can significantly enhance their critical current density. The effect is most pronounced in the high-field regime for flux flow perpendicular to the filament surfaces. In addition, the absolute values of J_c increase with decreasing filament spacing.

ACKNOWLEDGEMENT

The authors gratefully acknowledge the Francis Bitter National Magnet Laboratory where the high-field measurements were performed and the National Science Foundation for support of this research through grants DMR-76-01111 and DMR-74-22263.

REFERENCES

1. J. Bevk, paper published in this Proceeding and references cited therein.
2. M. Tinkham, paper published in this Proceeding and references cited therein.
3. J. Bevk, J.P. Harbison and J.L. Bell, J. Appl. Phys. $\underline{49}$, 6031 (1978).
4. F. Habbal, J. Bevk and G. Dublon, to be published.
5. A.M. Campbell and J.E. Evetts, Adv. in Phys. $\underline{21}$, 199 (1972).
6. R.E. Howard, M.R. Beasley, T.H. Geballe, C.N. King, R.H. Hammond R.H. Norton, J.R. Salem and R.B. Zubeck, IEEE Trans. MAG $\underline{13}$, 138 (1977).
7. J. Bevk, J.P. Harbison, F. Habbal, G.R. Wagner and A.I. Braginski, to appear in the Appl. Phys. Lett. Jan. 1980 issue.
8. C.R. Spences, P. Martinoli, E.D. Gibson, J.D. Verhoeven and D.K. Finnemore, Phys. Rev. B $\underline{18}$, 1216 (1978).

EFFECTS OF PINNING ON THE DECAY OF SUPERFLOW IN THIN SUPERFLUID FILMS

D. A. Browne* and S. Doniach
Departments of Physics and Applied Physics, Stanford University,
Stanford, CA 94305

I. INTRODUCTION

The presence of thermally excited vortex-antivortex pairs in a thin 2-dimensional superfluid (10's of Angstroms for ^{4}He films, 100's of Angstroms for dirty superconducting films) provides a mechanism for the decay of persistent currents in a closed ring of the film. The existence of the Kosterlitz-Thouless[1] transition temperature, T_{2D}, above which there is a finite density of free vortices in a "vortex plasma" state leads to a qualitative change in the decay mechanism as the film temperature T increases through T_{2D}. For $T > T_{2D}$ the decay rate is finite as the superfluid velocity, v_s, tends to zero, leading to a finite resistivity in the case of a superconducting film.[2] For $T < T_{2D}$, Huberman et al.[3] and Ambegaokar et al.[4] showed that for an ideal film on a smooth substrate the decay rate varies as a power of the superfluid velocity as a result of the current-induced unbinding of bound vortex pairs:

$$\frac{dv_s}{dt} \propto v_s^{\beta(T)} . \tag{1}$$

So the decay of a persistent current goes from a linear regime for $T > T_{2D}$ to a nonlinear regime for $T < T_{2D}$.
The purpose of this paper is to provide a preliminary account of an investigation into the effects of vortex pinning in modifying the form of Eq. (1) for $T < T_{2D}$ at large values of v_s.

II. VORTEX PINNING

As is well known from the physics of bulk type II superconductors, pinning of vortices at imperfections in the substrate provides a qualitative change in the behavior of a superconductor at finite supercurrents. If, following Anderson,[5] it is assumed that an average pinning free energy barrier E_p varies linearly with v_s, then the rate of escape of pinned vortices from pinning sites may be estimated using a simple kinetic model as:

$$\frac{dn_p}{dt} = n_p^0 \nu_0 \exp [-(E_p^0 + E_p^1 v_s)/K_B T] \tag{2}$$

---

*NSF predoctoral fellow; Research partially supported by NSF through the Center for Materials Research at Stanford University.

The solution of this equation in an initial regime where the velocity dependence of the pinning energy dominates, leads to $v_s(t) \sim v_s(0) - a \ln(t)$. Here it is assumed that once a vortex is un-pinned it can cross the sample and hence reduce the superflow by a flux quantum, so that $dv_s/dt \propto dn_p/dt$.

This "creep" behavior of the decay of superflow is to be con-trasted with the power law time decay which comes from solving Eq. (1). For a thin film superfluid, it may be expected that the non-linear dependence of the rate of decay of persistent current on v_s will show both types of behavior: for large v_s the unpinning effects will dominate through the exponential dependence in Eq. (2), while for smaller v_s the power law behavior of Eq. (1) should take over.

III. KINETIC EQUATIONS

In order to formulate the kinetics of the superflow decay in the presence of both depinning and vortex pair unbinding, we set up a pair of kinetic equations for the numbers n_+ and n_- of unbound and unpinned vortices available to traverse the specimen and lead to re-moval of quanta of circulation from the system. (+ and - refer to the chirality of the vortices relative to the direction of v_s.) The kinetic equations may be written:

$$\frac{dn_\pm}{dt} = R_p + R_c - \Gamma_p n_\pm - \Gamma_c n_+ n_- \tag{3}$$

where R_p and R_c denote the rates of depinning and pair-unbinding, and Γ_p and Γ_c denote the rates of re-pinning and re-binding of the free vortices.

The rate of decay of the supercurrent may be calculated in terms of the rate at which the free vortices drift to the wall and are destroyed there as

$$\frac{dv_s}{dt} = - \frac{h}{mW} v_\perp^d (n_+ + n_-) \tag{4}$$

where W denotes the film width and $v_\perp^d$ the drift velocity perpendicu-lar to the flow. At a given v_s it is assumed that $n_\pm$ is in a steady state so that $dn_\pm/dt = 0$ leading to

$$n_\pm [v_s(t)] = (\sqrt{\Delta} - \Gamma_p)/2\Gamma c \tag{5}$$

where $\Delta = 4\Gamma c(R_p + R_c) + \Gamma_p^2$. In the absence of pinning, Eq. (5) corresponds to the kinetic equation of Huberman et al.[3] Eqs. (4) and (5) have been solved by numerical integration using the forms assumed in Eqs. (1) and (2): $R_p \propto e^{-E_1 v_s/K_B T}$, $R_c \propto v_s^{\beta(T)}$, with

306

$v_1^d \propto v_s$ and noting that Γ_c is independent of v_s and that $\Gamma_p \ll \Gamma_c$. The resulting solutions were fit to the data of Ekholm and Hallock on the decay of superflow in thin ^{4}He films by using a non-linear least squares routine to vary four undetermined parameters. A resulting fit is shown in Figure 1.

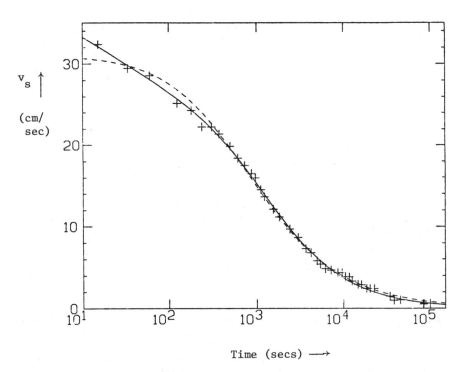

Time (secs) $\longrightarrow$

Figure 1. Fit of the model to data of Ekholm and Hallock[6] for superflow in a ^{4}He film of $\sim$ eight atomic layers thickness measured at 1.51°K. The dashed line indicates best fit using a power law only.

The initial decay is linear in log t and crosses over to a power law (i.e., exponential in log t) as v_s becomes smaller, The exponent $\beta(T)$ found is consistent with the values predicted by Huberman et al.[3] based on the Kosterlitz-Thouless theory of vortex pair binding. So far, only data at one temperature has been studied so that comparison of the temperature dependence of the fitted parameters with the above theoretical picture remains to be done.

We note a qualitative difference between the present picture and an alternative interpretation put forward by Donnelly and Roberts.[7] These authors suggest that the low v_s behavior will be dominated by a rebinding mechanism in which vortices cross barriers against the flow direction, leading to a decay rate $dv_s/dt \propto v_s$ for small v_s. This results in an exponential as opposed to power law behavior at intermediate to large times. However, it appears that the present model provides a better fit to Ekholm and Hallock's data in this time regime.

Acknowledgments: We are grateful to R.B. Hallock and R. Donnelly for a number of very stimulating discussions.

REFERENCES

1. M. Kosterlitz and D. Thouless, J. Phys. C. 6, 1181 (1973).
2. See review by B. Huberman and S. Doniach, this volume.
3. B. Huberman, R. Meyerson, and S. Doniach, Phys. Rev. Lett. 40, 780 (1978).
4. V. Ambegaokar, B.I. Halperin, D.R. Nelson and E.D. Siggia, Phys. Rev. Letts. 40, 783 (1978).
5. P.W. Anderson, Phys. Rev. Lett. 9, 309 (1962).
6. Ekholm and Hallock, Phys. Rev. Lett. 37, 1484 (1976), and Proceedings of L.T. - 15 (to be published).
7. R. Donnelly and P.H. Roberts, Proc. Royal Soc. (London), 271, 41 (1971).

PERCOLATION CRITICAL EXPONENTS FOR CONDUCTANCE
AND CRITICAL CURRENT IN TWO DIMENSIONS

C. J. Lobb and D. J. Frank
Division of Applied Sciences and Department of Physics
Harvard University
Cambridge, MA 02138

ABSTRACT

Using finite size scaling arguments on lattices containing up to 761 bonds, we estimate the critical exponents t and v for the normal-state conductance and the superconducting critical current density in a percolating two-dimensional square lattice. Our results suggest that $t = v = \nu$ in two dimensions, where ν is the mean cluster size exponent.

INTRODUCTION

The critical exponents for percolating systems are of considerable interest because, unlike the percolation threshold or mean field limit behavior, they should be the same for real continuum systems[1-5] as for theoretical lattice models[6-8]. We report the results of finite size scaling-renormalization group calculations for the conductance critical exponent t which we believe are superior to earlier results[9] because they consider a sequence of transformations of increasing cell size to minimize finite cell size errors[10,11]. In addition, we report the first finite size scaling calculation of the critical current exponent, which has recently been measured in two-dimensional Pb-Ge films[5] and estimated by another method.[12]

FINITE SIZE SCALING

Consider a square lattice of size L, with lattice spacing ℓ. Links are present with probability p, and absent with probability 1-p. For calculating conductance properties, these links are taken to have unit resistance. To calculate critical current properties, the links are assigned a unit critical current. As p increases from zero in an infinite lattice, the mean cluster size ξ increases, finally diverging as

$$\xi \sim \ell |p-p_c|^{-\nu} \qquad (1)$$

where $p_c = \frac{1}{2}$ for the square lattice, and $\nu \approx 1.35$ in two dimensions[10]. A finite lattice of size $b = L/\ell$ has a probability $p'(p,b)$ of being connected. We define $p^*(b)$ to be the probability at which $p' = p$, and $\epsilon \equiv p-p^*$.

The average conductance, $<G>$, of a finite lattice is

$$<G> = f(\epsilon, 1/b) \qquad (2)$$

where average means any power-like mean, such as the nth root of
the mean n[th] power. We assume that f is an homogeneous function of
its variables[13]

$$f(\varepsilon, 1/b) = \gamma f(\gamma^{-1/t}\varepsilon, \gamma^{-\nu/t}/b). \tag{3}$$

Letting $\gamma^{-1/t}\varepsilon = 1$, and taking $b \to \infty$, we get

$$<G> = \varepsilon^t f(1,0)[1 + \mathcal{O}(\xi/L)] \tag{4}$$

Thus we see that the conductance varies as ε^t for an infinite sample
when ε is small. Similarly, for $\gamma^{-\nu/t}/b = 1$, and $\varepsilon \to 0$,

$$<G> = b^{-t/\nu} f(0,1)[1 + \mathcal{O}(b^{1/\nu}\varepsilon)] \tag{5}$$

so that the average conductance at $\varepsilon = 0$ varies as $b^{-t/\nu}$ for
large b.

To summarize,

$$G \sim (p-p_c)^t \qquad \text{(infinite sample)} \tag{6a}$$

$$<G> \sim b^{-t/\nu} \qquad \text{(when } p = p*) \tag{6b}$$

Similarly, the critical current density J_c varies as

$$J_c \sim (p-p_c)^v \qquad \text{(infinite sample)} \tag{7a}$$

$$<J_c> \sim b^{-v/\nu} \qquad \text{(when } p = p*) \tag{7b}$$

We can thus calculate infinite sample exponents t and v by
looking at the average behavior of large finite samples.

METHOD OF SOLUTION

We work with nearly square lattices which have one fewer row
than columns, with equipotentials attached to the left and right
(see Fig. 1)[9,10,11]. For cells of this type, $p* = \frac{1}{2}$ independently
of b.[9] To calculate the conductance of a given cell, the program
removes dangling ends, reduces simple series and parallel combinations, and uses the Y-Δ transformation until the cell is reduced to
a single conductance. In the largest cells considered, where b = 14,
the program failed to reduce only 0.5% of the 30,000 cases studied.
This introduces a small known uncertainty into the estimate of <G>.[11]

To calculate the critical current of a cell, we proceed in the
same way, employing a rather simplified model. We assume that the
critical current of a parallel arrangement is the sum of the individual critical currents, that the weakest link gives the critical current of a series arrangement, and hence Y-Δ transformations can be
made as shown in Fig. 2. Using this model, we have studied up to
b = 20, where only 28 out of 40,000 cases failed to reduce. In all
cases, we calculated arithmetic, geometric and harmonic means of

conductance and critical current density, as well as standard deviations, which give the distribution widths. For b = 2, 3, we calculated the means exactly, by going through all of the possible combinations.

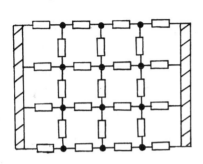

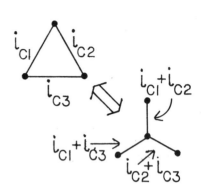

Fig. 1. Cell used for
b = 4 calculations.

Fig. 2. A Y-Δ transformation for critical currents.

RESULTS

Figs. 3 and 4 are log-log plots of 1/<G> vs. b and 1/<J$_c$> vs. b, for various means. As Eqs. (6b) and (7b) predict, the points on each graph fall onto parallel straight lines. The slopes of these lines imply that

$$t/\nu = 0.996 \pm 0.01 \qquad (8a)$$

$$v/\nu = 0.990 \pm 0.005 \quad . \qquad (8b)$$

The error bars include statistical uncertainties, and subjective estimates of error due to the differences between various means and the effects of including or not including data for small b in the fit. We believe that these results are consistent with the hypothesis t = v = ν,[14] as larger cells of this type tend to give higher estimates for t/ν[9,11] and v/ν. Within the errors present in calculating standard deviations, σ also varies roughly as b^{-1}, as expected.[10] Using the value ν = 1.356 ± 0.015,[10] we obtain t = 1.35 ± 0.02 and v = 1.343 ± 0.016.

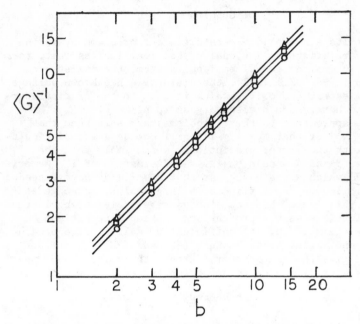

Fig. 3. Inverse mean conductance vs. cell size, for harmonic, geometric and arithmetic means (top to bottom).

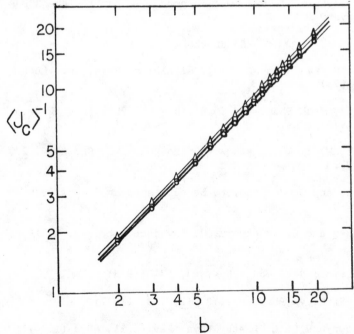

Fig. 4. Inverse mean critical current density vs. cell size, for harmonic, geometric and arithmetic means (top to bottom).

312

DISCUSSION

These results are applicable to different problems by making use of duality relations[7]. The dual of Eq. (6a) implies that, for a superconducting-normal two dimensional system, the resistance varies as $(p-p_c)^{1.35}$. Similarly, the dielectric breakdown voltage of a metal dielectric composite, which is dual to the critical current calculated here, should also vary as $(p-p_c)^{1.35}$.

Alternate approaches to these problems have suggested that either $t = v = v^{14}$ or that $t = v = 1^{12,15}$. Our data are difficult to reconcile with the latter predictions, which imply that the slopes in Figs. 3 and 4 should be $1/v \simeq 0.74$ instead of 1. Numerical simulations which seem to suggest that $t \simeq 1.1^{7,16}$ have depended on varying p while keeping L fixed at a large value, as suggested by Eq. (6a). This method has the disadvantage of requiring increasingly larger lattices as p approaches p_c to keep fluctuations and the first order term in Eq. (4) sufficiently small. Our approach fixes p at p* and varies L, as in Eqs. (6b) and (7b). Since both methods should give the same answer, further theoretical and experimental work is clearly needed to see which answer is correct.

ACKNOWLEDGEMENTS

We gratefully acknowledge useful discussions with Keith R. Karasek, David R. Nelson, W. J. Skocpol and M. Tinkham in the course of this work. This work was supported in part by the NSF through the Harvard MRL.

REFERENCES

1. B. Abeles, H. L. Pinch and J. I. Gittleman, Phys. Rev. Lett. 35, 247 (1975).

2. N. T. Liang, Yeuh Shan, and Shou-yih Wang, Phys. Rev. Lett. 37, 526 (1975).

3. C. J. Lobb, M. Tinkham, and W. J. Skocpol, Sol. St. Comm. 27, 1273 (1978).

4. L. N. Smith and C. J. Lobb, to be published in 1 Nov. 1979 Phys. Rev. B.

5. G. Deutscher and L. Rappaport, J. Physique Lett. 40, L-219 (1979).

6. S. Kirkpatrick, Rev. Mod. Phys. 45, 574 (1973).

7. Joseph P. Straley, Phys. Rev. B. 12, 5733 (1977).

8. B. P. Watson and P. L. Leath, Phys. Rev. B 11, 4893 (1974).

9. J. Bernasconi, Phys. Rev. B 18, 2185 (1978), and references cited therein.

10. Peter J. Reynolds, H. Eugene Stanley and W. Klein, J. Phys. A 11, L199 (1978).

11. C. J. Lobb and D. J. Frank, to be published in J. Phys. C.

12. D. A. Huse and R. A. Guyer, Phys. Rev. Lett. 43, 1163 (1979).

13. Joseph P. Straley, J. Phys. C 10, 1903 (1977).

14. M. E. Levinshtein, M. S. Shur and A. L. Efros, Sov. Phys. JETP 42, 1120 (1975).

15. P. G. DeGennes, J. Physique Lett. 37, L-1 (1976).

16. S. Kirkpatrick, Les Houches Lectures (1978), in "Ill-Condensed Matter", R. Balian, R. Maynard, & G. Toulouse, eds., (North-Holland, 1979).

Vortex Noise at the Superconducting Transition
in Granular Aluminum Films

R. F. Voss, C. M. Knoedler, and P. M. Horn
IBM Thomas J. Watson Research Center
Yorktown Heights, NY 10598

ABSTRACT

We present the results of a systematic study of resistance noise near the superconducting transition in granular Al films with sheet resistances $R_\square$ in the range 500 $\Omega/\square$ < $R_\square$ < 9000 $\Omega/\square$. In all samples we find a sharp peak in the noise magnitude vs temperature at temperatures slightly above the onset of dc resistance. The width of the noise peak is proportional to the width of the resistive transition which in turn scales with $R_\square$ in qualitative agreement with the predictions of Beasley et. al.[1] The noise is interpreted with a shot noise model as arising from random voltage pulses generated by the motion of free vortices.

INTRODUCTION

Strictly speaking, at finite temperatures a two dimensional superconductor is unstable with respect to the formation of free vortices. In the absence of an applied magnetic field, the vortices exist as elementary excitations of the superconductor with equal numbers having positive and negative vorticity. Free vortices can move in response to a current and contribute a finite resistivity to the superconductor.

However, it has recently been observed that thin film superconductors can have a magnetic screening length $\lambda_\perp = \lambda^2/d$ (λ is the London penetration depth and d is the film thickness) that is comparable to the size of the sample[1-3]. In this limit, vortices of opposite sign interact via an attractive logarithmic potential at macroscopic distances[4]. At temperatures below T_c vortices of opposite sign become bound in pairs[5]. The onset of resistance at T_c can then be associated with the unbinding of these pairs.

One of the essential features of the above model is the existence of free vortices above T_c but below the BCS temperature[1-3]. We have attempted to verify the vortex unbinding model by measuring the noise associated with free vortex motion in granular aluminum films.

EXPERIMENT

The films used in the experiment were flash evaporated onto glass substrates in an oxygen atmosphere using the procedures described by Abeles et. al.[6]. This technique produced films less than 100 Å thick with small grain sizes (less than 100 Å) and high sheet resistances, $R_\square$. The films were then scribed to allow four terminal measurements on sample areas of 1-2 mm by 0.3-0.8 mm.

0094-243X/80/580314-05$1.50 Copyright 1980 American Institute of Physics

The samples were immersed directly in liquid helium inside a double mu metal shielded dewar. The ambient magnetic field inside the dewar was less than 1.7×10^{-4} Oe. Individually shielded twisted pair leads coupled the sample to a special low noise FET preamplifier and to external current and voltage connections. The output of the preamplifier was coupled to a bandpass filter and ac voltmeter to allow estimation of the voltage noise spectral density in the frequency 10-100 kHz. A small dc current $(0.5-25\mu A)$ was applied to the sample and the dc voltage and RMS noise voltage were recorded by an IBM Series/1 computer as the temperature was lowered by pumping on the liquid He.

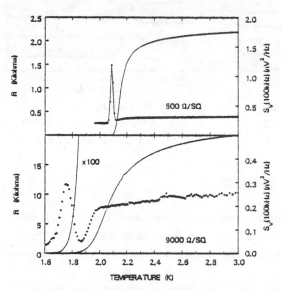

Figure 1. R and S_V(100kHz) vs temperature for a 500 $\Omega/\square$ sample and a 9000 $\Omega/\square$ sample.

Typical results are shown in Figure 1. The spectral density of the voltage noise at 100kHz, S_V(100kHz), and sample resistance are plotted vs temperature for a 510$\Omega/\square$ and a 9000$\Omega/\square$ sample. As the temperature is lowered the decreasing resistance initially leads to a decrease in the Johnson noise $(S_V(f)=4k_BTR)$. Just above T_c there is a sharp peak in S_V. This peak is a universal feature of our data. As the temperature is further lowered the noise decreases to a limiting value of about 1.6×10^{-18} V^2/Hz set by the preamplifier. Both the width of the resistive transition and the noise peak are strong functions of $R_\square$, with broad transitions occurring at large values of $R_\square$.

We have examined the dependence of the noise on dc driving current, applied magnetic field, and frequency. Figure 2 illustrates the dependence of the measured noise on applied dc current. At zero current the noise peak is absent and only the decrease in Johnson noise as the resistance changes is observed. This implies that the noise peak is "current induced" and can be considered as monitoring the fluctuations in sample resistance. As the current is increased the noise peak and the resistive transition become broader and shift to lower temperature. Similar effects are observed with the application of a magnetic field perpendicular to the plane of the sample as shown in Figure 3. Increasing the field from its ambient value of less than 1.7×10^{-4} Oe to approximately 0.1 Oe produced no change in the noise. With fields greater than 0.1 Oe the noise peak broadens and shifts to lower temperature. In the frequency range 10-100kHz the magnitude of the noise

316

was independent of frequency indicating that characteristic times for the fluctuation process were smaller than about 0.1 msec.

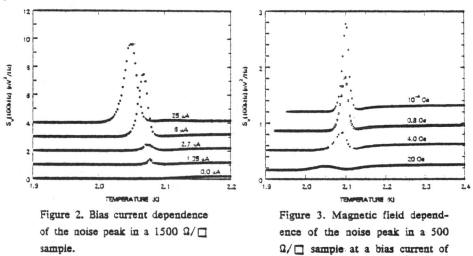

Figure 2. Bias current dependence of the noise peak in a 1500 $\Omega/\square$ sample.

Figure 3. Magnetic field dependence of the noise peak in a 500 $\Omega/\square$ sample at a bias current of 1.35 μA.

DISCUSSION

In the discussion that follows we interpret our measurements in terms of a vortex model. Although the physical mechanism may not be unique, the qualitative and quantitative agreement between the model and the data is extremely suggestive that the observed noise arises from free vortex motion.

Above some characteristic temperature T_c the bound vortex-antivortex pairs are in equilibrium with a gas of free vortices. In the presence of a driving current the members of a dissociated pair will be accelerated in opposite directions and will quickly reach a terminal velocity $v = J\Phi_0/\eta c$, where J is the two dimensional current density, Φ_0 is the flux quantum, c is the speed of light, and η is the viscosity the film presents to the moving vortex[7]. As these free vortices move a voltage pulse is observed at the contacts. This voltage remains until the vortex annihilates with a free vortex of the opposite sign or with the side of the sample, or becomes pinned on a defect. In order to estimate the duration of the voltage pulse it is necessary to know the viscosity coefficient η. η can be estimated by inducing free vortices with a magnetic field and measuring the flux flow resistivity ρ_F[7]. This procedure is complicated by the fact that at high temperatures with large $R_\square$ samples the flux flow characteristics are nonlinear[8]. Nevertheless, we estimate η at the temperature of the noise peak to be 2×10^{-16} gm/sec. This implies a vortex velocity at our lowest driving currents of about 5×10^3 cm/sec. Thus, we expect that the time between creation and annihilation of a free vortex to be small compared to the inverse of our measuring frequency.

On the time scale of our measurements the fluctuations in the number of free vortices produce narrow random voltage pulses similar to the current pulses in a thermionic diode.

If we assume independent motion (uncorrelated in time) that produces phase slips of magnitude 4π (2π for each member of the pair) the observed voltage is given by the Josephson relation $V = 2\Phi_0 r$, where r is the rate of phase slips. By analogy with the usual shot noise spectral density ($S_I(f)=2e<I>$), we estimate the spectral density to be

$$S_V(f) = 4\Phi_0 < V > \tag{1}$$

where $<V>$ is the average voltage drop across the sample. Equation (1) is valid only at low temperatures where the density of free vortices is small. When the density becomes sufficiently large, the mean free path decreases and the phase slips become considerably smaller than 4π leading to a sharp decrease in the magnitude of the noise. These ideas are compared with experiment in Figure 4 where we plot log S_V(100kHz) vs log $<V>$ for a variety of samples. In all cases the preamplifier background was subtracted and S_V(100kHz) and $<V>$ were measured with a constant driving current as the sample temperature was varied. At low temperatures (small $<V>$) the noise does indeed increase linearly with $<V>$. Furthermore, the noise is in general agreement with Eq. (1) (shown as a solid line), with the magnitude being slightly greater than predicted. It is useful to compare this data with typical flux flow noise measurements in Type II superconductors. A voltage shot noise is also observed but its magnitude is much larger (corresponding to coherent motion of 10^3-10^5 flux quanta) and the characteristic times are much longer (several msec)[9]. In the present case, at most a few flux quanta are moving coherently corresponding to a magnitude slightly greater than that predicted by Eq. (1). Presumably this is due to some short range order between the free vortices.

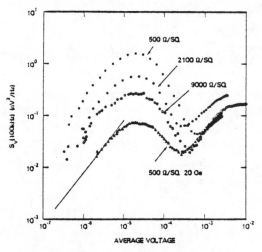

Figure 4. S_V(100kHz) vs $<V>$ for various samples. The prediction of the shot noise model, $4\Phi_0<V>$, is shown as the solid line.

As the temperature (and $<V>$) increases, the number of free vortices increases and, as anticipated above, the noise decreases. In all samples studied, the temperature at which the noise peaks corresponds to a sample resistivity of about 5 $\Omega/\square$. Using the dc conductivity as a measure of the number density of free vortices[2-3], we find that in all samples the noise peaks when the average linear separation between the vortices is approximately 9000 Å. It is important to note that this length remains fixed even though $R_\square$ and the width of the transition changes by more than an order of magnitude.

In this context the dependence of noise on magnetic field can be easily understood. The field introduces free vortices through the relation $H = n \, \Phi_0$, where n is the density of vortices. These additional vortices affect both the dc resistivity and the noise as discussed above. However, as shown in Figure 4, the position of the noise peak relative to $<V>$ (and $R_\square$) remains invariant. Even in an applied field the noise peaks when the separation between the vortices is about 9000 Å. Moreover, for applied fields greater than about 25 Oe the average separation between vortices is always less than 9000 Å, and in this limit the noise peak is suppressed. At present we have no understanding of the significance of this particular length scale. However, anomalous behavior is also observed in ac conductivity measurements when the correlation length exceeds 9000 Å[10].

REFERENCES

1. M. Beasley, J. Mooij, and T. Orlando, *Phys. Rev. Lett.* **42**, 1165 (1979).

2. S. Doniach and B. Huberman, *Phys. Rev. Lett.* **42**, 1169 (1979).

3. B. I. Halperin and D. R. Nelson, *J. Low Temp. Phys.*, to be published.

4. J. Pearl in *Low Temperature Physics LT9*, edited by J. Daunt, D. Edwards, F. Milford, and M. Yaqub, (Plenum Press, N.Y. 1965) p566.

5. J. M. Kosterlitz and D. Thouless, *J. Phys.* **C6**, 1181 (1973); and J. M. Kosterlitz, *J. Phys.*, **C7**, 1046 (1974).

6. B. Abeles, R. W. Cohen, and G. W. Cullen, *Phys. Rev. Lett.* **17**, 632 (1966).

7. Y. B. Kim and M. J. Stephen in *Superconductivity*, edited by R. D. Parks (Marcel Dekker, N.Y. 1969) Chapter 19.

8. P. M. Horn and R. D. Parks, *Phys. Rev.* **B4**, 2187 (1971).

9. D. J. Van Ooijen and G. J. Van Gurp, *Phys. Lett.*, **17**, 230 (1965).

10. A. T. Fiory and A. G. Hebard, preprint.

EFFECT OF NONEQUILIBRIUM PHONONS ON
SUPERCONDUCTING STATES WITH TWO COEXISTING ENERGY GAPS

André-Marie Tremblay *
Laboratory of Atomic and Solid State Physics
Cornell University, Ithaca, NY 14853

Gerd Schön
Institut für Theorie der Kondensierten Materie
Universität Karlsruhe, BRD

ABSTRACT

It is shown that under the influence of tunnel currents, superconductors may exhibit a "first order transition" to a state with
two coexisting energy gaps. An energy and number conserving approximation for the collision operator is used to explicitly take into
account in the theory the effect of nonequilibrium phonons. Quantitative predictions for experiments are presented.

1. INTRODUCTION

We have now reached, mainly through the study of radiation
stimulated superconductivity and of inhomogeneous states, the stage
where many "nonequilibrium phases" (nonequilibrium collective effects) may appear in superconductors, immediately bringing to the
forefront the problems of stability of dissipative states which are
nowadays under intense investigation[1] in the field of nonequilibrium statistical mechanics in general. Thanks to the work of
Eckern, Schmid, Schmutz and Schön[2] (ESSS) we have now a large number of cases where the stability of dissipative states has been
investigated, including some examples where detailed balance[1] is
violated.

Although the work of ESSS predicts many phenomena which can be
qualitatively checked with experiment, a quantitative comparison is
difficult, mainly because phonons were assumed to remain in equilibrium, a condition which we know is violated in most experimental
situations.[3]

In this paper, we return to one of the first examples (which
is now part of the more general picture of ESSS) where the ideas
of Schmid[4] on the stability of nonequilibrium superconducting
states were applied. In ref. 5 (hereafter I) it was shown that in
superconducting tunnel junctions, two values of the energy gap
could simultaneously be a solution of the gap equation. The results are in qualitative accord with the pioneering experimental
work of Dynes, Narayanamurti and Garno[6] and of Gray and Willemsen[7].

This paper reports on how the theory of I is modified when
nonequilibrium phonons are included in the simplest possible way.
This allows us to set limits on the domain of validity of the theory
of I and to make quantitative predictions in the regime where we
can show that nonequilibrium phonons only renormalize the temperature entering the Landau-Ginzburg equation. If these simple theoretical predictions can be checked quantitatively by experiments,
it will give strong support to the theoretically sound global

*Present Address: Université de Sherbrooke, Sherbrooke, Qué., Canada

0094-243X/80/580319-06$1.50 Copyright 1980 American Institute of Physics

picture emerging from the work of ESSS. However, if a quantitative
comparison with experiment is not successful, the theoretical calculation of at least the effect of nonequilibrium phonons will need
to be improved.

2. MICROSCOPIC THEORY

For convenience, we first summarize the results already obtained
in refs. 5 and 2. We consider a tunnel junction consisting of the
superconductor of interest (the probe) coupled to a second superconductor (the injector). We momentarily neglect the effect of nonequilibrium phonons. We also assume that,

a) the probe is thin enough that we may assume a uniform injection
over the thickness of the junction;
b) the gap of the injector Δ^i, in contrast to the gap of the probe,
is not appreciably perturbed by the tunneling process. This can be
achieved by using an injector which is much thicker than the probe.
Qualitatively, our results should also apply to a more symmetrical
case[7] but since it is hard experimentally to make the injector and
the probe identical, we prefer to study the case where they are
markedly different;
c) we restrict ourselves to temperatures T close to the transition
temperature T_c (Landau–Ginzburg region), $(\Delta, \Delta_i \ll T)$.

The equations describing such a system have been derived many
times. The gap equation is,

$$(\alpha - \beta\Delta^2)\Delta = -\chi\Delta - \xi^2\nabla^2\Delta \quad , \tag{1}$$

where ξ^2 is the usual Landau Ginzburg coherence length, $\alpha = (T_c - T)/T_c$,
$\beta = 7\zeta(3)/8\pi^2 T^2$ and the "gap control" (or anomalous term, or control
function) χ is defined by,

$$\chi = -\int_{-\infty}^{\infty} dE \, \frac{1}{E} \, N_1(E) \delta n(E) \quad , \tag{2}$$

where $\delta n(E)$ is the angular average (isotropic part) of the energy
dependent deviation of the distribution function from its local
equilibrium value. $N_1(E) \equiv \Theta(|E| - \Delta)|E|/(E^2 - \Delta^2)^{\frac{1}{2}}$ is the BCS density
of states and $\delta n(E)$ obeys a Boltzmann equation.[2] The collision
operator I_{ep} can be written down in the relaxation time approxima-
tion, $I_{ep}[\delta n(E)] = \tau_E^{-1} \delta n(E)$ where τ_E can be taken as a constant τ_o
equal to its value at $E = 0$ and $T = T_c$ because E and Δ are small
with respect to T. To order $(\Delta/T)^2$ the scattering-in term can be
neglected. Finally, the term representing the effect of tunnel injection can be derived using, for example, golden rule arguments.
Since only the part of $\delta n(E)$ which is odd in energy contributes to
χ in Eq. (2), we can write,

$$(\dot{n}_E)_D = 2B \left\{ N_1^i(E-eV)[n_T(E-eV) - n_T(E)] + (eV \leftrightarrow -eV) \right\} \quad , \tag{3}$$

$$B \equiv (8e^2 R\Omega N(0))^{-1} \quad ,$$

where R is the resistance of the junction, Ω the (effective) volume
of the probe, $N(0)$ the normal density of states and N_1^i the injector BCS density of states.

It was shown by ESSS that the most stable states in this situation were homogeneous so that the analysis of I applies under more general conditions. The global stability of the various homogeneous stationary states can be determined from the following potential (generalized free energy) which can be obtained from the stationary solutions of the Fokker-Planck equation [2,4] obeyed by our system,

$$F = -2N(0) \int d^3r \int_0^\Delta d\Delta' [\alpha - \beta\Delta'^2 + \chi(\Delta')]\Delta'. \qquad (4)$$

Since such a potential function (generalized free energy) exists, our system obeys the principle of detailed balance[1] and its behavior will be analogous to systems in thermodynamic equilibrium; in particular it will exhibit a first order phase transition when two minima of F correspond to the same value of the generalized free energy density[8].

To proceed any further, we need an explicit expression for χ, the gap control. The Boltzmann equation for the distribution function in the stationary homogeneous situation reduces to $\delta n(E) = \tau_0(\dot{n}_E)_D$. The quantity χ is computed using this equation and Eqs.(2), (3). The first order expansion in $\frac{eV}{T}$ of Eq. (3) is plotted in Fig. 1. This graph of $\delta n^{(1)}(E)$ is useful to understand the results given in analytical form in I.

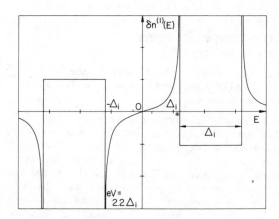

Fig. 1: The first order contribution $\delta n^{(1)}(E)$ to the quasiparticle distribution function describing an excess number of excitations (particle-like for $E > 0$ or hole-like for $E < 0$) as a function of energy.

Consider the solid line in Fig. 1 for the case $|eV| \sim \Delta_i + \Delta$. We can qualitatively understand why two solutions of the gap equation may simultaneously be possible, as follows. Suppose that $\Delta = \Delta_i$ is a self-consistent solution of the gap Eq. (1). Then the peak in $\delta n(E)$ at $1.1\Delta_i$ will be convoluted with the peak in $N_1(E)$ at $\Delta = \Delta_i$ and will give a large negative contribution to χ in Eq. (2). It is thus plausible that there also exists a solution with $\Delta > 1.1\Delta_i$, since in such a case the peak in $\delta n(E)$ at $1.1\Delta_i$ would not contribute to χ and a more positive χ is consistent with a larger gap (see Eq. (1)).

The effects of heating on $\delta n(E)$ will in most instances introduce a large but smooth background. If spikes similar to those depicted in Fig. 1 show up on this background then clearly the above qualitative picture of why there may exist two gap solutions will remain valid. On the other hand gap enhancement depends very much on the level of the background.

The effect of nonequilibrium phonons becomes important when the phenomenological "escape" time τ_{es} becomes much longer than the phonon scattering time τ^{ph}, i.e., when $\tau_{es} \gg \tau^{ph}$ where τ^{ph} can be expressed as a function of τ_o using the ratio of the normal electron and longitudinal phonon specific heats C_N^{el}, C^{ph} respectively[9],

$$\tau^{ph}/\tau_o = 35\zeta(3)C^{ph}/(4\pi^2 C_N^{el}).$$

Using the energy and number conserving approximation method of Eckern and Schön[9] we find that the effect of nonequilibrium phonons can be represented as simple heating when

$$1 \ll \tau_{es}/\tau^{ph} \ll (T/\Delta)(T/eV). \tag{5}$$

In such a case, the parameter α becomes α'[10].

$$\alpha' = \alpha + \delta\alpha_h = \alpha - 2.59 B\tau_o (eV/2T)^2 (\tau_{es}/\tau^{ph}). \tag{6}$$

Note that $\delta\alpha_h$ does not have any sharp step. By contrast, χ computed with $\delta n^{(1)}(E)$ has a step[5]. It is basically this step which leads to multiple solutions of the gap equation.

3. SIMPLE PREDICTIONS FOR EXPERIMENTS
3.1 Qualitative Aspects

We quote a few qualitative features of the theory, some of which have already been experimentally observed, some of which will hopefully be checked in future experiments.

a) The phase transition aspects of our theory have already been noted[5,2] and seem to agree with experimental findings[6,7]: at a certain voltage (see also Sec. 3.2), a low gap region (large injection current density) appears in the probe and grows relative to the larger gap region (low injection current density) as the total injection current increases. The expected hysteresis has also been observed[6,7]. This transition in the junctions is analogous to a liquid gas transition at constant pressure where the relative volumes are controlled by the total volume. The total injection current which controls the transition has no analogue in any of the other nonequilibrium first order phase transitions studied by ESSS.

b) There is no threshold current, conductance or quasiparticle density in our theory. The two coexisting gaps can be in principle observed at the threshold voltage in many kinds of junctions, even at very low injection current density, as long as the energy difference between the two coexisting gaps (see following section) is large enough to be resolved from relaxation time smearing effects and other similar complications.

c) The Chi and Clarke gap enhancement (to be published) and the coexisting gaps can be observed in principle in the same junction.

d) If heating effects are negligible, one of the two coexisting gaps may be enhanced with respect to the equilibrium gap.

e) The coexistence of a superconducting and a normal phase is possible, as can be seen using either the graphical methods of I and ESSS or an analytical method. Since this possibility is probably harder to see experimentally, we shall not give any more quantitative results on that matter.

Although the qualitative features described in paragraphs a) and b) have already been observed, observation of the phenomena described in paragraphs c), d), e) above would certainly give a stronger experimental support to our theory.

3.2 Quantitative predictions

Assume that Eq. (5) holds. Then Eq. (6) also holds. In the homogeneous case and when $|eV|$ is very close to $\Delta + \Delta_i$, one can find a simple analytical form for Eq. (2). The transition voltage is determined using the procedure outlined in Eq. (4).

This leads us to our first quantitative prediction,

$$|eV_o| = \Delta_i + 1/2(\Delta_s(\alpha') + \Delta_\ell(\alpha')). \tag{7}$$

The transition voltage eV_o can be determined experimentally. It should be related to the injector gap and to the experimentally determined values of the two coexisting gaps $\Delta_s(\alpha')$ and $\Delta_\ell(\alpha')$ as described in Eq. (7). Note that Eq. (7) and Eq. (8) that follows are valid only when the condition

$$\frac{B\tau_o}{\alpha'} \left(\frac{\Delta_s(\alpha')+\Delta_i}{2T}\right) \pi \left(\frac{\Delta_i}{\Delta_s(\alpha')}\right)^{\frac{1}{2}} \ll 1$$

is satisfied.

The temperature and conductance dependence of the two coexisting gaps consitute our second quantitative prediction. If Δ_i is roughly constant in the temperature range of interest and $\Delta_i \gg \Delta_s(\alpha')$ we have

$$\Delta_\ell(\alpha') - \Delta_s(\alpha') \sim \frac{R^{-1}}{(T_c-T)^{3/4}} + \frac{R^{-2}}{(T_c-T)^{7/4}}. \tag{8}$$

The last term depends on the square of the conductance (R^{-2}) and on τ_{es} and by assumption is smaller than the term proportional to the conductance.

4. CONCLUSION

Five qualitative predictions were given in Sec. 3.1 and two quantitative predictions in Sec. 3.2. Predictions concerning the absolute values of the observed gaps can be derived but they are less useful because they contain the parameter τ_{es}/τ^{ph} which may be harder to obtain experimentally. Nevertheless, it is useful to observe that our theory is not inconsistent with the fact that experimentally, the two coexisting gaps have values smaller than the equilibrium gap. If, as was the case in the theory presented in I, the condition $\dfrac{\tau_{es}}{\tau^{ph}} \left(\dfrac{\Delta_s(\alpha)+\Delta_i}{2T}\right) \ll \left(\dfrac{\Delta_i}{\Delta_s(\alpha)}\right)^{\frac{1}{2}}$

is realized, then the largest of the two coexisting gaps has a value larger than the equilibrium value. In practice, the above condition may not be satisfied.

It would be interesting to extend these ideas to low temperatures where a solution of the deterministic equation also leads to the possibility of a phase transition[5] but where a determination of the fluctuations, which we must know to determine the global stability, is more complicated than close to T_c.

If the predictions presented in this paper are verified, we are confident that our theory will also explain new experiments which have just been done[11].

Finally, guided by the analogies between the generalized free energy determining the stability of the nonequilibrium state and the usual thermodynamic free energy, one can speculate that future experiments may exhibit phenomena analogous to spinodal decomposition in fluids[12]. A rapid change of voltage in a junction is analogous to a rapid change of pressure in the fluid. The current and junction conductance are analogous respectively to the volume and temperature of the fluid.

It is a pleasure to acknowledge stimulating discussions with V. Ambegaokar, and correspondence with K. E. Gray and B. Huberman. This work was supported in part by the U.S. Office of Naval Research, Technical Report No. 3.

REFERENCES

1. H. Haken, Rev. Mod. Phys. 47, 67 (1975).
2. U. Eckern, A. Schmid, M. Schmutz and G. Schön, J. Low Temp. Phys. 36, 643 (1979).
3. A. Rothwarf and B. N. Taylor, Phys. Rev. Lett. 19, 27 (1967).
4. A. Schmid, Phys. Rev. Lett. 38, 922 (1977).
5. G. Schön and A.-M. Tremblay, Phys. Rev. Lett. 42, 1086 (1979).
6. R. C. Dynes, V. Narayanamurti and J. P. Garno, Phys. Rev. Lett. 39, 229 (1977).
7. K. E. Gray and H. W. Willemsen, J. Low Temp. Phys. 31, 911 (1978).
8. We are neglecting changes in the free energy density of the injector and of the detector.
9. U. Eckern and G. Schön, J. Low Temp. Phys. 32, 821 (1978).
10. Even when $\tau_{es} \ll \tau^{ph}$, the term of order $(eV/T)^2$ in Eq. (3) contributes to gap reduction (see Ref. 5). We restrict ourselves to the case $\tau_{es} \gg \tau^{ph}$.
11. I. Iguchi, D. Kent, H. Gilmartin, and D. N. Langenberg, Bull. Am. Phys. Soc. 24, 329 (1979).
12. J. W. Cahn, Trans. Metall. Soc. AIME 242, 166 (1968); J. S. Langer in Fluctuations, Instabilities, and Phase Transitions, edited by T. Riste (Plenum, New York, 1975), p. 1. We should like to thank Professor W. I. Goldburg for suggesting these references.

FLUCTUATIONS AND THE DETERMINATION OF CRITICAL CURRENTS IN GRANULAR MICROBRIDGES

T. F. Refai and R. A. Peters
Catholic University of America
Washington, D.C. 20064

S. A. Wolf and F. J. Rachford
Naval Research Laboratory
Washington, D.C. 20375

ABSTRACT

The reduction of measured critical currents in granular microbridges can be understood as an effect of Langer-Ambegaokar-McCumber-Halperin type thermally activated phase slips. Single fluctuation events which lower the critical current were detected at various rf frequencies and amplitude modulation rates at temperatures well below the transition of the microbridge. Good agreement was found between theory and experiment.

INTRODUCTION

Our study of the thermal fluctuation effects in ultra-thin granular weak links demonstrate the existance of large thermal fluctuation effects at reduced temperatures of approximatly half the critical temperature T_c. These effects are seen because the free energy of a granular weak link can be comparable to $k_B T$ over a greater than usual range of currents and temperatures. The effect of thermal fluctuations on the critical currents of the granular weak links was investigated as a function of temperature, rf excititation frequency, and amplitude modulation frequency.

A single fluctuation event can induce a premature transition from a uniform superconducting state to a dissipative state. Due to a critical current hysteresis (Fig. 1) at the temperatures of interest, the sample will remain in a dissipative state even though the applied current is less than the critical current. Such fluctuation induced transitions will result in an apparent critical current below the "true" (mean field) value. The apparent critical current is also a function of modulation frequency since the slower the rf current amplitude is modulated the more time is available for a possible fluctuation induced transition. Hence slower modulation rates result in lower measured critical currents. This effect is illustrated in Fig. 1. By measuring the critical current as a function of modulation frequency, it is thus possible to infer the role of fluctuations on the critical current.

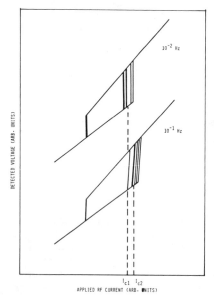

DETECTED VOLTAGE (ARB. UNITS)

10^{-2} Hz

10^{-1} Hz

I_{c1} I_{c2}
APPLIED RF CURRENT (ARB. UNITS)

Fig. 1 A tracing of x-y recorder plots showing multiple sweeps of detected voltage vs rf drive current at two modulation frequencies at a temperature of 1.631K. A critical current hysteresis is seen and as well as a scatter in position of the superconducting to dissipative state transitions. I_{c1} is the average critical current for the 10^{-2} Hz trace, and I_{c2} is the average critical current for the 10^{-1} Hz trace.

We find that the measured critical currents are strongly influenced by thermal fluctuations of the type described by the Langer-Ambegaokar-McCumber-Halperin (LAMH) model[1-3]. Our results provide a quantative confirmation of the LAMH model at temperatures far below T_c. The theory provides a method of determining the true critical current in the presence of fluctuations. Corrections to the critical current can be large at typical x-y recorder rates. For this sample we note a 20% reduction in critical current at a reduced temperature of 0.6.

EXPERIMENTAL

The weak link was produced by sputtering a 240 A thick film of niobium on a 1 mm diameter quartz rod. A microbridge was sculptured in this film by conventional photolithography and anodization producing a weak link 1 micrometers long and 40 micrometers wide, and approximately 35 A thick. Weak links prepared in this way have a granular structure consisting of isolated grains in a niobium oxide matrix.

In this experiment, the rf was triangularly modulated and inductively coupled to the weak link. Because the coupling was weak, relatively large rf currents were used to drive the sample. A combination of mu-metal, superconducting and normal metal shields reduced stray rf pick-up to levels which were at least eight orders of magnitude smaller than the drive amplitude. A spectrum analyzer was used as a tuned receiver to detect and display the signal as a function of rf amplitude at fixed rf frequencies.

Measurments were obtained at rf frequency and temperature combinations where a critical current hysteresis could be observed. The modulation frequency was varied from 10^{-2} Hz to 10^3 Hz. The averaged measured critical current increased as the modulation frequency increased. For slow modulation frequencies (≤ 0.1 Hz) an x-y recorder was used to plot the I-V curve from which the critical currents were measured. For fast modulation frequencies the critical currents were obtained directly from the spectrum analyzer display. The critical current at each modulation frequency was obtained from the average of approximatey ten traces.

THEORY

Langer and Ambegaokar[1] (LA) developed a theory to explain the onset of resistance in superconducting filaments below T_c produced by fluctuation induced phase slips. The detected voltage in such samples was found to be proportional to the thermally activated phase slip rate, Γ, which can be expressed by the equation

$$\Gamma = \Omega \exp(-\delta F/k_B T) \tag{1}$$

where Ω is an attempt rate prefactor assumed by LA to be a constant, δF is the free energy necessary to produce a phase slip in the filament, and k_B is the Boltzman constant. In the absence of a current through the sample, the free energy term can be expressed as the product of the free energy density (condensation energy) and the volume of superconductor which goes normal upon the generation of a phase slip. This volume is proportional to the filiment crossection, σ, times the coherence distance, $\xi(T)$,

$$\delta F_0(T) = \frac{\sqrt{2}\, H_c^2(T)}{3\,\pi}\, \sigma\, \xi(T). \tag{2}$$

In the presence of a normalized current density, j, the free energy, δF, is decreased by a factor f(j), $\delta F = \delta F_0 \times f(j)$.

McCumber and Halperin modified the LA model substituting a temperature and current dependent prefactor

$$\Omega(T,j) = \frac{L}{\xi(T)}\, \frac{\sqrt{3}}{2\pi^{3/2}\tau(T)\sqrt{k_B T}}\sqrt{\delta F_0} \times g(j) , \tag{3}$$

where the current dependence is contained in the factor g(j), and where L is the length of the microbridge. General agreement was found with the theory by many experimental groups studying the critical current onset at low dc currents and very near T_c.[4-7] However T_c

328

had to be considered an adjustable parameter in the fit and small variations in T_c could change the predicted result by many orders of magnitude.

To apply the LAMH model to calculate an average transition rate, $\Gamma(j)$, eq.(1) and (3) were evaluated numerically for one quarter of the the rf cycle by approximating the rf quarter cycle by 20 constant current steps taken at equal time intervals. For each step a $\Gamma_s(j)$ was calculated. The transition rate averaged over a quarter rf cycle, $\Gamma(j)$, is then the sum of the Γ_s or $\Gamma(j) = \sum \Gamma_s(j)$. Next, the rf amplitude is increased and a new $\Gamma(j)$ is obtained. If the rf current amplitude is constant, the probability, P, of having one or more transitions in a time Δt is given by:

$$P = 1 - e^{-\Gamma(j)\Delta t} . \qquad (4)$$

Since the rf current amplitude was triangularly modulated, j was an increasing function of time. This modulation was approximated by assuming that j increased in a stepwise fashion, where the width of the step was Δt. After finding Δt from the modulation frequency and current range, the probability of a transition is found from:

$$P = 1 - e^{-\sum(\Gamma(j)\Delta t)} = 1 - e^{-(\sum\Gamma(j))\Delta t} . \qquad (5)$$

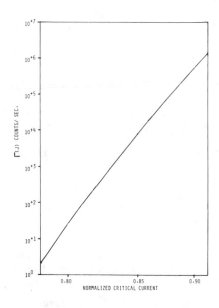

Fig. 3. A plot of the average transition rate (j) vs the normalized current j

To compare predictions from the LAMH model with experimental data, a table of $\Gamma(j)$ vs j was calculated, similar to that shown in Fig. 2. It was assumed that there was only one active phase slip site in the weak link so that $L/\xi(T)$ in Eq. 3 was put equal to one. The average critical current for a given modulation frequency represents a 50% chance of having a transition at that temperature, Δt, and j combination. To compare the experimental data to the theoretical predictions, $j_c(T)$ and δF were iteratively adjusted to fit the modulation frequency dependence of the average critical current. A variation of δF changes both the shape and the position on the temperature axis of our fit while, to first order, a variation in j_c changes only the position. If δF and j_c are both varied for best fit, the result is a change in the slope. The dashed line shows the "best fit" obtained in this way for a 20%

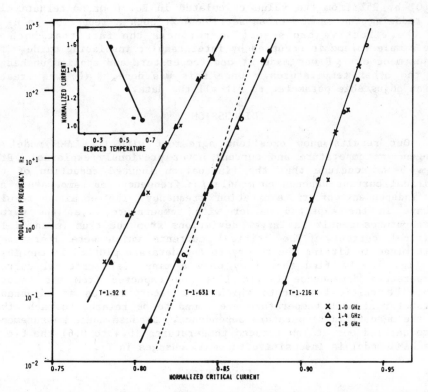

Fig. 3. A plot of data (points) and theory (solid lines) with the logarithm of modulation frequency vs the normalized critical current for three temperatures and three rf frequencies. The dashed line illustrates the effect of a 20% change in the free energy term in Eqs. 2 and 3. The "true" critical current,inferred from the fit at each temperature, is plotted in the inset versus reduced temperature. The solid line in the inset is a best fit to the mean field critical current temperature dependence.

change in δF. These calculations predict that the critical current should be independent of the rf excitation frequency but should depend on the modulation frequency and the temperature.

The free energy (Eq. 2) was calculated using the thermodynamic critical field equation,

$$H_c(0) = \sqrt{\frac{3}{2}} \; \phi_0 / \pi^2 \xi_0 \lambda(0) \qquad (6)$$

where ϕ_0 the flux quantum, and $\lambda(0)$ is the modified London penetration depth[8] given by $\lambda(0) = (\lambda_L(0)^2 \xi_0)^{1/3}$. To obtain a good fit to the data it was found necessary to reduce δF by reducing

$H_c(0)$ by 25% from the value calculated in Eq. 6 or, alternatively, by reducing the sample cross-section 44%. Such a reduction in H_c or in the effective cross-section reflects the fact that much of the sample volume is occupied by intergranular insulating oxide. The adjustment of δF was made at one temperature and applied unchanged at the other temperatures. Once this was done, $j_c(0)$ was treated as an adjustable parameter to fit all the data.

DISCUSSION

Our results show excellent agreement with the LAMH model at ranges of temperature and current never previously explored. From Fig. 3 we conclude that the fluctuation induced reduction of the critical current depends on modulation frequency and temperature and is independent of rf excitation frequency. The obtained results behave in the expected manner with temperature, i.e. the warmer temperatures result in larger deviations from the true (mean field) critical current. The critical currents which were iteratively determined in fitting the theory to the data are plotted in the inset of Fig. 3. We find that they obey a mean field critical current temperature dependence (solid line) as expected from the theory. Thus the critical currents which were determined as an adjustable parameter at each temperature are found to be related to each other by the mean field temperature dependence. Because these measurements were carried out at low reduced temperatures (0.4 to 0.6) the fit to the LAMH model is insensitive to small changes in T_c.

CONCLUSION

We find that fluctuations can appriceably reduce the measured critical current in hysteretic weak superconductors at temperatures well below T_c. In this work, fluctuations were found to result in a substantial reduction of the critical current of an ultra-thin granular sample. Studies of the critical currents in weakly superconducting systems allow sensitive tests of fluctuation theory. Although the LAMH theory was developed to describe the fluctuation induced onset of the critical current near T_c, we find excellent quantative agreement in our application of the theory well below T_c. We have developed a procedure to calculate the true critical current in the absence of fluctuations.

REFERENCES

1) J. S. Langer and Vinay Ambegaokar, Phys. Rev., <u>164</u>, 498 (1967).
2) D. E. McCumber and B. I. Halperin, Phys. Rev., <u>B1</u>, 1054 (1970).
3) G. Schoen and V. Ambegaokar, Phys. Rev., <u>B19</u>, 3515 (1979).
4) R. S. Newbower, M. R. Beasley, M. Tinkham, Phys. Rev., <u>B5</u>, 864 (1972).
5) W. W. Webb and R. J. Warburton, Phys. Rev. Letters, <u>20</u>, 461 (1968).
6) J. R. Miller and J. Pierce, Phys. Rev., <u>B8</u>, 4164 (1973).

7) J. E. Lukens, R. J Warburton, W. W. Webb, Phys. Rev. Letters, <u>25</u>, 1180 (1971). J. E. Lukens, J. M. Goodkind, Phys. Rev. Letters, <u>20</u>, 1363 (1968)
8) <u>Introduction to Superconductivity</u>, M. Tinkham, McGraw-Hill, New York, 1975, pp. 74-75.

ATTENDEES

Joseph C. Amato
Colgate University
Hamilton, NY 13346

B. Bandyopadhyay
Rutgers University
Serin Physics Laboratory
Frelinghuysen Road
Piscataway, NJ 08854

Stewart E. Barnes
DPMC
Ecole de Physique
32 Boulevard d'Yvoy,
1211 Geneve, SWITZRLAND

C.M. Bastuscheck
Physics Dept. Clark Hall
Cornell University
Ithaca NY 14853

Malcom R. Beasley
Stanford University
Department of Applied Physics
Stanford, CA 94035

J.L. Berchier
Universite de Geneve
Dept. Physique, 24q E. Ansermet
1211 Geneve SWITZERLAND

David J. Bergman
Physics Dept.,
Tel-Aviv University
Tel-Aviv, ISRAEL

Joze Bevk
Harvard University
Division of Applied Sciences
9 Oxford St.
Cambridge, MA 02138

Richard G. Brandt
Office of Naval Research
1030 E. Green St.,
Pasadena, CA 91106

R. Mark Boysel
Physics. Dept.
Ohio State University
Columbus, OH 43210

Robert Buhrman
Clark Hall
Applied Physics
Cornell University
Ithaca, NY 14853

G. Lawrence Carr
Physics Dept.
Ohio State University
Columbus, OH 43210

Jhy-Jiun Chang
Dept of Physics & Astronomy
Wayne State University
Detroit, MI 48202

T. Chui
Rutgers University
Serin Physics Laboratory
Frelinghuysen Road
Piscataway, NJ 08854

John Claassen
Code 5263
Naval Research Laboratory
Washington, DC 20375

Tord Claeson
Dept. Applied Physics
Stanford University
Stanford, CA 94305

J.R. Clem
Iowa State University
Dept. of Physics
Ames, Iowa 50010

M.C. Cross
Bell Laboratories
600 Mountain Avenue
Murray Hill, NJ 07974

Edward J. Cukauskas
Code 5263
Naval Research Laboratory
Washington, DC 20375

E. Dan Dahlberg
Physics Dept.
University of Minnesota
Minneapolis, MN 55455

Edison Z. da Silva
H.H. Wills Physics Laboratory
Royal Fort,
Tyndall Avenue
Bristol BS81TL

A. Davidson
T.J. Watson Research Ctr.
P.O. Box 218
Yorktown Hghts., NY   10598

Bascom S. Deaver, Jr.
Physics Dept.
University of Virginia
McCormick Rd.,
Charlottesville, VA   22901

Tel Aviv University
Attn: Guy Deutscher
Department of Physics & Astronomy
Ramat-Aviv, Tel Aviv, ISRAEL

Stanley A. Dodds
Dept. of Physics
Rice University
Houston, TX   77001

G.J. Dolan
Bell Laboratories
Room 1D304
600 Mountain Avenue
Murray Hill, NJ   07974

G.B. Donaldson
Dept. of Applied Physics
John Anderson Bldg.
University of Strathclyde
Glasgow G4 ONG, SCOTLAND

S. Doniach
Dept. of Applied Physics
Stanford University
Stanford, CA   94305

E.A. Edelsack
Office of Naval Research
Code 427
800 No. Quincy Street
Arlington, VA   22217

Ora Entin-Wohlman
Physics Dept.
Tel-Aviv University
Tel-Aviv, ISRAEL

F. Paul Esposito
Dept. of Physics
Univ. of Cincinnati
Cincinnati, OH

Charles M. Falco
Solid State Science Division
Argonne National Laboratory
Argonne, IL   60439

Thomas Fariss
Physics Dept.
University of Virginia
McCormick Road
Charlottesville, VA   22901

J.L. Feldman
Code 6339
Naval Research Laboratory
Washington, DC   20375

R.A. Ferrell
Institute for Theoretical Physics
University of California
Santa Barbara, CA   93106

D.K. Finnemore
Iowa State University
Dept. of Physics
Ames, Iowa   50011

Anthony Fiory
Bell Laboratories
Murray Hill, NJ   07974

Daniel S. Fisher
1D-266 Bell Labs
600 Mountain Ave.,
Murray Hill, NJ   07974

Simon Foner
Francis Bitter National Magnet Lab.
MIT, 170 Albany St., NW 14-3117
Cambridge, MA   02139

J.C. Garland
Ohio State University
Dept. of Physics
174 W. 18th Avenue
Columbus, Ohio 43210

John Gavaler
Westinghouse R&D
Churchill Boro
Pittsburgh, PA 15235

Arup K. Ghosh
#480, Brookhaven National Lab
Upton, NY 11973

Bernard Giovannini
DPMC, 32 bd d' Yvoy
Universite de Geneve
1211 Geneve 4, SWITZERLAND

Rolfe E. Glover, III
University of Maryland
Dept. of Physics
College Park, MD 20742

A.M. Goldman
University of Minnesota
School of Physics
116 Church Street, SE
Minneapolis, MN 55455

D.M. Grannan
Physics Dept.
Ohio State University
Columbus, Ohio 43210

K.E. Gray
Bldg. 223
Argonne National Laboratory
Argonne, IL 60439

D.U. Gubser
Code 6338
Naval Research Laboratory
Washington, DC 20375

Michael Gurvitch
Bell Laboratories
Rm 1D-410
Murray Hill, NJ 07974

Fawwaz Habbal
Harvard University
Div. of Applied Sciences
9 Oxford St.
Cambridge, MA 02138

Arthur F. Hebard
Bell Laboratories
Room 1D-460
600 Mountain Avenue
Murray Hill, NJ 07974

David F. Heidel
Physics Dept.
Ohio State University
Columbus, OH 43210

R.A. Hein
National Science Foundation
1730 K Street, NW
Washington, DC 20006

Paul M. Horn
IBM, Thomas J. Watson Research Ctr.
P.O.Box 218
Yorktown Hghts., NY 10598

B.A. Huberman
Xerox Palo Alto Research Center
Palo Alto, CA 94304

John J. Hudak
Dept. of Defense
R553 9800 Savage Rd.
Ft. Meade, MD. 20755

Y. Imry
Dept. of Physics
Tel Aviv University
Tel Aviv, ISRAEL

L. Ishol
Naval Coastal Systems Center
Panama City, Florida

Aloke Jain
Dept. of Physics
State Univ. of NY at Stony Brook
Long Island, NY 11794

Alan Kadin
Dept. of Physics
State University of NY at
  Stony Brook
Long Island, NY 11794

Clyde W. Kimball
Physics Dept.
Northern Illinois University
Dekalb, IL 60115

E. Scott Kirkpatrick
IBM Research Center
Yorktown Heights, NY 10598

T.M. Klapwijk
Harvard University
Gordon McKay Lab
9 Oxford Street
Cambridge, MA 02138

Barry M. Klein
Code 6684
Naval Research Laboratory
Washington, DC 20375

Christina Knoedler
IBM, Thomas J. Watson Research
  Center
P.O.Box 218
Yorktown Hghts., NY 10598

Paul M. Kogut
Serin Physics Lab
Rutgers University
Piscataway, NJ 08854

Robert Laibowitz
IBM Research Center
P.O. Box 218   19-032
Yorktown Hghts., NY 10598

W.J. Lamb
Dept. of Physics
Ohio State University
Columbus, OH 43210

J.R. Leibowitz
Physics Department
Catholic University of America
Washington, DC 20064

M. Levy
Dept. of Physics
Univ. of Wisconsin, Milwaukee
Milwaukee, Wisconsin 53201

P. Lindenfeld
Rutgers University
Serin Physics Laboratory
Frelinghuysen Road
Piscataway, NJ 08854

Chris J. Lobb
Harvard University
Div. of Applied Sciences
29 Oxford St.
Cambridge, MA 02138

James Lukens
Dept. of Physics
SUNY, Stony Brook, NY 11794

P. Martinoli
University de Neuchatel
Institut de Physiks
R.A.L. Brequet 1 - UNI
CH-2000 Neuchatel, SWITZERLAND

W.L. McLean
Rutgers University
Serin Physics Lab
Frelinghuyser Road
Piscataway, NJ 08854

J.E. Mooij
Lab. Technical Physics
Larentzweg 1
Delft
THE NETHERLANDS

Richard Newrock
University of Cincinnati
Dept. of Physics
Cincinnati, OH 45221

R. Orbach
University of California
Dept. of Physics
Los Angeles, CA 90024

336

Zvi Ovadyahu
Brookhaven National Laboratory
Bldg. 480
Upton, NY 11973

Bruce R. Patton
Ohio State University
Dept. of Physics
174 W 18th Avenue
Columbus, OH 43210

S. Perkowitz
Dept. of Physics
Emory Univ.
Atlanta, GA 30322

F.J. Rachford
Code 5293R
Naval Research Laboratory
Washington, DC 20375

N.A.H.K. Rao
Dept. of Physics
Ohio State University
174 W 18th Street
Columbus, OH 43210

T.F. Refai
Physics Department
Catholic University
Washington, DC 20064

J. Rosenblatt
I.N.S.A.
Rennes, 20, avenue des
Buttes de Coesmes
35031 Rennes Cedex,
FRANCE

Steven T. Ruggiero
Ginzton Laboratory
Stanford University
Stanford, CA 94035

D. Sanchez
Section de Physique
32 bd d'Yvoy
1211 Geneve 4 SWITZERLAND

Kurt Scharnberg
Inst. Ang. Physik
Univirsitat Hamburg
Jungiusstrasse 11
D-2000 Hamburg 36
WEST GERMANY

A.I. Schindler
Code 6000
Naval Research Laboratory
Washington, DC 20375

Albert Schmid
Institute for Theoretical Physics
University of California
Santa Barbara, CA 93106

J.T. Schriempf
Code 6330
Naval Research Laboratory
Washington, DC 20375

Ivan Schuller
Solid State Science Div.
Bldg. 223, Argonne National Labs
Argonne, IL 60439

Brian B. Schwartz
School of Science
Brooklyn College
Brooklyn, NY 11210

Campbell Scott
Physics Dept. Clark Hall
Cornell University
Ithaca NY 14853

S.T. Sekula, Solid State Division
Oak Ridge National Lab
P.O. Box X,
Oak Ridge, TN 37830

M.V. Sienko
Department of Chemistry
Cornell University
Ithica, NY 14853

Eugen Simanek
Dept. of Physics
Univ. of California
Riverside, CA 92521

Mark R. Skokan
Code 5263
Naval Research Laboratory
Washington, DC   20375

Richard Steiner
Physics Dept.
University of Virginia
McCormick Road
Charlottesville, VA   22901

J.W. Straley
University of Kentucky
Dept. of Physics
Lexington, KY   40506

Myron Strongin
Brookhaven National Laboratories
Dept. of Physics
Upton, NY   11973

D.G. Stroud
Dept. of Physics
Ohio State University
Columbus, OH   43210

Max Swerdlow
5704 Lenox Road
Bethesda, MD   20034

D.B. Tanner
174 W 18th Ave.
Columbus, OH   43210

Michael Tinkham
Harvard University
Physics Department
Cambridge, MA   02138

A.M. Tremblay
Laboratory for Atomic & Solid State Physics
Cornell University
Ithica, NY   14850

C.C. Tsuei
P.O. Box 218
IMB Thomas J. Watson Reseach Center
Yorktown Hghts., NY   10598

Richard F. Voss
IBM, Thomas J. Watson Research Center
P.O.Box 218
Yorktown Hghts., NY   10598

John L. Warren, ER152
MS-J309, Div. of Mat. Sci.
Dept. of Energy   .
Washington, DC   20545

Gene L. Wells
Physical Review Letters
Brookhaven National Laboratory
Upton, NY   11973

Jeffrey O. Willis
Los Alamos Scientific Lab.
P.O. Box 1663 MS 764
Los Alamos, NM   87545

Stuart A. Wolf
Code 6338
Naval Research Laboratory
Washington, DC   20375

James T. Yeh
IBM Thomas J. Watson Research Ctr.
Yorktown Hghts., NY   10598

AIP Conference Proceedings

		L.C. Number	ISBN
No.1	Feedback and Dynamic Control of Plasmas	70-141596	0-88318-100-2
No.2	Particles and Fields - 1971 (Rochester)	71-184662	0-88318-101-0
No.3	Thermal Expansion - 1971 (Corning)	72-76970	0-88318-102-9
No.4	Superconductivity in d-and f-Band Metals (Rochester, 1971)	74-18879	0-88318-103-7
No.5	Magnetism and Magnetic Materials - 1971 (2 parts) (Chicago)	59-2468	0-88318-104-5
No.6	Particle Physics (Irvine, 1971)	72-81239	0-88318-105-3
No.7	Exploring the History of Nuclear Physics	72-81883	0-88318-106-1
No.8	Experimental Meson Spectroscopy - 1972	72-88226	0-88318-107-X
No.9	Cyclotrons - 1972 (Vancouver)	72-92798	0-88318-108-8
No.10	Magnetism and Magnetic Materials - 1972	72-623469	0-88318-109-6
No.11	Transport Phenomena - 1973 (Brown University Conference)	73-80682	0-88318-110-X
No.12	Experiments on High Energy Particle Collisions - 1973 (Vanderbilt Conference)	73-81705	0-88318-111-8
No.13	π-π Scattering - 1973 (Tallahassee Conference)	73-81704	0-88318-112-6
No.14	Particles and Fields - 1973 (APS/DPF Berkeley)	73-91923	0-88318-113-4
No.15	High Energy Collisions - 1973 (Stony Brook)	73-92324	0-88318-114-2
No.16	Causality and Physical Theories (Wayne State University, 1973)	73-93420	0-88318-115-0
No.17	Thermal Expansion - 1973 (lake of the Ozarks)	73-94415	0-88318-116-9
No.18	Magnetism and Magnetic Materials - 1973 (2 parts) (Boston)	59-2468	0-88318-117-7
No.19	Physics and the Energy Problem - 1974 (APS Chicago)	73-94416	0-88318-118-5
No.20	Tetrahedrally Bonded Amorphous Semiconductors (Yorktown Heights, 1974)	74-80145	0-88318-119-3
No.21	Experimental Meson Spectroscopy - 1974 (Boston)	74-82628	0-88318-120-7
No.22	Neutrinos - 1974 (Philadelphia)	74-82413	0-88318-121-5
No.23	Particles and Fields - 1974 (APS/DPF Williamsburg)	74-27575	0-88318-122-3